MEDICINE, MOBILITY, AND POWER IN GLOBAL AFRICA

MEDICINE, MOBILITY, AND POWER IN GLOBAL AFRICA

TRANSNATIONAL HEALTH AND HEALING

EDITED BY

HANSJÖRG DILGER,
ABDOULAYE KANE,

AND

STACEY A. LANGWICK

Indiana University Press
Bloomington and Indianapolis

This book is a publication of

Indiana University Press
601 North Morton Street
Bloomington, Indiana 47404-3797 USA

iupress.indiana.edu

Telephone orders   800-842-6796
Fax orders   812-855-7931

Library of Congress Cataloging-in-Publication Data

   Medicine, mobility, and power in global Africa : transnational health and healing / edited by Hansjörg Dilger, Abdoulaye Kane, and Stacey A. Langwick.
   p. cm.
   Includes index.
   ISBN 978-0-253-35709-0 (cloth : alk. paper)
   ISBN 978-0-253-22368-5 (pbk. : alk. paper)
   ISBN 978-0-253-00532-8 (eb)
   1. Medical care—Africa. 2. Health services accessibility—Africa. 3. Traditional medicine—Africa. I. Dilger, Hansjörg. II. Kane, Abdoulaye. III. Langwick, Stacey Ann.
   RA545.M47   2012
   362.1096—dc23   2012005731

   1 2 3 4 5   17 16 15 14 13 12

CONTENTS

ACKNOWLEDGMENTS

This book is a product of the intellectual excitement the three of us shared together as faculty in a vibrant and dynamic Center for African Studies at the University of Florida in the early 2000s. In 2006, with the support of the University of Florida we organized a small working conference on transnationalism and medicine in Africa. The complexity of the issues and our desire to continue the conversation there gave rise to this volume. A few of the presentations given at that conference provided the seeds for chapters in this book. Others have joined us since then. While we editors are now each in different universities and on two different continents, we have treasured the excuse working on this volume provided to continue our conversations on a regular basis.

We would like to extend a very special thank-you to Leonardo Villalón, director of the Center for African Studies at the University of Florida 2003–2011. He supported both us and this generative international conversation. We thank the students in Professor Dilger's graduate seminar "Mobility and Health in Africa," which led up to the conference in the fall of 2006. We also appreciate the range of support that we received for the original conference from Kenneth Sassaman, Allan Burns, Corinna Greene, and Ikeade Akinyemi. We benefited from the generous funding of the International Office at the University of Florida. Susan Reynolds Whyte was a gifted and generative discussant at the conference. We owe a special thank-you to her for her invaluable input. We thank Julie Livingston, Brenda Chalfin, and Luise White for their intellectual interventions. The Department of Political and Social Sciences at Freie Universität (Berlin) and the Department of Anthropology in Cornell University granted funding for the preparation of the book. Carla Dietzel provided invaluable administrative support in managing deadlines and submissions as well as excellent skills in layout.

Edited volumes are always a process and we thank the authors for their patience. Dee Mortensen understood the value of the conversation that this volume catalyzes and was a skillful editor. We thank Marisa Maza for the cover work, and Jeff Bercuvitz for hosting the three of us in Ithaca for a critical meeting of the editors. We hope that in the coming years this volume will generate more conversations and scholarly exchange on the transnationalization of health, medicine, and healing in and beyond Africa.

MEDICINE, MOBILITY, AND POWER IN GLOBAL AFRICA

INTRODUCTION

Transnational Medicine, Mobile Experts

Ethnographic and historical work on healing and medicine in Africa reveals a great deal about politics and power; social organization and economic conditions; global regimes of value and local practices of valuing bodies, kin, and community. Medicine is significant not only for its therapeutic effects on individual bodies, whether biological, symbolic, spiritual, or otherwise mediated. Medicine and healing, as Steven Feierman (1985) argues, have also long been implicated in the organization and transformation of social and communal life in the sub-Saharan African region—and vice versa. Therefore, on a larger scale, as medicinal substances, therapeutic practices, and healing practitioners (as well as the institutions, technologies, policies, and ethical frameworks to which they adhere) circulate, they shape myriad aspects of social, political, and economic life. This volume takes the mobility of medicines, patients, and experts as its primary object of investigation. Few studies of the postcolonial transnationalisms that shape medicine in or out of Africa have included both "traditional" and "modern" medicines in their accounts. Yet the histories of "traditional" medicine, religious healing, and biomedicine are intertwined, and all indicate the importance of regional and inter-regional movement.

That "mobility is power" is an old truism in African healing. Even in precolonial times, healing powers were assumed to increase significantly with the movements of healers and medicinal products across often wide regional distances (Comaroff 1981). Traditional African therapies and healers traveling from afar have long claimed heightened potency (Digby 2004), while biomedicine spread throughout the continent as a result of missionization, colonization, and international development (Vaughan 1991). Equally, military conquests as well as the establishing of labor markets, urban centers, and the associated infrastructures of mobility in colonial settings paved the way for the spread of epidemic diseases and mobile pathogens (Feierman 1985: 85f.); this in turn effected medical interventions and long-term changes in local social and moral orders (Ranger 1992: 247) and facilitated the incorporation of Africa into the emerging capitalist world order.

The authors in this volume train attention on the transnational mobilities of therapies and therapeutic experts as they shape life, health, and healing for contemporary Africans. Together, these chapters catalyze new ways of understanding the imaginations, networks, movements, and practices—as well as the hopes, disillusions, and "failures"—that comprise contemporary globalized medicine. In so doing, they describe some of the forces shaping contemporary human experiences of affliction and healing that have often gone unacknowledged in studies more tightly organized around specific medical systems or geographic locales.

We begin from the belief that accounting for globalization today requires a careful examination and historicization of mobility as an effect of power. This includes official movements—of international development experts, international migrants, consultants, essential medicines, WHO guidelines and national policy documents—as well as smuggled remnants of pharmaceutical prescriptions, remittances from distant relatives, and the circulation of traditional healers and medicines. We also attend to the "side effects" of biomedical programs—from the resistance to Western childhood vaccines in Niger to the end of the indigenous pharmacy industry in Nigeria. We describe the disconnects between public health notions of responsible behaviors, including moral ways of thinking and acting, and the situated ethics of the everyday struggles of men and women in Africa. Attention to the ways that Africans seek to gain control of their bodies and the meanings of their afflictions leads us to illustrate some of the more complicated dynamics that influence contemporary international health. It challenges the sometimes simplistic assumptions that underlie health interventions and globalized health priorities of basic treatment and care in resource-poor settings. And it calls for scholarship that resists being another "derivative" of African suffering (Hunt 1999).

Similarly, the unofficial movements of healers and medicines from Africa to Europe (and vice versa) bring to light a subtler picture of medicine and health in Africa—from Somali healers who use new telecommunications technology to attend to clients in Scandinavia to Senegalese migrants who organize to provide their home village with ambulances. Furthermore, the circuits of exchange and the medical modernities they engender are diverse, as illustrated through the example of Chinese doctors in Kenya. We argue that neither a faithful epidemiological profile of Africa nor a rigorous account of the landscape of therapeutic options and the context of health-seeking behaviors can be conceived without attention to both official and unofficial movements of medicines and experts in and out of Africa. The multidirectional trajectories and transnational relations depicted in this volume have demonstrable impact on the health of Africans, the shape of illnesses seen in Africa, and the kinds of healing practices and options found in Africa and among the African immigrant communities in Europe and America.

In addition, this analytical focus highlights the importance of other objects of study. Authors in this volume consider the politics of pharmaceuticals, international property rights, biobureaucracies, medical humanitarianism, and new communication technologies such as the internet and cell phones. Furthermore, they are concerned with the massive influx of resources for diseases such as HIV/AIDS, as well as the concurrent draining of "local" capital and the growing (but often limited) efforts of governments and international agencies to establish universal access to biomedical services and to impose the socially transformative effects of public health programs. In aggregate the following chapters illustrate both the interconnectedness and the imbalances that have characterized the formation of the global world order over the last few decades.

Global Restructuring and the Emergence and Transformation of "Transnational Medicine"

While globalization is not new, the way it operates in the late twentieth and early twenty-first centuries is distinctive (Cooper 2005). The work in this volume attends to this distinctiveness in two ways. First, some of us argue that international financial organizations and health development programs have formulated a specific notion of globality in practice. Second, the political and economic agreements that structured independence as well as the regulatory forms that define the postcolony have influenced the marking and meaning of territorial boundaries and determined the specific sorts of territorial crossing that define contemporary social, economic, and political relations. We argue that the forms of regulation—legal and economic as well as moral and political—implemented in the name of postcolonial development define the past 40 years as a particular era.[1] Both of these arguments suggest that the rise of "development" as a dominant discourse producing "Africa," and its effects on relations among African nations as well as between Africa and the rest of the world, have generated a unique historical moment worthy of careful and sustained analytic attention (Ferguson 1990; Escobar 1995).

From the late 1970s onward, the internal and external problems faced by African states, along with the subsequent introduction of structural reforms in the name of economic development, have had dramatic impact on health and health care. The time period of the 1980s and '90s was characterized by the privatization and commercialization of health care, concurrent inadequacies in state expenditures for the provision of health-related services, the (re)emergence of epidemic diseases such as HIV / AIDS and tuberculosis, and the increased social and physical mobility of African health professionals and other parts of African populations within and beyond the continent.

The processes that have been contained in the ongoing reconfiguration of African health care systems and health-seeking practices across national and continental borders imply a wide range of engagements and developments, of opportunities and restrictions. First, the movements of things and people over the past four decades have transformed health care options on the continent, leading to the attenuation of resources within public health systems as well as the diversification and stratification of medical landscapes. On the one hand, the social, political, and economic transformations—as well as periods of civil war and political oppression in some parts of the continent—during the 1970s, '80s, and '90s have catalyzed the migration of African men and women to Europe, the U.S., and other destinations in Africa. The human, financial, and social resources in numerous communities were consequently compromised. Furthermore, in state hospitals and clinics throughout the continent, the absence of drugs, equipment, and medical personnel in the wake of reduced government funding—and the concurrent commercialization and privatization of medicine and health care—have restricted overall access to biomedical services (Turshen 1999). These shortages have reinforced existing social, economic, and physical inequalities, particularly in rural areas. Finally, the emergence and reinforcement of new forms of poverty and structural dependencies in the context of recent globalization processes have refigured vulnerabilities and risks in relation to health, as well as to gender, age, and locality. These contemporary configurations of vulnerability and risk increasingly extend into transnational and migratory settings.

On the other hand, the trans- and intracontinental movements of people, resources, and ideas have been accompanied by the emergence of a wide range of social, institutional, and cultural configurations that allow African citizens to deal with health-related challenges and to make sense of, and respond to, individual and collective suffering. Thus, the widely ramified migratory flows across the globe have been associated with the (re)investment in and the (re) building of community-based health care systems in various parts of Africa, supported by both personal remittances from migrants and public donations and loans. Not only capital for health but also health care workers and medical technologies are on the move. Medical researchers, entrepreneurs, and healers offer their services to the growing market of clients and consumers in private clinics and healing centers, and specialized medical services such as in-vitro fertilization are becoming available for the wealthy parts of African populations, thus expanding the therapeutic itineraries of those with greater resources (Hörbst, this volume). Moreover, along with the increased diversity of religious, traditional, and biomedical healing practices, syncretistic forms of healing and treatment emerge and are further modified and reconfigured in the transfer of "African" healing practices into other parts of the world.

Second, the growing economic liberalization and privatization of health care systems in many parts of Africa have been inseparably intertwined with shifts in international health policies and the emergence of new forms of epidemic disease and new modes of intervention. The multiple governmental and non-governmental programs and health care projects have, at times, reinforced inequalities and inequities on the continent. At the same time, however, the growing (potential) availability of financial resources on all levels of social and political organization—as well as the ideas, images, and practices that are contained in the increased presence of international development and humanitarian intervention—have produced new forms of subjectivity and experience in relation to health as well as emerging understandings of citizenship, empowerment, and health activism. The challenging and paradoxical subject positions contained in the globalization of therapeutic markets in and beyond Africa—and the frustration with government policies and international experts that are observed in some parts of the continent—shed light on both people's efforts to make sense of the social and moral crises associated with globalization and modernity, and on the social relationships that have remained central in people's search for health and healing in and beyond Africa (Dilger and Luig 2010; Masquelier, this volume).

In accounting for the transnational movements of medicines, health policies, and bureaucratic technologies, and the mobility of therapeutic experts and forms of expertise, this volume draws together three strands of anthropological and social science literature.

NEOLIBERALIZATION

The recent shifts in the field of health and medicine within and beyond the continent have to be understood with regard to the way in which neoliberal reform processes and global development have affected the relationships between African states, communities, and civil society organizations. Thus, liberalization and market reforms have (1) enhanced the mobility of human labor and skills despite the efforts of receiving countries to control migration flows, (2) diversified the field of health politics within and across the borders of most African states, (3) transformed African governments' capacities to provide health services for their citizens, and (4) shifted their position

in transnationalized configurations of governance and health care and created the context for (transnational) civil society organizations and corporate
entities to fill the gaps in health care systems (cf., Ferguson 2006). In some
cases, the concerted "dispossession" of African states through international
policies, trade regulations, and new funding mechanisms for health care in
the wake of structural adjustment and globalized systems of governance can
be described as a process of "emptying out space" for new forms of capital,
statecraft, and social and cultural legitimacy (Peterson, this volume). At the
same time, however, these dynamics highlight the alleged failure of African
governments to deal thoroughly with the growing challenges of poverty and
newly arising health problems, a "failure" that stands in stark contrast to the
claims of many postcolonial governments that free health care is the obligation of a legitimate state.

TRANSNATIONALISM AND GLOBALIZATION

The reconfigurations in the field of health and medicine in and beyond
Africa have to be understood in relation to the literature on transnationalism and globalization that has shaped debates in anthropology and African
Studies over the last decades. While globalization literature has played a
preeminent role in highlighting the manifold and multidirectional flows and
entanglements that have become entrenched in the deterritorialization, circulation, and appropriation of ideas, objects, and practices in an interconnected
world (Appadurai 1990, 1996), this literature has also been criticized for being
in some instances ahistorical, as well as for its tendency to naturalize and
culturalize neoliberal reconfigurations and people's exposure to and experiences with global power relations (Kearney 1995; Edelmann and Haugerud
2007). Taking these critiques into account, the contributions to this volume
highlight the necessity of looking at the multiple ways in which health and
medicine in and beyond Africa continue to be shaped in relation to state-based
bureaucracies and power structures—and vis-à-vis a wide range of social and
political actors and relations that have shaped people's struggles over identity,
belonging, and solidarity within and across national borders (cf., Glick Schiller
2004; Aretxaga 2003). Furthermore, while the chapters in this book emphasize the "newness" of some of the health-related phenomena in global and
transnational settings, they also consider that these processes are embedded
in longstanding histories of health care, politics, and social relationships in
colonial and postcolonial Africa. The authors have therefore analyzed these
phenomena with regard to the continuities as well as the ruptures taking place
in the context of globalization and transnational mobility. One of the issues

this commitment to history raises in Africa is the fact that national boundaries and ethnic affiliation do not always map neatly over one another. The resulting frictions complicate analytical references to transnationalism and insist on the importance of articulating the particular meaning(s) of transnationalism within Africa and beyond.

CONTEMPORARY MEDICINE AND HEALTH CARE

Finally, the contributions in this book are to be read in relation to recent debates in the subfield of medical anthropology, and with regard to the way in which ethnographic approaches to medicine and health in Africa may create a unique perspective on large-scale processes like neoliberalism, transnationalism, and globalization. Over the last decade, medical anthropologists have identified the multiple power relations, dependencies, and inequalities that have shaped and restricted people's well-being and access to health services in a globalizing world (Baer, Singer, and Susser 1997; Farmer 2003). Furthermore, they have highlighted the multiple opportunities and challenges that emerge as a result of individual and collective suffering and that are to be seen not only as a reaction to, but as being *constitutive* of global and transnational processes and configurations. Thus, medical anthropologists have argued that the increased presence and global circulation of medical technologies—as well as the emergence and identification of new biological conditions or epidemic diseases like HIV / AIDS—have played a major role in emerging forms of sociality, governance, and citizenship within and across national and continental borders (cf., Rabinow 1992; Petryna 2002; Rose and Novas 2005; Ecks 2005). Furthermore, they have argued that an ethnographic perspective may reveal the multiple struggles over meaning, identity, and belonging that have come to characterize the micro-politics of health and medicine in a globally and transnationally interconnected world (cf., Rose 2007; Biehl, Good, and Kleinman 2007; Nichter 2002; Dilger and Hadolt 2010).

Taken together, these three bodies of literature blur the boundaries between medical anthropology and the larger field of social and cultural anthropology. Work at this intersection challenges the subdiscipline to account for the diverse ways in which health and medicine—understood as a complex set of substances, ideas, symbols, and relationships—have become implicated in transnational and global forms of politics, ethics, mobility, and development (Ong and Collier 2005; Lock and Nichter 2002). With this book, we aim to build on these dynamic disciplinary debates by bringing Africa to the heart of the conversation. On the one hand, we will draw on longstanding arguments in Africa-related medical anthropology which have emphasized that health and healing on the continent cannot be understood outside of the history of social, cultural, economic, and political relations (Feierman and Janzen 1992; Janzen 1978; Whyte 1997; Luedke and West 2005). On the other, the literatures cited above concerning neoliberalization; transnationalism and globalization; contemporary medicine and health care have been written mostly in relation to North and South American, European, and East Asian contexts (for exceptions see Nguyen 2005; Whyte 2009). We bring these debates to bear on health and medicine in sub-Saharan Africa. In the remainder of this introduction we want to describe the specific objects of analytical attention that emerge from such a transnational approach to health and medicine in and beyond Africa and how this approach is exemplified by the chapters in this volume.

Mobility, Expansion, and Containment

One of the most challenging questions for anthropology in the past decades has been how to study contemporary forces that articulate their work on a global scale. Ethnographic studies of globalization in Africa have tended to have two foci: (1) the ways in which the goods, ideas, and media of the world have brought modernity (or, as some have preferred, "alternative" or "parallel modernities") to African villages and towns (e.g., Larkin 1997; Piot 1999) and (2) the effects that international financial organizations have had on specific locales and practices (e.g., Ferguson 1999). These studies have been productive in that they have grounded claims about globalization in specific actions, ideas, people, institutions, and movements. Furthermore, several authors have illustrated how global exchanges and migrations enact Africa as politically and economically marginal to the global economy and yet how this "margin" remains critical to the workings of the so-called West (e.g., Kapur and McHale 2005; Manuh 2005).

The chapters in this volume are inspired by these studies. By focusing on medicine, healing, and mobility, however, they also suggest a third way of accounting for "globalization" and "Africa" ethnographically. The authors in this volume approach mobility in ways that integrate not only the movement of people as labor migrants, refugees, traders, doctors, healers, patients, experts, and others going to and from Africa but also describe the movement of health-related resources, ideas, finances, and objects—both afflicting and healing—that are important elements of migrants' identities and health practices between home and host countries. Furthermore, while mobility has often been perceived as a disruptive social experience for the individuals involved, the contributions in this volume—focusing on mobility and its influence on the health care choices of Africans established "at home" as well as abroad—elaborate the themes of connectivity, multidirectionality, and return as important aspects of African mobility in relation to health and health care.

Mobility has become one of the predominant characteristics of our time (Appadurai 2001). The globalization of the world economy and the revolution of transportation and information technologies have contributed to increasing the number of people crossing borders and engaging in transnational practices by engendering flows of money, goods, ideas, images, and people between poor(er) and rich(er) countries. As the contributions in this volume confirm, Africa and Africans are active participants in these global flows. The use of the term "flow" should not be taken to imply that the different forms of mobility are fluid and uninterrupted. In fact, however, human mobility from the so-called "developing" countries to more industrialized countries may be restricted and controlled by increasingly tough immigration laws. The changes in African postcolonial patterns of mobility are a response to the increasingly unwelcoming attitudes of former colonial (as well as non-colonial) powers that began attracting significant numbers of migrants from the former colonies during the 1950s to help with post–World War II reconstruction.

The usual explanation of why people in Africa move has focused on economic disparities between sending and receiving places (MacGaffey and Bazenguissa-Ganga 2000; Adepoju 1991; Arthur 2000). The push and pull factors that were defined by these studies tend to focus on "states of emergencies" and do not give a full picture of the multiple mobilities in which the economic, social, and religious dimensions of movement become blurred. Some healers or *marabouts* are better off in Africa and travel only at the request of their patients or disciples. Similarly, the Malian couples who are seeking treatment for infertility outside Mali (Hörbst), or the wealthy patients and retirees going to Europe for medical reasons (Kane), do not match the category of desperate young Africans consumed by the desire to enter Europe or North America where they envision a prosperous future (Ferguson 2002). Furthermore, the Chinese doctors who perceive African countries like Kenya as a land of economic and financial opportunities (Hsu) can be used as a counter-argument to the classic theory of the "push and pull factors."

The contributions in this book focus on the multiple forms of mobility that are not usually captured by an exclusive focus on economic disparities and/or *human* mobility. Some of them show that traditional medicines have provoked the mobility of both patients and healers. Well-known healers are attracting patients from neighboring villages, towns, and countries. Tiilikainen describes how hundreds of patients from neighboring countries cross borders to seek treatment in Somalia. The movements of patients, healers, and medical experts within Africa and between Africa and the West has increased in recent years due to the increase in migration flows and the co-presence of a variety of forms of healing in both sending and receiving countries.

On another level, the transnational practices in which Africans living outside their countries of origin are participating include the flow of medicine in various forms (herbs, pills, blessed water, prayers, audiocassettes of holy scripture recitations) and the displacement of inflicting agents (witches, *jinn,* spirits, winds). Some of the contributions in this volume analyze how technologies and methods of communication are used to enable a faster movement of ideas, concepts, and things, making "healing and afflicting at a distance" possible. These new technologies of communication affect not only the movement of things and ideas but also social relations between migrants and their families left at home. Tiilikainen presents various cases in which treatment for Somali refugees in the diaspora in northern Europe is provided by using modern technologies of communication. The participation of family members in proxy forms of treatment is thereby made critical. The relatives are the intermediaries between patients in the diaspora who are not able to travel to Somalia and local healers—whose diagnosis and treatment rely on what family members report to them. Similarly, Mohr's contribution shows a high degree of coordination between leaders of independent and Presbyterian churches in Ghana, on the one hand, and indigenous leaders, believers, and patients in the United States on the other.

The presence of religious and cultural perceptions of illness and healing among Africans in the diaspora (see Tiilikainen, Mohr, Carvalho, Kane, Hsu) should not automatically be understood as a rejection of biomedical healing practices per se. The existence of opposite flows of biomedicine from diaspora locations to home communities attests to the growing interest in "modern" forms of healing practices. The suitcases filled with biomedicine that Tiilikainen and Kane report in their respective chapters indisputably place biomedicine on the long list of things circulating between Africans abroad and their hometowns and villages (see also Krause 2008). As a matter of fact, such remittances of medicine have become critical to many poor people left to fend for themselves in a context of neoliberal policies that make them more vulnerable.

Finally, a growing number of international institutions are operating in Africa to deal with the negative effects of globalization on "the poor." They intervene in social sectors, such as health and education, that have been undermined by structural adjustment programs. These institutions participate in local, national, and global levels of action. They move staff, medicine, and experts from one location to the other. It is important to include in the multiple mobilities the institutional movement of state agencies, multilateral organizations, non-governmental organizations, and self-help associations. Institutional mobility includes both the installation of satellite institutions in Africa and the mobility of staff and experts travelling back and forth between headquarters and various targeted destinations. The mobilization and mobility of experts in times of emerging epidemics are central to the mission of multilateral institutions like the World Health Organization (WHO) (Janzen). The ability to move health experts from France to rural areas in Senegal is the fundamental objective of Fouta Santé, a self-help institution created by Senegalese migrants from the Senegal River Valley currently living in France.

The combination of these kinds of mobility and the various interventions they engender in the African health systems result in the emergence of new assemblages and their embedded frictions. The travel of healers to global cities and medical experts to rural and urban Africa are all symbols of the complexity of the global era, in which multiple mobilities are connecting the local and the global, the urban and the rural, and "Africa" to the "out of the way" places. Anthropologists who are used to studying the "places out there" find themselves in need of new approaches and methodologies to account for the unexpected interconnectedness between "exotic places" and global cities that emerges through the practices and experiences of migrants and mobile experts. The multi-sited approach is gaining currency in the discipline, pointing to the need to rethink the old ways of doing ethnography that depend analytically on a fixed locality. Most African villages today reflect Charles Piot's idea of a "remotely global" place, a term that highlights the connections villages have with faraway places through traveling villagers (Piot 2002). On the other side of the coin, the presence of shrines in Portugal among the Bissau Guineans is a good example suggesting that the globalization of "the local" may also expand to the former "centers" of the world system. Carvalho's chapter gives the powerful image of shrines and the healers called *jambakus* or *mouros* traveling from rural communities to European cities, where they symbolize the existence of plural global perspectives. It is thus not only "Western" powers, beliefs, and understandings that are mobile (and, to be sure, leading to a certain degree of cultural homogeneity); particular "African" cultural forms circulate broadly as well. As they are brought to Western urban settings, they connect diasporas to their "homes" and contribute to a different sense of the global. The concept of traveling culture developed by Clifford can be useful in comprehending the attempt to replicate some cultural forms, practices, and understandings—such as those associated with affliction and healing—in a host social setting (Clifford 1997). The contributions to this book show, each in its own right, multiple connections between a locality and the surrounding world dictated by various rationalities, desires, and commitments. They also attest to the blurring of clear-cut distinctions between "the local" and "the global" and show that globality is produced with regard to specific (locally perceived and experienced) configurations of mobility, connectedness, and ways of seeing the world.

Assemblages, Frictions, and Desires

Medical humanitarianism, public health vaccination campaigns, religious organization, international health policy making, medical technologies, and biosciences all pose anthropological problems that at times exceed ethnographic tracings of the movement, migrations, and boundary crossings of people and things. In their influential volume, *Global Assemblages,* Ong and Collier (2005: 5) have argued that globalization is not so much a specific process requiring description and explanation "as a problem-space in which contemporary anthropological questions are framed." Inspired in part by Foucault's notion of *assemblage,* Ong and Collier's volume brings the dynamics of marginalization, regionalization, inequities, postcolonialism, etc. to the fore through a focus on how phenomena are "territorialized in assemblages." As political, economic, technological, and ethical regimes are enacted in specific places at specific times, they establish both the channels and the gaps that come to constitute globalization. In much of the scholarship on globalization, "Africa" itself has emerged as a gap, as the place left behind. This phenomenon requires more explicit theorization. As Peterson argues in this volume, "Africa is being rigorously 're-inscribed' in the world via trade, development, and economic policies that suggest an importance greater than simple marginalization." Africa is not outside of the assemblages that make up this later modern moment, for assemblage is about power, and Africa is not outside the regimes of power that give rise to the way that the world may be known and apprehended.

At a broader level, the abstraction of Africa itself garners meaning and potency through the workings of global governance. If global power is best marked by its effects, then most foundational of these is a world constituted through scales—the global, the regional, the national, and the local. From the perspective of governance, Africa is an administrative unit. Studies of globalization, then, require attention to scale, or to what Langwick (this volume) calls "scalar developments." Janzen's chapter also raises the question of where we find "Africa" in studies of globalization and where we find "the global."

He juxtaposes emergency campaigns against Ebola virus in central Africa, the obstacles to the circulation of African medicines, and the debilities and traumas of Africans who migrated to the U.S. to escape war in their home countries. Dilger and Masquelier illustrate alternative assemblages, regimes of knowledge, ethics, and technologies that make up bodies and persons in ways that sometimes articulate with dominant biopolitical ontologies and some-times do not. In areas of the world that have been neglected by international and national efforts, that have not had the opportunity to or have refused to witness the universality of particular forms of knowledge, alternative forms of expertise arise. Migrant workers become "specialists" in the distribution of pharmaceuticals, and healers lay claim to cures for Ebola and AIDS. In addi-tion, the desires and pleasures, freedoms and risks articulated through other forms of knowledge and other kinds of bodies call to Africans abroad as well as at home. Traditional medicines, as mentioned above, move from Africa to Portugal (Carvalho), France (Kane), and Finland (Tiilikainen).

Attention to the workings of power and their limits draws attention to the distribution of expertise. Who can claim knowledge of places and of the bodies, illnesses, and medicines within them? Which sorts of expertise are evoked by specific technological regimes, ethical requirements, and institu-tional needs? The forms of knowledge and kinds of practices that incite global phenomena are forged within knowledge-making practices that make claims to the universal. Anthropologists can be part of this study, as illustrated in Janzen's chapter, where anthropologists and public health workers are called on to act as translators of biomedical knowledge and bridge builders between medical teams and the people among whom they work. Careful ethnography also holds out the possibility of posing questions in the times and places where "universal" knowledge comes into being in particular places and practices (Tsing 2004). Building on an ethnographic approach to the study of "frictions" and tensions that inhere in the global, the contributions in this book argue that the management of health and illness in the context of globalization—be it from the perspective of individuals, families, or institutions—involves more than establishing access to health-related knowledge and resources under con-ditions of inequality and poverty.[2] Health and illness are managed through the very ruptures, differences, and contestations that are mobilized and acted upon in the myriad attempts to enable, control, and tame the universalizing flows[3] of medicine, politics, economics, and science across national and conti-nental borders. In a similar vein to recent studies on modernity and the occult, the authors in this book argue that not only the individualizing of blame but also the steep increase of social and economic inequalities in contemporary Africa have refigured the moral meaning that people make of affliction and differences in bodily states. As Todd Sanders (2001) has argued with regard to Tanzania, moral discourses on occult practices of wealth accumulation provide a socially embedded answer to people's questions about who profits from current transformations, at whose expense, and for what purpose. Such discourses and practices may at times offer a way for individuals, families, and communities to establish some sense of control over the multiple (visible and invisible) forces that have come to shape their lives in the context of globalization and structurally adjusted modernity.

The chapters in this volume present examples of how differences, frictions, and tensions are experienced, negotiated, and produced in relation to health and medicine in and beyond sub-Saharan Africa. Some of the chapters focus on the ways in which international, national, and local institutional efforts to establish access to health care in different regions of the continent have been met by resistance, non-compliance, or simply disinterest on the part of local populations. These reactions lay open the complex and often paradoxical moral challenges that are implicated in the mobilization of resources, ideas, and practices in the wake of neoliberal reforms processes and experiences of inequality. The chapters by Masquelier and Janzen demonstrate how individuals, families, and communities in Niger and Central Africa have become distrustful of the health interventions of state institutions and international health organizations, which are experienced as excessive and partially abusive. Thus, while public health systems in sub-Saharan Africa in the wake of structural adjustment and neoliberal reform processes have become increasingly weakened, the perceived impotence and deficiencies of governments in providing health care for their citizens are called into question in cases such as: emergencies like Ebola, preventive campaigning like vaccinations, and responses to "more important" diseases like HIV/AIDS and tuberculosis. As has been argued with regard to global health interventions in general (Lakoff and Collier 2008), the linking of health issues with notions of biosecurity has enabled the excessive mobilization of national and international resources and state power, particularly in those cases where health care becomes a question of emergency, security, and humanitarian necessity.

The actual practices, ideas, and experiences that evolve from specific localities in relation to such interventions are more than a simple (non)compliance with or (non)adoption of the different policies, politics, and norms that are articulated by the bureaucratic regimes of global and national health actors in often remote settings. As the two cases in Tanzania show, the ethnographic focus on transnational health interventions reveals the boundaries and paradoxical relations contained in the making of global health subjects (Langwick), as well as the limitations and fragility of biopower in the context of neoliberally orchestrated health interventions (Dilger). Also as argued in the case of the introduction of health insurance initiatives in Senegal (Wolf), the moral challenges that people face with regard to institutional setups are experienced as being detached from social control, balanced reciprocity, and emotional bonds.

Finally, the case studies in this volume reveal that transnational configurations of medicine and health have led to the—sometimes contradictory—production and articulation of subjectivities, desires, and intimacies which are imagined and articulated in and through the flows of people, technologies, and resources across national and continental borders. The contribution by Hörbst highlights the way in which assisted reproductive technologies in Mali—which have long been marginalized in global perceptions of fertility and population development in sub-Saharan Africa—have evoked particular desires and intimacies among women and men of the urban middle classes which become simultaneously bound up with *and* detached from kinship obligations and gender norms in Bamako. Other chapters in the book describe how the hopes and desires that are contained and articulated in migratory pathways away from and toward Africa may be called into question by the experiences and politics of social, economic, and racial difference in the migrants' host countries, as well as by the challenges of developing identities and (gendered) ways of being that are often strikingly different from migrants' experiences and expectations in their home countries (Tiilikainen, Hsu, and Mohr). At the same time, however, these challenges and experiences in migratory settings—which may also be experienced by families and communities in the home countries (Kane)—have become inseparably intertwined with the negotiating and building of new relations, practices, and healing configurations that establish meaning, belonging, and trust in often unpredictable ways. Thus, experiences and politics of difference and exclusion in transnational settings have become intrinsically linked to contemporary issues such as the mobilization of plants, resources, and technologies away from and toward Senegal (Kane); the need for purification and ritualization of persons and landscapes in rural Guinea and urban Portugal (Carvalho); and the making of morally and spiritually purified masculinities in urban Philadelphia (Mohr).

While frictions, tensions, and conflicts have come to be intrinsic to the emergence of health interventions and medical assemblages in a transnationally interconnected world, the chapters in this volume demonstrate that the outcomes of these processes are often unpredictable, unstable, and not necessarily "welcome." Global health interventions and people's efforts to establish access to health and health care in transnational settings have a generative impact on nations, communities, kin, and individual subjects. Furthermore, bilateral and multilateral health development collaborations have established their own mechanisms of training people and institutions in relation to shifting global priorities, with their own rituals for accounting and remuneration (Wolf). However, both the successes and the failures of health interventions depend on responses of accommodation, refusal, acknowledgement, disregard, and strategizing that cannot be thought independently of the originally intended effects. They thus may become generative of other forms of knowledge and being and in turn have an effect on original interventions and configurations. It is the strength of an ethnographic perspective to reveal what remains excluded and hidden in the imaginations and expectations articulated in policy papers, health missions, and biobureaucratic regimes, by taking seriously the grappling and struggling of people and institutions in producing, managing, and coming to terms with the zigzag movements of actors (human as well as non-human), ideas, practices, and moral-ethical-scientific configurations in globally connected settings.

Chapter Summaries

SCALE AS AN EFFECT OF POWER

This first section considers how it is that the global is apprehended in practice and how we as scholars can approach it. In aggregate these chapters argue that thinking about global power necessitates thinking about the construction of scales. The first five chapters examine the specific practices through which the global (e.g., global subjects, knowledge, ethics, institutions, interventions, etc.) comes into being in relation to the national, the local, and the individual. They illustrate that the global (and therefore globalization) is no less located in place than these other scales of action; it is, however, distinguished by relation to them.

Stacey Langwick's chapter focuses on the conceptualization and formation of a "new" category of health expert—the traditional birth attendant (TBA)—which has occupied global and regional health politics in the "developing world" from the early 1970s onward. The chapter argues that the emergence of the TBA illustrates how the design and implementation of health interventions imagine and materialize the world as a set of nested administrative units—the global, the regional, the national, and the local. Langwick argues that the notion of the TBA as a global actor present in "all traditional societies" originally emerged through universalizing practices of cross-cultural health research. The personal and professional traits of the "locally distinct" health expert came to be defined through the preparation of global health

documents and the subsequent meetings they engendered between representatives of global health organizations on the one side and the delegates of
national and regional governments in various locations of the world on the
other. The TBA acquired particular meaning as a cost-efficient solution to
the health labor shortage during the second half of the twentieth century. By
demonstrating how the TBA, as a global type elicited out of various local cultural forms, becomes incorporated in health outreach work in rural areas of
Tanzania; and by describing the obligations, desires, and biographies of actual
TBAs; Langwick illustrates the nature of global subject formation.

Hansjörg Dilger's chapter tells of the f(r)ictions involved in global subject
formation in the context of the global health industry. His chapter examines
the social context in which shifting AIDS policies work on Tanzanian lives.
Examining national and international efforts to address HIV/AIDS, he notes
a move from fear-based messages to empowerment-based "projects" over the
past two decades. The current "empowered individual" is rational and self-
governing, juggling a range of demands, hopes, and aspirations. Messages
about HIV prevention and about care for loved ones with HIV/AIDS have
grown subtler, now differentiating target audiences by gender, age, education, and profession. Even in these more complex depictions, however, the
image of the empowered individual portrayed in public health initiatives cannot capture the fullness of Tanzanian lives. Dilger therefore contrasts the work
of these constructions with a portrait of the demands on rural Tanzanians
in Mara negotiating the patrilineal traditions of caring for widows and sick
wives, as well as of urban Tanzanians with HIV who turn to a Neo-Pentecostal
church for healing and support. The effects of biopower, as illustrated in the
global production and circulation of empowered individuals making personal
choices to prevent HIV and care appropriately for those with AIDS, are limited in Tanzania, he argues, because global regimes of truth and knowledge
interface with a state and with a group of non-governmental organizations
which "have only limited ability to establish and exercise biopolitical authority (also in its more beneficial form) in a *pervasive* way." Other regimes of
power—family and church for instance—remain central to the way that HIV/
AIDS is apprehended and to the forms of support and care that people with
AIDS have.

While Dilger looks at the circulation of technologies of the self, *Angelika
Wolf* turns to the circulation of financial models and instruments. She examines the emergence of community-based health insurance programs in Africa.
Wolf takes models of health insurance as a global object, discussing in particular the import of both the English and the German models into the developing world in the shape of health organizations. Local adaptations of these

models of mutual health insurance are heralded as one solution for protecting the poor from the expenses of health care as structural adjustment programs insist on the reduction of state expenditure on health. She discusses two forms of securing future access to health care in Diourbel, Senegal. First, a rich case study illustrates the benefits and constraints of the mutual health organizations, which subsidize 50 percent of the cost of services and medications in government hospitals. Not everyone finds these organizations worth the monthly expense, however, because government hospitals are often not well stocked with even the essential medicines that they are supposed to carry. Therefore, some in Diourbel prefer to invest in one of the many available savings associations. They can draw on these funds more flexibly for support during times of illness or other difficulties. Each of these techniques for ensuring access to health care when in need illustrate a broad shift in the forms of ethical responsibility for those with fewer resources. Wolf argues that both of these schemes are bureaucratic and financial technologies whose core effect is to insist on solidarity among the poor as a solution to economic inequality rather than solidarity between citizens of diverse economic standing.

John Janzen's chapter explores what he calls "Afri-global medicine." By juxtaposing three explorations—of humanitarian responses to Ebola outbreaks in Central Africa, of the obstacles to the development and broad circulation of indigenous medicines, and of Somali communities and the organizations working for their health and well-being—Janzen tells us that African health and healing are deeply implicated in the global at every turn. The movement of people and medicines, as well as the dual action of the humanitarian imperatives and the global trade policies that have together framed African health, compels ethnographic accounts that appreciate how the lives of Africans and their experiences of all forms of healing (including traditional medicine) are shaped by broader social, historical, and political conditions.

Globality is not only, in all places, a process of (re)filling health systems with new institutional arrangements, practices, and meanings, but also a process of emptying out. *Kristin Peterson's* chapter places the humanitarian imperatives of AIDS treatment in Nigeria in the broader contexts of the imperatives of capital. She seeks to complement anthropological work on globalization that traces the flows of finance and manufacturing capital by examining the places from which these flows of capital begin. Drawing attention to both extractive industries and "policy-driven capital" Peterson theorizes dispossession through an analysis of pharmaceutical capital in Nigeria and its ties to oil, debt, and military economies. She asks: "As it is widely recognized that the African continent continues to provide raw material in the form of oil, minerals, and cash crops to the rest of the world in crumbling and non-reproducible ways, can there be an analysis of an emptied-out space as the left-behind effect of such movement?" Peterson argues that the 1986 International Monetary Fund's (IMF) structural adjustment program (SAP) initiated a massive "emptying out" of existing health institutions and pharmacies and disabled drug manufacturing in Nigeria. The SAP's requirements for currency devaluation, wage decreases, state privatization and dismantling, and so on, devastated the practice of pharmacy in the country. She reports that by 1996, ten years after structural adjustment implementation, nearly two-thirds of the pharmaceutical manufacturing industry had bottomed out. As this dismantling of local generic production is combined with the mass introduction of proprietary ARV drugs and the imposition of an anti-generic intellectual property law, it became possible for U.S. proprietary drugs to thrive—at extremely high costs.

ALTERNATIVE FORMS OF GLOBALITY

While health interventions are often initiated by national governments and global health institutions, these large-scale actors are only *one* part of the global health picture. This section focuses on the manifold ways in which alternative forms of medicine and health-related globality are produced and negotiated by health professionals, religious leaders, and the health initiatives of individual men and women "on the ground." The section starts with the chapter by *Viola Hörbst,* who focuses on a much-neglected debate on medicine and health in sub-Saharan Africa: the introduction of cutting-edge medical technology and the way privatization and economic liberalization have created new opportunities for health professionals and the more wealthy parts of African populations. While infertility has become a significant challenge for women and men in Mali (with an estimated 23.6 percent of women suffering from secondary infertility and 10.4 percent from primary infertility), the internationally acclaimed "right to reproduction" hasn't been integrated into the country's health sector, which from the 1980s onward has focused on primary health care, equity of access, and "priority diseases." Hörbst shows how private practitioners in Mali—most of whom were trained abroad—have come to use their transnationally embedded professional channels and expertise in making assisted reproductive technologies available to their more wealthy urban middle-class clients. She also discusses the experiences, troubles, and dilemmas that men and women in Mali go through in conceiving a child: the issue of infertility is often surrounded by secrecy and the pressures of relatives who are expecting offspring from the newlywed couple, and husbands and wives have to negotiate mutually acceptable ways of coming to terms with the infertility diagnosis, and of undergoing assisted reproductive treatment if they choose that path. This in turn may challenge religiously and socially acclaimed gender hierarchies and may lead to new forms of dialogue and intimacy among married couples.

As private practitioners and health professionals have become engaged in the introduction of reproductive technologies in Mali, transnational migrants and migrants' associations have in a different way come to challenge and transform health systems and health practices in West Africa and beyond. *Abdoulaye Kane* shows how the dynamics of migration between Senegal and France have given rise to multifaceted and multidirectional flows of medicines, money, patients, and healers between the two countries; and how these flows are intrinsically tied up with processes of social and economic differentiation in the migrant's host countries and home communities. He argues that Haalpulaar males from the first generation of immigrants to France—many of whom came from rural areas in northeast Senegal and had limited educational backgrounds—have in particular become increasingly distrustful of the French health system and have lost much of the admiration for biomedicine that originally shaped their attraction to the West in the early 1960s. And just as the unfulfilled health needs of migrants in France engender a growing flow of plants, healers, *marabouts*, and overall medical expertise from the rural sending areas in Senegal, Haalpulaar men and women have also become invested in improving the health conditions and health care structures in their home areas in Senegal. Apart from individual efforts to send medications and pay for the medical treatment of relatives, the young generation of migrants especially has become engaged in organizing medical missions to Senegal and also providing resources for more sustainable health infrastructure in the country.

Religious leaders are not only exploring entrepreneurial opportunities and attending to the health needs of individual women and men in transnational settings; they may also have considerable influence on the everyday workings of public health and medicine in African countries—and on the religious and moral landscapes in which they are embedded. *Adeline Masquelier* draws on the case of Malam Awal, a Sufi preacher from Nigeria who arrived in Niger in the mid-1990s when the country had already gone through several years of economic, political, and media liberalization. While Islam and Muslim practice in Niger in the early 1990s had become strongly influenced by the strictly reformist movement Izala (which was dedicated to the promotion of religious rationalism and the eradication of "wrongful" *maraboutic* traditions), Awal's preaching focused on the importance of local healing traditions and the central concern of Muslim teaching and practice with ritual control over the occult. The strong appeal Awal's teachings had among wide segments of Niger's population also extended into the domain of public health and politics when he began to engage in a campaign against polio vaccination in the early 2000s. His claims about vaccinations being a conspiracy of the

Nigerien government and international (Christian/Western) organizations to eradicate the "heirs of true Islam" fell on fertile ground among a population where rumors and perceptions concerning state inefficiency and its failure to provide health care had become widely acknowledged.

Adam Mohr analyzes the reproduction of spiritual healing practices originating in Ghana among the Ghanaian diaspora in North America. He documents the evolution of Ghanaian Presbyterian and Pentecostal churches in the United States. One of the most important components of the Presbyterian churches both at home and in the diaspora seems to be healing and protecting against demonic attacks. The role of a particular Ghanaian priest and his family network in the duplication of local forms of religious healing in America is presented as critical. The practices of religious healing are centralized and involve the intervention of priests from Ghana. The institutional organization of Ghanaian churches in the North American context and their ability to maintain connections with mother churches in Ghana is highlighted. One of Mohr's important findings is how the changes in gender roles among the Ghanaian immigrant community in America affect the participation of men and women as patients in spiritual healing. In Ghana, it is primarily women who are afflicted, because they are exposed to social tensions and are in a weaker social position in a patriarchal society. In the United States, the increased opportunities for women to work, particularly in the health industry as nurses, means that they may earn more money than their male counterparts, putting the latter in a difficult position where they have to assume roles that are associated with "women's work" in Ghana. These changes in gender roles lead, Mohr argues, to men feeling emasculated and insecure, explaining their comparatively higher rates of "being possessed" by malevolent forces and of participation in religious healing practices in the U.S.

MOVING THROUGH THE GAPS

The chapters in this section address the movement of experts and patients trying to fill the gaps of the global health system—which is based primarily on biomedical approaches and understandings. *Marja Tiilikainen's* chapter looks at the mobility of Somali patients in the diaspora with regard to their home country. Tiilikainen examines the way Somalis in the diaspora organize themselves in a transnational space to benefit from the therapeutic skills of healers in the Horn of Africa. She analyzes the various instances in which Somali refugees abroad seek treatment from religious healers on the continent. It is usually in cases of mental distress or incurable diseases that Somalis in the diaspora return home to seek the services of indigenous healing practitioners. Tiilikainen explores the idea of transnational health care bringing together patients in the diaspora and healers at home through a variety of forms and mediums. She shows that transnational health care includes not only *people* who cross borders while they search for suitable treatment but also the transfer of advice, treatments, and medicines across space. The cases she follows show clearly that border-crossings may be made through travel, of bodies or suitcases; through memory; or in virtual space and time, with telephone calls, faxes, and the internet.

While Tiilikainen's chapter is about the mobility of Somali refugees and medicines in and out of their home country, *Elisabeth Hsu*'s chapter examines the motivations of Chinese doctors to migrate *to* East Africa. She uses the life stories of several Chinese doctors to describe their patterns of mobility and connectedness. The existence of what Hsu calls East–South mobility challenges the general assumption that mobility is unidirectional from South to North or from East to West. The push and pull factors motivating people's movements are not only related to contrasting levels of economic development in receiving countries but also people's movements driven by opportunities available in economic niches that exist in specific places. She shows how Kenya, and Africa in general, are perceived by Chinese doctors as places where they can make money to pursue their dreams in other destinations or to return back home. This movement of Chinese doctors to Africa is part of a general trend of globalizing forms of healing that pose as alternatives to the Western dominant biomedical style of medical practice. Hsu uses extended life stories to give valuable insights on the migration experiences of Chinese doctors in East Africa by exploring their motivation to leave China; their mobility patterns; their connectedness to home; their paths of professional and social insertion in Kenya; and their relations with the Kenyan authorities, the Chinese embassy in Nairobi, and their patients.

As the last chapter in this section, *Clara Carvalho*'s study looks at the way local health practices in Guinea Bissau are being brought into Portugal, Spain, and France by transnational migrants, and how this transfer of healing practices corresponds with the need to reproduce shrines in Portugal for healing purposes. Carvalho presents a multi-sited ethnography, following the cases of several traditional therapists on their migrant circuits as they cross the borders of not only distant countries but also of distinctive meaning systems and contrasting cosmogonies. She analyzes the reproduction of local forms of healing in the context of Guinean migration to Portugal, and how the Guinean local forms of healing are being transplanted by the *mouros* and the *jambakus* in European countries. This account gives a sense of the complexity of ritual practices in Guinea Bissau, where shrines and ritual practitioners are related to one another in a hierarchical manner. Carvalho focuses on the *jambakus* because, though they are one category of diviners and ritual experts among many in their home country, this category is the only form that she found replicated in the transcontinental context. The *jambakus* recreate shrines in Europe to maintain connections with spirits, ancestors under the supervision of local traditional authorities. Carvalho presents the transnational spread of Guinean healing forms as part of the globalization process that needs to be understood as a multilevel movement in which the dissemination of plural therapeutic practices transmitted by migrant populations along their migrant circuits plays an important part.

Together, the chapters in this volume consider globalization and Africa, specifically focusing on the movements of healers, patients, doctors, bureaucracies, policies, statistics, and medicines associated with various aspects of health care. They underscore both the interconnectedness and the imbalances of these linkages as they are realized in an era of neoliberal reforms. By examining the kinds of mobility that define the contemporary moment, we argue for the historical nature of globalization and the multiple valances of transnationalism. Neoliberal reforms in Africa have shaped the conditions of life, the management of affliction, and the strategies for survival of people, both on the continent and in the diaspora. By examining the everyday encounters of Africans and their practical efforts to communicate, care for loved ones; relieve discomforts; address misfortunes; and attend to the health and future of communities, nations, and regions, this volume illustrates how global connections are brought to life in and beyond Africa.

Notes

1. This argument is inspired by Fredrick Cooper and Ann Stoller's (1989) and Jane Guyer's (1993) arguments that certain colonial regulatory reforms serve to characterize that era.

2. In this work we are inspired by Anna Tsing's concept of "friction." In her book *Friction: An Ethnography of Global Connection* (2004), Tsing explores the multiple ways in which global connections "come to life" in everyday encounters and interactions between different scales and units of global social organization; and how frictions and tensions have become an integral part of the "makeshift links across distance and difference that shape global futures—and ensure their uncertain status" (2004: 2). The focus on frictions, tensions, and differences, Tsing argues, allows us to understand how specific configurations of economy, politics, and knowledge—and the contested relations between and within these particular fields of social organization—are being and have been produced in specific ethnographic settings through a particular set of global connections and power relations. This focus also allows us to take account of the unexpected, the unstable, and the unpredictable aspects of globalization processes—in short, the "messiness" of cultural production in a globally interconnected world which has become

embedded in the multidirectional motions of goods, ideas, money, and people across national and continental borders.

3. By "universalizing flows" we mean to highlight an understanding of how certain forms of knowledge—or, even more specifically, methodological techniques—are universalizing, i.e. make claims to the universal.

4. For similar arguments, see Comaroff and Comaroff (1993), Geschiere (1997), and Meyer (1995). In addition, for a summarizing critique of recent studies of "the occult" in Africa and the necessity of adopting a historically informed perspective in the study of religious organization and practice, see Ranger (2007).

5. The most explicit case for the relative excessiveness of governmental as well as non-governmental funds for specific health problems is probably HIV/AIDS. The recent focus by international funding bodies on a (potentially unsustainable) treatment apparatus has led to an increasing fragmentation and internal imbalance in many African countries' health systems (see, e.g., Sullivan 2011).

References

Adepoju, A. 1991. "South–North Migration: The African Experience." *International Migration* 29: 205–221.

Appadurai, Arjun. 1990. "Disjuncture and Difference in the Global Cultural Economy." *Public Culture* 2 (2): 1–24.

———. 1996. *Modernity at Large: Cultural Dimensions of Globalization.* Minneapolis: University of Minnesota Press.

———, ed. 2001. *Globalization.* Durham, N.C.: Duke University Press.

Aretxaga, Begoña. 2003. "Maddening States." *Annual Review of Anthropology* 32: 393–410.

Arthur, John. 2000. *Invisible Sojourners: African Immigrant Diaspora in the United States.* Westport, Conn.: Praeger.

Baer, Hans A., Merrill Singer, and Ida Susser. 1997. *Medical Anthropology and the World System: A Critical Perspective.* Westport, Conn.: Bergin & Garvey.

Berger, Peter L., and Samuel Huntington. 2002. *Many Globalizations: Cultural Diversity in the Contemporary World.* Oxford: Oxford University Press.

Biehl, Joao, Byron Good, and Arthur Kleinman, eds. 2007. *Subjectivity: Ethnographic Investigations.* Berkeley: University of California Press.

Clifford, James. 1997. *Routes: Travel and Translation in the Twentieth Century.* Cambridge, Mass.: Harvard University Press.

Comaroff, Jean. 1981. "Healing and Cultural Transformation: The Tswana of Southern Africa." *Social Science and Medicine* 15b: 367–387.

Comaroff, Jean, and John L. Comaroff. 1993. "Introduction." In *Modernity and Its Malcontents: Ritual and Power in Postcolonial Africa,* ed. Jean Comaroff and John L. Comaroff, xi–xxxvii. Chicago: University of Chicago Press.

Cooper, Frederick. 2005. *Colonialism in Question: Theory, Knowledge, History.* Berkeley: University of California Press.

Cooper, Frederick, and Ann Stoler. 1989. "Introduction: Tensions of Empire— Colonial Control and Visions of Rule." *American Ethnologist* 16 (4): 609–621

Digby, Anne. 2004. "'Bridging Two Worlds': The Migrant Labourer and Medical Change in Southern Africa." In *Migration and Health in Southern Africa,* ed. Robin Cohen, 18–26. Cape Town, South Africa: Content Solutions.

Dilger, Hansjörg, and Bernhard Hadolt, eds. 2010. *Medizin im Kontext. Krankheit und Gesundheit in einer vernetzten Welt.* Frankfurt am Main: Peter Lang Verlag.

Dilger, Hansjörg, and Ute Luig, eds. 2010. *Morality, Hope, and Grief: Anthropologies of AIDS in Africa.* Oxford: Berghahn Books.

Ecks, Stefan. 2005. "Pharmaceutical Citizenship: Antidepressant Marketing and the Promise of Demarginalization in India." *Anthropology and Medicine* 12 (3): 239–254.

Edelmann, Marc, and Angelique Haugerud. 2007. "Development." In *A Companion to the Anthropology of Politics,* ed. David Nugent and Joan Vincent, 86–106. Malden, Mass.: Blackwell Publishing.

Escobar, Arturo. 1995. *Encountering Development: The Making and the Unmaking of the Third World.* Princeton, N.J.: Princeton University Press.

Farmer, Paul. 2003. *Pathologies of Power: Health, Human Rights, and the New War on the Poor.* Berkeley: University of California Press.

Feierman, Steven. 1985. "Struggles for Control: The Social Roots of Health and Healing in Modern Africa." *African Studies Review* 28 (2–3): 73–147.

Feierman, Steven, and John Janzen, eds. 1992. *The Social Basis of Health and Healing in Africa.* Berkeley: University of California Press.

Ferguson, James. 1990. *The Anti-Politics Machine: "Development," Depoliticization, and Bureaucratic Power in Lesotho.* Minneapolis, Minn.: University of Minnesota Press.

———. 1999. *Expectations of Modernity: Myths and Meanings of Urban Life on the Zambian Copperbelt.* Berkeley: University of California Press.

———. 2002. "Of Mimicry and Membership: Africans and the 'New World Society.'" *Cultural Anthropology* 17 (4): 551–569.

———. 2006. *Global Shadows: Africa in the Neoliberal World Order.* Durham, N.C.: Duke University Press.

Geschiere, Peter. 1997. *The Modernity of Witchcraft: Politics and the Occult in Postcolonial Africa.* Charlottesville: University Press of Virginia.

Glick Schiller, Nina. 2004. "Transnationality." In *A Companion to the Anthropology of Politics,* ed. David Nugent and Joan Vincent, 448–467. Malden, Mass.: Blackwell Publishing.

Guyer, Jane. 1993. "'Toiling Ingenuity': Food Regulation in Britain and Nigeria." *American Ethnologist* 20 (4): 797–817.

Hunt, Nancy Rose. 1999. "STDs, Suffering, and Their Derivatives in Congo-Zaire: Notes Towards an Historical Ethnography of Disease." In *Vivre et penser le sida en Afrique/ Experiencing and Understanding AIDS in Africa,* ed. Charles Becker, Jean-Pierre Dozon, Christine Obbo, and Moriba Touré, 111–131. Paris: Codesria, IRD, Karthala.

Janzen, John M. 1978. *The Quest for Therapy in Lower Zaire.* Berkeley: University of California Press.

Kapur, Devesh, and John McHale. 2005. *Give Us Your Best and Brightest: The Global Hunt for Talent and Its Impact on the Developing World.* Cambridge: Center for Global Development.

Kearney, Michael. 1995. "The Local and the Global: The Anthropology of Globalization and Transnationalism." *Annual Review of Anthropology* 24: 547–565.

Krause, Kristine. 2008. "Transnational Therapy Networks among Ghanaians in London." *Journal of Ethnic and Migration Studies* 34 (2): 235–251.

Lakoff, Andrew, and Stephen J. Collier, eds. 2008. *Biosecurity Interventions: Global Health and Security in Question.* New York: Columbia University Press.

Larkin, Brian. 1997. "Indian Lovers and Nigerian Lovers: Media and the Creation of Parallel Modernities." *Africa* 67 (3): 406–440.

Lock, Margaret, and Mark Nichter. 2002. "Introduction: From Documenting Medical Pluralism to Critical Interpretations of Globalized Health Knowledge, Policies, and Practices." In *New Horizons in Medical Anthropology: Essays in Honour of Charles Leslie,* ed. Mark Nichter and Margaret Lock, 1–34. London: Routledge.

Luedke, Tracy J., and Harry G. West, eds. 2005. *Borders and Healers: Brokering Therapeutic Resources in Southeast Africa.* Bloomington: Indiana University Press.

MacGaffey, Janet, and Rémy Bazenguissa-Ganga. 2000. *Congo-Paris: Transnational Traders on the Margins of the Law.* Bloomington: Indiana University Press.

Manuh, Takyiwaa, ed. 2005. *At Home in the World: International Migration and Development in Contemporary Ghana and West Africa.* Accra, Ghana: Sub Saharan Publishers.

Meyer, Birgit. 1995. "'Delivered from the Powers of Darkness': Confessions about Satanic Riches in Christian Ghana." *Africa* 65 (2): 236–255.

Nguyen, Vinh-Kim. 2005. "Antiretrovirals, Globalism, Biopolitics, and Therapeutic Citizenship." In *Global Assemblages: Technology, Politics, and Ethics as Anthropological Problems,* ed. Aihwa Ong and Stephen J. Collier, 124–145. Oxford: Blackwell Publishing.

Nichter, Mark. 2002. "The Social Relations of Therapy Management." In *New Horizons in Medical Anthropology: Essays in Honor of Charles Leslie,* ed. Mark Nichter and Margaret Lock, 81–111. London: Routledge.

Ong, Ahiwa, and Stephen J. Collier, eds. 2005. *Global Assemblages: Technology, Politics, and Ethics as Anthropological Problems.* Oxford: Blackwell Publishing.

Piot, Charles. 1999. *Remotely Global: Village Modernity in West Africa.* Chicago: University of Chicago Press.

———. 2002. "Des cosmopolites dans la brousse." *Les Temps Modernes* 57 (620–621): 240–260.

Petryna, Adriana. 2002. *Life Exposed: Biological Citizens after Chernobyl.* Princeton: Princeton University Press.

Rabinow, Paul. 1992. "Artificiality and Enlightenment: From Sociobiology to Biosociality." In *Zone 6: Incorporations,* ed. Jonathan Crary, 234–252. Cambridge, Mass.: MIT.

Ranger, Terence. 1992. "Plagues of Beasts and Men: Prophetic Responses to Epidemic in Eastern and Southern Africa." In *Epidemics and Ideas: Essays on the Historical Perception of Pestilence,* ed. Terence Ranger and Paul Slack, 241–268. Cambridge: Cambridge University Press.

———. 2007. "Scotland Yard in the Bush: Medicine Murders, Child Witches, and the Construction of the Occult: A Literature Review." *Africa* 77 (2): 272–283.

Rose, Nikolas. 2007. *The Politics of Life Itself: Biomedicine, Power, and Subjectivity in the Twenty-First Century.* Princeton: Princeton University Press.

Rose, Nikolas, and Carlos Novas. 2005. "Biological Citizenship." In *Global Assemblages: Technology, Politics, and Ethics as Anthropological Problems,* ed. Aihwa Ong and Stephen Collier, 439–463. Oxford: Blackwell Publishing.

Sanders, Todd. 2001. "Save Our Skins: Structural Adjustment, Morality, and the Occult in Tanzania." In *Magical Interpretations, Material Realities: Modernity, Witchcraft and the Occult in Postcolonial Africa,* ed. Henrietta L. Moore and Todd Sanders, 160–183. London: Routledge.

Sullivan, Noelle. 2011. "Mediating Abundance and Scarcity: Implementing an HIV/AIDS-Targeted Project within a Government Hospital in Tanzania." *Medical Anthropology* 30 (2): 202–221.

Tsing, Anna Lowenhaupt. 2004. *Friction: An Ethnography of Global Connection.* Princeton: Princeton University Press.

Turshen, Meredith. 1999. *Privatizing Health Services in Africa.* New Brunswick, N.J.: Rutgers University Press.

Vaughan, Megan. 1991. *Curing Their Ills: Colonial Power and African Illness.* Cambridge: Cambridge University Press.

Whyte, Susan Reynolds. 1997. *Questioning Misfortune: The Pragmatics of Uncertainty in Eastern Uganda.* Cambridge: Cambridge University Press.

———. 2009. "Health Identities and Subjectivities: The Ethnographic Challenge." *Medical Anthropology Quarterly* 23 (1): 6–15.

PART 1

Scale as an Effect of Power

The Choreography of Global Subjection: The Traditional Birth Attendant in Contemporary Configurations of World Health

Stacey A. Langwick

This chapter is about how transnational collaborations elicit a global subject. It takes the Traditional Birth Attendant (TBA) as the site for unraveling the movements critical to an African globality. The TBA, as it was forged in the health crises of the second half of the twentieth century, is both a radically localized figure and a completely global product. Anthropologists have recognized that health development and humanitarianism are powerfully evocative spaces from which to examine the forms of violence as well as the kinds of liberation tied up in the obligations and ethics of medical interventions (Fassin 2008; Nguyen 2005; Peterson forthcoming; Redfield 2005, 2006, 2008). The marginality of the TBA within biomedical discourse—the suspicions as well as the hopes it generates, the controversies as well as the solutions it sustains—leads our attention in a different direction than ethnographies of other global medical interventions do, however (for example, in this volume see chapter 4 by John Janzen). The TBA recasts how we think about global subjectivity. As global health governance elicits the world as a set of nested administrative units—the global, the regional, the national, and the local—the subject is formulated as one more level of administration.

The imagined TBA profiled in the international health development documents of the World Health Organization (WHO) maps neatly over the iconic "Third World woman" of the feminist texts examined by Mohanty (1986) in her classic essay "Under Western Eyes." Mohanty argues that the Third World woman depicted in "Western" feminist scholarship is distinct in her homogeneity from the flesh-and-blood historical women who live varied lives in Africa, Asia, and Latin and South America. The average Third World woman emerges through the universalizing methodologies of cross-cultural analyses. By formulating women as a stable category and marking only the "Third World difference" these studies maintain the West as a privileged referent or norm. The TBA who peoples the pages of the policy documents, public health guidelines, training manuals, and other texts that comprise so much of international health development work is a specialized version of the Third World woman. She is generated through the intersection of two sets of universalizing knowledge practices concerning gender and medicine. She illustrates how the differences central to Mohanty's "gendered worldings" both enable and are enabled by distinctions between biomedical knowledge and other forms of knowledge about bodies, health, and healing.

Stacy Leigh Pigg (1997a, 1997b) takes up a similarly discursive argument when she accounts for both TBAs and Traditional Medical Practitioners (TMPs) as products of international health development discourse. The concept of tradition, as it is unpacked by Pigg, does work similar to Mohanty's Third World difference. In the United States or Western Europe there may be homebirth midwives, even direct entry midwives, but there are, in the current framework, no longer TBAs. Even the process of identifying TBAs marks an area as the Third World. Pigg examines development agency reports and policy statements in Nepal in order to describe the translations that render a range of birthing practices in Nepal as "traditional." The documents Pigg examines articulate TBAs as practitioners "found in most societies" who are trusted custodians of cultural knowledge. In so doing, they establish a binary division of reproductive knowledge—traditional and modern—that is implicitly ranked. Pigg argues that this conceptual move "position[s] development institutions as the locus of authoritative knowledge while devaluing other, local forms of knowledge" (1997a: 233).

In this chapter, I build on these textual analyses by exploring the institutional work that generated the materials grounding the WHO's concept of the TBA, and the effects of the circulation of these materials. The genesis and movement of these documents reveal more than biomedicine's role in the "discursive colonization" of women's bodies in the developing world; they also reveal the constitution of a particular vision of the world itself. Literature is central to the practices of development organizations that render the world as scalar and thereby manageable. This effect of literature is less evident inside of texts, however, and more evident in the consequences of their production and circulation. The making of TBAs serves as one example of the ways in which development's iterative bureaucratic processes—and the letters, minutes, reports, and manuals they involve—conceive a world that can be apprehended as a collection of regions, which are themselves collections of nation-states, which are themselves collections of communities, which are themselves collections of individuals. Diverse areas and peoples become parts of wholes.

The evocation of and training of TBAs illustrates how "world health" is continually formulated as a practical framework for articulating problems and imagining solutions.[1] Within these programs the global appears to be common sense, and international development appears to be a necessary, even ethical, intervention. While the effectiveness of programs involving TBAs has been hotly debated (especially as effectiveness is often defined strictly in terms of maternal mortality statistics)[2], the work to develop these programs generates effects outside the realm of reproductive health care. For this reason, I argue, controversies over the value of the TBA in health programs have not seemed to reduce programming related to the TBA. If anything, with the outbreak of AIDS, international interest in and training for TBAs has increased.

While international development literature depicts TBAs as an already always-available resource to be tapped, in truth the making of the TBA as an articulate global subject has required an enormous amount of work. While I approach the making of the TBA as a global actor through the WHO, their records make it clear that the TBA makes sense only within a specific assemblage of actors. For instance, the background document for the 1973 Consultation compiled reports from over 40 ministries of health as well as both the published work of scholars and personal communications concerning their research. The meeting itself included observers from UNICEF, the United Nations Population Fund (UNFPA), the Population Council, the International Planned Parenthood Federation (IPPF), the International Council of Nurses (ICN), the International Confederation of Midwives (ICM) / International Federation of Gynaecology and Obstetrics (FIGO) Joint Study Group, and a consultant from the London School of Hygiene and Tropical Medicine (N2/180/3 130B[3]). Collier and Ong (2005: 14) argue that one "function of the study of assemblages is to gain analytical and critical insight into global forms." This is a study of assemblage both to account for the TBA as a global actor in health development and to explore how the global itself—what Tsing (2005) has called "globality"—is constituted.

The WHO is an ideal site to examine what the work of gathering data, assembling experts, establishing linkages, and coordinating commitments generates. The WHO describes itself as "the directing and coordinating authority for health within the United Nations system."[4] It facilitates, motivates, and shapes the work of others. In short, it generates the institutional collaborations and the technical, ethical, and political assemblages necessary for the world health that it purports to address. WHO initiatives concerning TBAs reveal the forms of difference most relevant to constructions of world health, as well as the techniques of managing difference within administrative scales. The history of the TBA, with its explicit marking of the traditional, throws into particularly strong relief frictions between local specificity and universal categories of behavior, practice, and experience. I examined WHO archival files from the late 1960s, when traditional birth attendants and traditional medicine became organizing concepts within the WHO, until 1987, when efforts concerning TBAs were solidified as part of the Safe Motherhood Project. I read the findings of my archival research through my experience conducting ethnographic research on traditional healing, including the work of TBAs, in Tanzania since 1998.

Discerning TBAs

Women who specialized in assisting other women with birth caught the attention of the WHO as early as 1955. At this time, participants in the Technical Discussions of the Sixth Session for the WHO Regional Committee for the Western Pacific Region debated the potential contributions of "domiciliary midwifery." They reached no consensus, however, as "almost diametrically opposite conclusions were arrived at by the participants with respect to the importance of domiciliary midwifery in the development of rural health services and whether or not efforts should be made to give training to unqualified midwives while undertaking at the same time the preparation of qualified midwives" (quoted in WHO 1973: 2 file N2/180/3 Jkt 2).

Two years later the topic of training "indigenous midwives" appeared on the agenda of the Tenth Session of the WHO Regional Committee for South East Asia. A paper presented at this meeting reflected the continued ambivalence of the biomedical personnel and policy makers working with the WHO. While noting that "with the development of scientific knowledge and the acceptance of more advanced obstetrical services, the indigenous midwife has, in many countries, gradually lost her place," regional health policy makers felt that "[t]he countries of South East Asia . . . with their vast populations, the variations in the cultural development of their many communities, and their present inability to train a sufficient number of fully qualified midwives, are obliged, for the time being, to look to the indigenous midwives for service to women in childbirth in wide areas of their rural communities" (quoted in WHO 1973: 2 file N2/180/3 Jkt 2). In 1972, during the planning meetings for the first WHO conference to focus on non-biomedically-trained midwives, a definition of the TBA was initially hammered out. This definition has remained basically unchanged: "a person who assists the mother during childbirth and initially acquired her skills by delivering babies herself or through apprenticeship to other traditional birth attendants" (WHO 1992).

These early records of the WHO reveal the problem of describing a TBA in the abstract to be no less challenging than identifying one in the field (N2/180/3). During the Planning Committee meeting for the "Studies of the

Activities of the Traditional Birth Attendant," which would be one of the foundational pieces of research for WHO work with TBAs, members debated who might be included under the rubric of the TBA.

> From material already examined, it is obvious that there will be a problem of defining exactly who is a TBA. Dr. Rosa [Chief Medical Officer, Maternal and Child Health, World Health Organization] suggested her as one who has practiced before being trained, as opposed to auxiliary nurses and midwives. Another criteria [sic] might be to identify TBAs as those who are self-employed. A clear definition and delineation will have to be established to avoid confusion with other personnel. Should the category also include all those who deliver members of their own families? (June 27, 1972. N2/180/3 71A)

Despite these difficulties, for the publication of the WHO's first guide to the training of Traditional Birth Attendants the authors managed to develop a profile of a TBA. She came to be:

> . . . an older woman, almost always past menopause, and who must have borne one or more children herself. She lives in the [most often rural] community in which she practices. She operates in a relatively restricted zone. . . . Many of her beliefs and practices pertaining to the reproductive cycle are dependent upon religious and mystic sanctions. . . . The Traditional Birth Attendant is often an accomplished herbalist, whose knowledge and use of herbs, roots, and barks may be quite extensive. . . . Typically, [she] is illiterate and has no formal training. (Verdersese and Turnbull 1975: 7)

A functional, if at times contentious, description of the TBA emerged though these and other regional meetings and the resulting documents. By the late 1970s, TBAs appeared as part of WHO guidelines for achieving "health for all by the year 2000," a call that animated their focus on primary health care (WHO 1978a, 1978b). TBAs had come to be seen as a cadre of community leaders who could address the perceived need for rapid expansion of health care services in economically constrained countries. They held a particularly hopeful role, promising "better" birth assistance to rural women and thereby reducing maternal mortality rates.

Training Distinctions

October 19, 1998. The Maternal and Child Health Coordinator, Mama Chikawe, and Assistant Coordinator, Mama Chibwana, travel from the district hospital in Newala to a Rural Health Center in Kitangari, a village about

30 kilometers north across the Makonde Plateau in southeastern Tanzania. They intend to supervise a training session for TBAs. The session will continue for five days. These two nurses from Newala, however, will only be able to supervise the first two days of the training because the district hospital has only one vehicle and there are a number of different projects that compete for the use of it.

Familiar with this Health Center after years of supervisory visits, they walk directly into a large white room with a cement floor. Along the far wall under the only windows in the room is a long low bench on which sit seven village leaders who hold official positions in the political structure. To their right, along an adjacent wall, a number of women squat on the floor. Each of them has arrived this morning from one of five different villages in the area to participate in the training workshop. These women look up to a table and four chairs. The Newala guests and I are shown to the chairs, and the Health Center nurses who are conducting the training stand next to the table to begin their introductions.

After introductions, the trainers dismiss the women who will be trained as TBAs, asking them to return the following day. The midwives gather together outside and prepare lunch for themselves on charcoal stoves. Meanwhile, the remainder of this first day of training is addressed to the village leaders. The District Maternal and Child Health Coordinator stands up and lectures, emphasizing that the maternal mortality rate in Tanzania, particularly in the southern part of the country where we are, is distressingly high. She then stresses the importance of keeping accurate records. The local leaders still perching on the bench under the windows respond by expressing their concerns about transportation and the difficulties of getting a woman in labor to a health facility for assistance.

Later the same day, a series of pictures is held up by the nurses and shown to the village leaders. While walking back and forth in front of her attentive audience, one of the nurses makes explicit the lessons to be drawn from each of the pictures. In the first picture, the important points, according to the nurse-trainer, are that the family illustrated has only two children; the mother is pregnant; and they are eating healthy food. The second picture depicts a girl and an older woman. Pointing to each of the figures in turn, the trainer asserts that girls below the age of 16 and women over the age of 35 should not get pregnant. If they do, she continues, they should be sent to the Newala District Hospital for maternity care. They should not under any circumstances give birth at home, even under the care of a trained TBA. The trainer uses the third picture, an illustration of an exhausted-looking woman surrounded by many children, to impart the lesson that one should not get pregnant too frequently or have too many children. The nurse-trainers continue in the same way to elaborate on the message encoded in each of the dozen or so pictures in order to illustrate the Safe Motherhood Initiative's criteria for a healthy, safe, and hygienic birth.

October 20, 1998. The lessons for TBAs begin. Large grass mats are spread on the cement floor and the women sit on these while leaning against the wall. The trainers in blue uniforms still stand in front of them or sit on chairs behind the table. I choose to sit on the mats with the TBAs. After a long conversation about healthy food, a woman next to me changes the subject. She asks the nurse conducting the training about the use of medicines. Medicine, the nurse answers, is not bad. However, a woman should always go to the hospital to get safe, clean medicine. She should not use the medicine of *wakunga wa jadi* (traditional midwives).[5]

This workshop was one instance of the implementation of an internationally designed and nationally organized project to train two TBAs in every village in Tanzania. Through this ambitious project, the Tanzanian government ostensibly made its greatest effort to incorporate traditional practitioners into the biomedically designed national health care system. The incorporation of TBAs into the national health development plans required that the Tanzanian state discern differences among "indigenous practitioners." The nebulous distinction between the biomedical practitioners and all other healers (whether "charlatans" or persons with "good intentions"), who had served as a foil for biomedicine since the beginning of the twentieth century, came to be slightly more refined through the separation of traditional midwives and traditional healers. Traditional midwives were to be outreach workers, helping in the fight to reduce the maternal and infant mortality figures that contributed to Tanzania's ranking as one of the least developed counties in the world. Through the Safe Motherhood Initiative (SMI), which started in 1987, the Tanzanian government strove to train 32,000 TBAs. To understand this significant effort we must step backward in time.

In 1961 the newly independent Tanzanian government inherited a dispersed group of health care facilities. Colonial health services had focused primarily on urban areas, and the colonial government had relied on mission stations to offer clinical care in rural areas. Biomedicine, in the context of colonialism and missionization, had not been held accountable to a national public.[6] At independence the new administration found itself with health care facilities that were radically inadequate to care for all of its citizens. In its response, it invoked the TBA and other lay health workers as keys to a rapid extension of biomedical care through existing indigenous networks. The TBA emerged as a biomedical helper, an outreach worker, a stopgap measure. She was never conceptualized as a colleague in imagining the new nation's goals in relation to health, healing, and birth, or in formulating the structures of medicine and care to which the government might be held accountable. In fact, while the rhetoric of valuing indigenous knowledge and tapping what Feierman (1990) has called "peasant intellectuals" dovetailed with socialist development objectives, the ministry of health remained suspicious of any focus that drew already too-scarce resources away from clinics. They feared that the international community would offer TBAs as a cheap (and second-rate) solution to the health care crisis. As a result, before the SMI, efforts to identify and train TBAs in Tanzania were scattered. Below, I examine the work done to make TBAs coherent figures leading up to their incorporation in the SMI, and the increased prominence that this initiative lent to their role in global health. Interestingly, much of this work occurred outside of Tanzanian borders, even outside of Africa.

This bias may have been partly an effect of personal histories. Ms. Verdersese, the consultant who prepared the original background paper for the 1973 Consultation, was a former Western Pacific Regional Office (WPRO) regional officer. Dr. Maglacas, who came to be the point person for all TBA activities within the WHO, was from Malaysia.[7] The professional and personal connections that WHO staff had in the Western Pacific, along with the prominence of China and to some extent India in global conceptualizations of traditional medicine, appear to have made regions and countries in Asia more accessible and feasible sites for the elaboration of the TBA. As we will see below, both the Africa Regional Office (AFRO) and individual African countries were slow to respond to the requests of the World Health Organization Headquarters (WHO HQ). The reasons for this were likely many (technological, bureaucratic, financial, etc.). The WHO struggled to involve those in Africa in their conceptualization and mobilization of TBAs. Reading archives in reference to global initiatives to recruit and train TBAs throughout Tanzania reveals an irony in the making of this traditional global subject. While the effort to train 32,000 TBAs in Tanzania purportedly tapped particularly local subjects "confined to their community," TBAs existed as such only because of a great deal of work done elsewhere.

Emergency and Emergence

The WHO files indicate that the information about Africa sought for the background document for the 1973 Consultation meeting that laid the groundwork for the definition and profile of a TBA (as described above) was limited. The report by the WHO AFRO arrived at headquarters too late to be incorporated into the broader background paper. Consultation participants received the report as an appendix to the background document (WHO 1973). WHO staff had culled the literature and contacted scholars and development workers in order to extract some information that would help them include Africa in the profiles compiled for the meetings. Upon the recommendation of Dr. Bannerman—the Programme Manager for the Traditional Medicine unit and himself Ghanaian—the organizers invited a health officer from Ghana to represent the Africa Regional Office (AFRO) in the actual gathering (Planning Committee Meeting, November 9, 1972: 112).[8]

The real work for this consultation—the hundreds of pages of paper in the archive concerning this gathering—was in the planning. In particular, two aspects of planning this "consultation" took up most of the time of the WHO staff and consultants: (1) preparing the report on which the members of the consultation would comment and that would thereby serve as a common point of reference for discussions; and (2) the invitations. The former established the first broad foundation for claims to a worldwide actor known as the TBA, and the latter indicated who had the right to shape this actor.

The first objective of the 1973 consultation meeting was, "To explore sources of information and to collect and review data on traditional birth attendants in order to develop a profile of traditional birth attendants [*sic*] roles, their place in society, their beliefs and practice" (Planning Committee Meeting Minutes, November 23, 1972: 114). The background documentation compiled and prepared by Ms. Verdersese, a Nurse Consultant for the WHO and an ex-officer of the WPRO, gathered together country-specific statistical and narrative information on TBAs from published materials, unpublished documents, and personal communications. A substantial section of the 165-page document sent to all participants contained a multi-page chart identifying key characteristics of the 76 countries reviewed. These characteristics included the "local" name for the actor who might be translated as a TBA, whether or not there were national laws permitting untrained persons to attend births, if there were training programs for these "indigenous midwives," and what sorts of incentives they received for attending training.

The consultation document illustrates some of the tensions that shaped the category of TBA as it rose to prominence in health development circles, tensions between the needs of international development and the realities of people in a variety of places in the world. The note on the top of the AFRO regions chart, for instance, reads:

> In most African countries there is no legal status accorded to the TBA. The MCH [Maternal and Child Health] component of the overall health planning is drawn up without reference to the TBA, even though it is known that the bulk of midwifery care is done by the TBA. Some of them have some "training" on the job by their pre-decessors. Others are just ordinary mothers probably of more than 2 children who are called up in case of delivery. (N-190–3 Jkt 2: 119, WHO 1973: 9)

The Tanzanian example and many others in the initial WHO compilation reveal the difficulties in articulating the relationship of the profiled TBA to those attending birth in a variety of locations. The process was fraught with inconsistencies and the results were unruly.

Even the title of a person who might be called a TBA drew a question mark in the study. In Tanzania, people speak 127 different "local" languages. However, due to British colonization between the First World War and 1961 and its effects on colonial Tanganyikan and Zanzibarian education, law, and international relations, English became one of the official national languages in the newly independent conjoined country called Tanzania (Kiswahili being the other national language).[9] The Tanzania entry in the study captured the ambiguity this diversity caused by noting the title of such specialists as "Traditional Midwives?" with a question mark (see table 1).

This entry also reveals that the new category of the TBA in Tanzania brought the "old traditional midwife" together with young girls in primary school—who often had no experience giving birth themselves or having helped others give birth but who had been tapped to receive some basic training in midwifery. Thirty years later this conflation of older women with young women trained in some basic care continued to create friction within TBA training programs. The nurses facilitating the training session described above remarked on their frustration when dealing with the older women, who often refused to accept the authority of biomedical knowledge. These nurses favored the younger women, who had significantly less experience and who came to the training hoping to learn skills to help them build a practice. Indeed, the relations of TBAs with clinics through southeastern Tanzania reveal that many of those who most successfully serve as extensions of the clinic are women whose expertise concerning birth and delivery was built through biomedical health programs (Langwick 2010).

This issue of age and education has plagued TBA projects in many parts of the world. When responding to a report concerning TBA programs in Jordan, the Regional Director of the Eastern Mediterranean Regional Office

Country or Territory	Title	Legal Status	Identity or Register	Training Programme	Certificate of Licence to Practice	Incentives	Supervision — Yes or No	Observations — By whom?
Tanzania	Traditional Mid-wives (?)	—	—	Yes (3 months)	—	—	—	Plans are on hand to increase the numbers of "Village Midwives" (young girl (sic) in primary school or old traditional midwife selected by each village and given a 3 month training, after which she returns to her village to carry on her work) so as to have one Village Midwife at each health centre and later at each village dispensary.

Table 1.1. Table excerpted from Consultation on the Role of the Traditional Birth Attendant in Family Planning, p. 10 in File N-190-3 Jkt 2: 120.

(EMRO) noted that a much higher percentage of women in the 30–50 year age range were trained than those who were over 60 years old. He concluded: "It shows again that the best point of concentration is the under 50 years olds, with progressively advanced training. The over 50 years old TBA's will die out soon anyway" (N2/180/3 EMR letter dated May 31, 1979).

A number of anthropological studies have examined how global policy and practice impose abstract categories of being onto locales. These forms of imposition may be repressive or generative, but much of the work on global health agrees in seeing a struggle between abstraction and particularities, between policy and practice, between the global and the local.[10] While the formulation and management of these divisions has been important to the knowledge practices of health development organizations and their global imaginings, accounts emphasizing these binary tensions gloss over some of the important world-making work of global health. Articulating the global requires not only the gathering of examples and the abstraction that imagines a planet-wide condition. It also requires a subsequent series of iterations that establish the global in relation to its definitive others—the regional, the national, and the subject. As Dr. Bannerman, the WHO Programme Manager for Traditional Medicine, and Dr. Maglacas in the Division of Human Manpower Development (HMD) noted in a memo to a number of collaborators at the UN, World Bank, and other international organizations: "a Consultation Meeting has meaning only if it is followed up at national and regional levels by mutually supporting activities that are consistent with the policies agreed upon" (N2/445/16 Jkt 1, letter sent September 4, 1984). Understanding the iterative nature of health development is central to understanding the construction of world health and the role of health development work (and, I would submit, development work more broadly) in global governance. This chapter describes the subtle and complicated generation of a scalar world through international health development projects promoting TBAs.

Paper and People

The first phase of WHO work created a profile of the TBA and a rationale for her centrality to an emerging global biopolitics. In the late 1970s, while continuing to gather reports on TBAs and birth practices, the WHO began to focus also on disseminating the information that they had compiled in an effort to support program planning. Four main projects followed the 1973 Consultation report and grounded WHO's efforts to formulate the TBA as a global resource.

1. 1975: *The Traditional Birth Attendant In Maternal and Child Health and Family Planning: A Guide to Her Training and Utilization,* by Maria de Lourdes Verdersese, Nurse Consultant, and Lily M. Turnbull, Chief Nursing Officer, Division of Health Manpower Development (WHO Offset Publication No. 18).

2. 1979: *Traditional Birth Attendants: A Field Guide to Their Training, Evaluation, and Articulation with Health Services,* by Beverley du Gas, Amelia Mangay-Maglacas, Helena Pizurki, and John Simons (WHO Offset Publication No. 44).

3. *Traditional Birth Attendants: An Annotated Bibliography on Their Training, Evaluation, and Articulation with Health Service,* (HMD / NUR/79.1), and Supplements I and II of the bibliography, 1979–1982.

4. 1981: *The Traditional Birth Attendant in Seven Countries: Case Studies in Utilization and Training,* ed. Amelia Mangay-Maglacas and Helena Pizurki (WHO Public Health Papers No. 75).

In project after project, information was gathered from very specific locales and read as representative. These projects defined the TBA as already everywhere and imagined her as a target for intervention (as the title of one USAID paper during this period concisely stated, "Reaching the Rural Poor: Indigenous Health Practitioners Are There Already").[11] By the early 1980s, the thrust of WHO efforts concerning TBAs had turned to the creation of appropriate technology (e.g., "the TBA kit," including a debate over timers for TBAs to use to time contractions) and of bureaucratic tools to facilitate integration into national health systems (e.g., flow charts), as well as to the coordination of TBA training with longstanding development initiatives (even those outside of health, e.g., adult education and literacy).

The universalizing methods of public health that shaped each of these projects cannot fully account for their power and utility. Research is also a technology of international health governance. These four grounding documents both concretize the relations necessary to their making and establish new relations through their circulation. As each document travels it not only represents a knowledge-making project, but it also becomes a central actor in bureaucratic practice. The lifeblood of bureaucratic workings are paper and people.

Recent ethnographies of bureaucratic practice have shed light on the complicated power dynamics within the relations that are often glossed as transnationalism or globalization when they relate to development.[12] In describing the rise of a development industry broadly, Ferguson notes the constitutive role of the work of "employing expatriate consultants and 'experts' by the hundreds, and churning out plans, programs, and, and most of all, paper, at an astonishing rate" (1990: 8). Susan Reynolds Whyte (2011) focuses even more specifically on the importance of paper and the forms of inscription that it enables in medical research. Inspired by these calls to pay ethnographic attention to paper as a mediating substance, I read the WHO archive ethnographically (Hunt 1999) with a focus on who is cc'd on letters and memos, who receives the initial mailing of reports, which documents are mailed in response to questions or requests, and what documents are sent back in exchange for the initial documents. The circulation of paper begins to mark those who are "in the loop." It enacts relations not only among WHO offices (headquarters in Geneva, regional offices, and field offices) but also between the WHO in all these forms and ministries of health, scholars, and biomedical personnel "on the ground"; national development agencies such as USAID; and international NGOs such as IPPF, Margaret Sanger Institute, and various branches of the UN. The movement of paper delimits the geographic scope and marks the level (inter-regional, regional, national) of the project.

In contrast to people, paper can span multiple distances simultaneously and relatively cheaply. People cannot always move, and one person cannot be in multiple places at once. Limited resources and busy schedules, among other things, restrict the mobility of people at all levels. Paper, therefore, is a particularly powerful and critical medium for global relations. Yet the movement of paper cannot be divorced from the movement of people. Documents are shaped by and in turn shape the movement of people. The mobility of WHO HQ staff, consultants, temporary advisors, and observers from international organizations contrasts sharply not only with the (im)mobility of TBAs but also with the (im)mobility of people in regional and national offices. These contrasts are themselves generative. Headquarters' staff, temporary advisors, and consultants travel across continents, regional staff travel across countries, field staff travel to cities, and TBAs travel to trainings within districts or villages. The paths traveled by paper and the different mobilities of people render the global, regional, national, and in this case the "traditional" more than administrative categories; these movements render them scales of action.

The WHO Division of Human Manpower Development (HMD) catalyzed the initial efforts concerning TBAs and later came to coordinate all activities related to them. The HMD staff—particularly Lily Turnbull and Dr. Amelia Maglacas, who in succession took up the cause of TBAs within the WHO—organized their efforts and future goals by envisioning a series of phases.[13] Phase I involved collecting data about TBAs and preparing the background document described above. Phase II was the 1973 Consultation meeting itself and the report on this meeting. Phase III was longer and more involved, requiring the development of workshops for groups of countries in one or more regions; this repeated the Phase II consultation process but with the main objective focused on the field trials or implementation of training programs. Subsequent phases were not as consistently numbered, but they involved the preparation of guidelines, training manuals, and manuals to train the trainers, with an emphasis on evaluation, supervision, and policy development. The HMD staff argued the logic and necessity of each step on the basis of the last. In this way, the movement between projects generated an extension of time. The use of documents in multiple trainings and the looping back over material in different locations and at different times marked the progress of their efforts. It is this progressive time, time that lengthens out, which supports spatial extension. The regional, the national, and the local unfold as politically and bureaucratically salient spaces, as already well-known facts are repeated and practices configured for another setting.[14]

Tracing how descriptions, reports, and case studies move out of "locales" while guidelines, categories of behavior, good practices, mission teams, and consultants move into "locales" opens up ways of questioning the spatial and temporal nature of global health governance. In 1974 a series of regional and inter-regional workshops (Phase III) built explicitly on the 1973 Consultation (Phase II). After receiving the 1973 Consultation report and learning of the interest of the WHO HQ in TBAs, the Regional Office for the Americas (AMRO) rushed an inter-office memorandum to the Director General of the WHO with a proposal for a regional "Seminar on the Utilization and Training of Traditional Birth Attendants in Maternal and Child Health and Family Planning." In this memo, Dr. J. L. Garcia Gutierrez argues that such a TBA seminar would be the next logical step in efforts to reach the rural poor in the Americas. His memo marks their proposal as congruent with the goals for health care coverage development made by the Ministers of Health of the Americas in the Ten Year Health Plan for the region, and as an immediate response to the calls issued by the recent work groups on the "Organization of Rural Health Services and the Utilization of the Auxiliary" that his office sponsored. The first Phase III regional seminar for 15 countries in the Americas was held in San Salvador, El Salvador, in September and October 1974 (N2/180/3 AMR). In the same year, the South East Asia Regional Office (SEARO) and WPRO offices hosted an inter-regional conference for four countries in Manila, the Philippines. Regional and field staff from AMRO, SEARO, and WPRO also attended meetings involving their respective regions. The Chief Nursing Officer in HMD HQ sent multiple copies of the reports from the meetings in El Salvador and the Philippines to the Regional

Director in the AFRO office, who was preparing the "study group" on TBAs to be held in Brazzaville, Congo, in December 1975 (N2/27/1, discussed further below). The WHO sponsored an "Inter-regional Consultation on Traditional Birth Attendants" in Mexico City in December 1979, which was specifically designed to follow up on the 1973 Consultation and update information on TBAs around the world.[15]

In such bureaucratic practice (unlike, for instance, in scientific practice) repetition rather than novelty is recognized as generative. The Regional Nursing Adviser for the AFRO Regional Director eloquently illustrated this fact in a memo to the Chief Nursing Officer in the WHO HQ arguing for a regional workshop in Africa. She wrote:

> The subject of training, utilization and supervision of the Traditional Birth Attendants is not new in the Africa Region. What is new is the momentum which it has gained due to the increased recognition of the contribution this category of health worker can make toward a more extended health delivery system in rural areas. Secondly, the acceptance of the fact that 80–90 per cent of the deliveries in many countries in Africa are done by Traditional Birth Attendants. (N2/180/3 AFR letter dated November 5, 1974)[16]

On many of the regional proposals sent to HQ, key arguments or phrases are marked, checked, or underlined. The reader in HQ noted the repetition of key language and the tracing of dominant genealogies. The first proposal from the Regional Officer in the AFRO office offered the following justifications for the training of TBAs:

1. The "Report of Review and Analysis of Information and Data on Traditional Birth Attendants," Geneva, 13–20 March 1973.
2. For 10 years UNICEF has been providing assistance to various countries of the Region for the training of traditional birth attendants[.] "Report on UNICEF/WHO Co-ordination meeting," Brazzaville, 15 June 1973.
3. Although there is an overall increase in the number of hospital deliveries as reported by the countries of the Region, it is an established fact that the majority of women deliver at home with traditional birth attendants who have had no training and who work without any supervision. (N2/180/3 AFRO memo dated May 15, 1974)

Each point received a hand-marked check. Circulating documents like this thus served as guides, building blocks, and shortcuts.

While the proposal from AFRO clearly illustrated this bureaucratic principle of repetition, the Chief Nursing Officer in the HMD HQ responded by
suggesting that the AFRO Regional Director consider leaning even more heavily on published material. She encouraged her not only to locate this seminar
in line with the WHO's broader efforts, but also to use WHO background
documents to prepare participants and more efficiently achieve the objectives
of the study group.

> The suggested objectives are all very pertinent to the subject but I
> wonder whether you can expect the participants to achieve them in a
> five day workshop. The background documents will provide a frame-
> work and both general and specific information on most of the objec-
> tives which might mean that your group could move through c, d, e,
> and f, following an approach similar to that used by the participants at
> the inter-regional meeting in the Philippines. (N2/180/3 AFR memo
> dated April 11, 1975)

Within the WHO network, the use of background documents concern-
ing TBAs to "provide a framework" was a common strategy for promoting the
necessary iterations of "both general and specific information." The EMRO
Regional Director reported the circulation of a document entitled "The
Traditional Birth Attendants in MCH and Family Planning" (WHO Offset
Publication No. 18) to the Acting Director General in Geneva.

> It was used in the seminars on Training and Utilization of Traditional
> Birth Attendants held in Pakistan and Sudan, and in the last meeting
> of the Regional Expert Advisory Panel of Nurses on the Nurses' Role
> in Primary Health Care, as providing examples of the utilization and
> training of traditional health workers. . . . Copies have been given to
> interested national nurse/midwifery teachers . . ." (N2/180/3 Jkt 3
> memo dated November 2, 1976)[17]

Thus, in this international project the movement of memoranda, reports,
and guidelines between headquarters and regional offices and between
regional offices and national field offices is what guided the recapping of specific facts, goals, and objectives, the replication of certain procedures, and the
duplication of organizational structures across the globe.

Desiring Nations

The establishment of the region and the nation as scales of action is
reinforced when repetition of language—certain phrases, lists of priorities,

descriptions of the problem, and assessments of resources available for a solution—generates institutional change. In 1979, Dr. Maglacas, a Senior Scientist for Nursing, Division of Health Manpower Development, became the focal point for information about TBAs within the WHO and the catalyst for activities within the regions and countries relating to TBAs. Dr. Maglacas's appointment and her efforts to continually collect up-to-date information on TBAs created in turn a sense of need at country-level WHO offices for a designated person to gather and disseminate information on TBAs. For example, in 1981, Ms. Gentles, the WHO Nurse Educator in the Department of Post Basic Nursing, replied to Dr. Maglacas's request for information about TBA training in Zambia by reporting that a joint Ministry of Health/UNICEF evaluation of the impact of TBA training had been planned three years earlier, but that they had not yet been able to implement it. With her reply, however, she enclosed the following three documents:

- A 1977 WHO national office report on a "Pilot Project for Establishing the Training and Roles of Traditional Birth Attendants" by Dr. S. H. Brew-Graves WHO Medical Officer, Maternal and Child Health. (The WHO field office conducted this study upon the request of the Zambian Ministry of Health, which had suspended the training of TBAs in 1976 "because the results were generally unsatisfactory" [Brew-Graves 1977].)

- The *Training Guide for Traditional Birth Attendants* developed by and used by the Ministry of Health, Lusaka, Zambia.

- The Certificate of Attendance given by the Zambian Ministry of Health to people who completed a TBA training course.

The same year, in a WPRO seminar on TBAs, "[p]articipants were urged to call the attention of their governments to the inclusion of TBAs in the context of individual country policies and plans for national FP [family planning] and health programmes" (N2/180/3, Maglacas's travel report to the International Seminar on Traditional Birth Attendants in Family Planning, June 11–13, 1981, Manila).

Ms. Gentles's correspondence with Dr. Maglacas is an example of how global work depends on local responsiveness. Regions and nations do not always respond to the provocations of global actors. This was illustrated most clearly in the WHO archive through the story of a failed WHO/UNESCO/UNICEF literacy project for TBAs. In 1981, WHO and UNESCO agreed to cooperate on a literacy initiative. That same year, Dr. Maglacas, who had been given responsibility for this project within the WHO, requested that the SEARO Regional Director "seek . . . the interest of any country that might be willing to have WHO's collaboration in integrating a literacy component into TBA training programmes." Field officers from India and Thailand responded. She foresaw the need for national commitment. She reasoned that because "literacy is highly based on the language of the country . . . the undertaking of many of the activities will be by nationals and the assessment would be done by nationals, WHO and UNESCO." Even before knowing the country in which the pilot project would take place, she began to plan a mission trip that would assess the ability of the country selected to carry out the project and to discern the commitment of officials in the country. In 1982, the Director General of Health Services in Bangladesh agreed that "the Government is interested to have our collaboration in the joint UNESCO/WHO proposal for the "Strengthening of training programmes for Traditional Birth Attendants through the incorporation of a literacy component" (N2/180/3 SEARO WHOGRAM dated April 29, 1982).

In 1983, Dr. Maglacas traveled to Bangladesh with representatives from UNESCO and UNICEF to discuss "the nature" of this proposal and to "establish the feasibility requirements and plan of action for trial" (N3/180 Travel Report Summary, March 7, 1983). In the country the mission team met regional program officers as well as national officials in the Ministry of Health. Dr. A. Islam became the point person for the Ministry of Health in Bangladesh and worked in concert with the UNICEF and WHO field offices there. In the acknowledgments of the report from the mission team, they noted, "The proposed plan could not have been achieved were it not for Dr. Islam's situational knowledge and information about TBAs and his readiness to indicate what was feasible and what methods will work" (N2/180/3 A. Mangay-Maglacas, J. G. Kim, and Nuhad Kanawati, "Report of a Mission on Strengthening of Existing Training Programmes for Traditional Birth Attendants in Bangladesh through the Incorporation of a Literacy Component," February 16–22, 1983).

A series of meetings and preliminary negotiations established the details of the pilot project. At a certain point it was necessary for the Bangladeshi government to respond with a very simple request for a consultant. This request was never forthcoming. UNESCO would have provided the funds, and the WHO the consultant. Dr. Maglacas's letters, memos, and telegrams requesting that someone in the Bangladesh government declare their interest in and desire for this project grew increasingly frustrated and terse. In order for the project to move forward, for the global plans to be meaningful, the government of Bangladesh had to articulate its desire, to manifest agency—even if it was in the briefest of letters or a telegram. The failure of this project despite a substantial investment of energy and will at the global level exposes the mechanisms through which the nation is constituted as a critical administrative unit, a necessary scale of action.

Managing Variation

At least part of the work of the iterative style of bureaucratic practice is that it circumscribes variation through scalar developments. A level such as the region is concretized as similarities are established and difference is attributed to the next, slightly more fragmented unit, such as the nation. This is the work of consultations. When the AFRO study group was presented with the WHO's argument concerning the value of the TBA and her usefulness in expanding health care services, a "stimulating discussion" followed. Thirteen participants—six of whom were from ministries of health; seven of whom were from medical schools or midwifery institutes; and all of whom were senior nurse-midwives, midwives, public health nurses, or maternity nurses—debated the role of the TBA. In addition, one international observer, the WHO Chief of Medical Education from Geneva, six regional officers from the WHO AFRO office, and a short-term consultant from the Department of Sociology at the University of Ibadan in Nigeria participated in the study group. As they talked,

> It became clear that there was some resistance to the acceptance of traditional birth attendants into the health team. Participants gave the impression that the concern in creating countries was to replace traditional birth attendants in the shortest possible time by a category between traditional birth attendants and professional midwives. After further discussion, the group reached the consensus that it was concerned exclusively with traditional birth attendants as defined in the document INF.07. . . . After some discussion, it was agreed that the traditional birth attendant has a role to play in the delivery of primary health care. (AFR/MCH/71)

Despite this "consensus" the evaluation at the end of the group's four working days indicated that the objectives of the study group were "found directly relevant to the Region" by only 77 percent of the participants, "directly relevant to participants' countries" by 70 percent of the participants, and "directly relevant to participants' present and future activities" by 62 percent of the participants. In other words, a significant percentage of the participants who were identified as the individuals who would most logically coordinate any effort to train TBAs in their home countries did not see the relevance of this topic to their work. Yet their willingness to repeat the profile and role of the TBA and imagine it abstractly within the scope of regional or global health governance garnered the reported consensus.

The iteration of specific language, policy, and procedures through meetings and trainings first designed in Geneva, London, and New York and then repeated in continental centers and finally in country capitals works to manage difference.[18] Alterity becomes quickly reduced to the specificities allowed by the given level of structure. Global projects articulate difference between regions; regional projects articulate difference between nations; national projects articulate difference between communities. In the AFRO study group, as in all the consultations that succeeded the 1973 Consultation, countries comprised the unit of organization and therefore became the level of salient variation. The situation and practices of TBAs in Senegal came to be compared to those in Nigeria, Tanzania, and other African countries. Any distinction between local conditions and the generalized principles, profiles, and procedures articulated in WHO documents described *national* differences. Through these seminars and the trainings they aimed to motivate, Africa and Tanzania became intelligible as scales of action.

Administering Subjects

At a country level, one of the most salient and noteworthy iterations is that of the list of tasks that a TBA is supposed to master at each birth phase interval. The guides place emphasis on hygiene, nutrition, timing of birth, sterilization of the tool used to cut cord, signs of danger, and referral to hospital. They also introduce TBAs to additional responsibilities concerning sanitation, nutrition, vaccinations, first aid, and family planning. The 1979 publication listed above as one of the foundational documents grounding international efforts concerning TBAs elaborates the "definition of functions and tasks of the TBAs." In so doing, this document rationalizes the link between globally articulated definitions and the TBA evoked in villages around the world. It reads: "the clear specification of tasks is necessary as a basis for determining both the learning objectives against which individual performance is to be measured and the kinds of effect it is reasonable to expect the training programme to have on health" (du Gas, Mangay-Maglacas, and Simons 1979: 22).

As the "functions and tasks" as well as the desires and intentions of the TBA are repeated in regional consultations, national meetings, and village trainings, "health" of the population is linked with the actions of individual women attending births. The subject becomes the last level of iteration.

In Tanzania, the Safe Motherhood Project has supported the most significant initiatives to train TBAs in Tanzania. However, it is also possible to trace other scattered efforts by mission hospitals, the Red Cross, and smaller nongovernmental efforts concerned with maternal and child health. This support trickled down unevenly to district hospitals and local dispensaries in a variety of ways. Sometimes the Ministry of Health carried out formal trainings like the one I describe above. The time of district nurses, however, is precious, as all but the best of the referrals hospitals in the country are very short-staffed. In addition, a variety of public health projects ranging from family planning to sanitation to child health to AIDS call district nurses away from the hospital. Even if the district staff make the training of TBAs a priority, they must find days when the hospital vehicle is free (and in repair), and allocate money for fuel, a driver, and the nurses' per diems. These obstacles delayed the training many times over the course of months before I finally observed it. While trainings happened infrequently, in practice, clinic and dispensary staff developed individual relationships with women who assisted or who wanted to assist women to deliver in areas far from clinical care. Amina, a TBA in the Newala district, had developed an exemplary relationship with the dispensary nearest her home in this way. Although she first learned midwifery skills from her mother in-law, who had "delivered many children," she chose to deliver all eight of her pregnancies in a hospital. She herself was born in 1947. When I interviewed Amina in the Malatu dispensary, there was some debate as to whether she had attended a formal TBA training. Whether or not she had the opportunity to attend a Ministry of Health training, she has explicitly and vocally taken on the language and objectives of her biomedical counterparts. My open-ended questions about her practice elicited answers that were startlingly similar to the Ministry of Health training manual for TBAs. She focused on sanitation, hygiene, identifying dangers, and referrals to biomedical staff.

Amina and her work ethic illustrate the internalization of supervisory and evaluative structures discussed at global, regional, and national levels. A TBA who performs within the framework of health services is initially instigated through training and perpetuated through supervision and evaluation. Ideally, however, the subject will incorporate the structure of the supervision and evaluation within their own ethic. As we were talking, Amina evaluated appropriate TBA practice in the process of telling me about helping a less experienced midwife. She reflected on the situation she found when responding to an emergency call. When she arrived, the other midwife was sitting on the floor (rather than up off the ground) and appeared to be inactive. She did not know what to do when the woman she was assisting failed to expel her placenta after the birth of her newborn child. The fellow midwife looked for Amina, walking to her house several times, but when she failed to find her she merely sat with the troubled new mother. When Amina returned home and was alerted by her neighbor, she went to the new mother's house and found the midwife in this position. In addition, the newborn child was not cleaned or dressed, and there was evidence that he had been placed naked on the dirt floor. Upon entering this scene, Amina's immediate responses were to change her clothes, wash her hands, reprimand the midwife for not insisting that this woman be brought to the health center, and most importantly, take action to remove the placenta. Amina told the story as follows:

> Truthfully, this has occurred to me [that a younger TBA might have to get advice from an older TBA]. The reason is that my companions are beginning [novices]. I mean, I have come upon them [practicing]. I entered [in on an incident] last year. I was in the fields. I did not know that a certain woman was giving birth. She went to my colleague who is in between here and there [pointing]. This woman gave birth at 8 o'clock in the morning. Me, I was in the fields. I returned from my fields at 11:30 in the morning. A young person called on me at my house and [told me], that my midwifery colleague from over there had come [to my house]. She did not find me; she came a second time, and a third. "Indeed, [said this youth] we met each other [several times]. Mama, you are needed." [I asked,] "Me, by who?" [This youth responded by] saying [that] my sister had given birth. [Adding] "Now I do not know if she calls you, but there is another midwife [who has tried to call you]." Aah. [I wondered] what was happening? I entered inside [my house] to change my clothes [and] wash my hands. I left. I met this [other] midwife. She was sitting on the ground and the patient was lying in bed and she had put the child in between them. [I asked] "Why did you call me?" At this point, indeed, I saw the child. [I continued] "Now the mother is which person? Say if you are the mother." A person in the room said, "me." [Turning to her I asked] "Now, you, why [did you call me]? Is there a nurse here?" She says, "there is a problem." I did not understand, [so I asked] "what is the problem?" [She] says, "My placenta has not come out?" It has not come out? Now, what if I had been in the fields and I had slept and returned in the evening? [Turning to the other midwife, I ask] "Why have you not told them to go to the clinic? The ones there can reduce your anxiety." Indeed, this is the reason the clinic was built. In each village the health center [is staffed with] someone who will attend to illnesses in a room [in the health center]. Me, I entered the room. I put on my clothes. I washed my hands. I grabbed the placenta, pulling it slowly. Slowly, it came out. [Then I said to the family in the room] "You folks come here. Watch her. First, [I know] you are tired; she delivered late. Watch [her] now. And this child does not yet wear clothes, and he has been put down on the ground in the dirt. Come mama, my dear, won't you and this *mganga* [referring to the other midwife as a "healer"] talk together about what needs to be done?

In giving this account, Amina clearly illustrates which practices she thinks should be respected and which ones should not. She highlights some of the reasons that many biomedical practitioners argue that untrained midwives are dangerous and hesitate to fully support TBA training and incorporation into the national health care structure. In describing her own actions she articulates the behavior and the thinking, the functions and the tasks, of a good TBA. She puts into action the lists crafted in global exchanges, regional consultations, and national meetings. She exemplifies the last iteration. She completes the distinctions between the global, the regional, the national, and the subject. She makes them meaningful.

Scalar Developments

The WHO as an assembling body with an explicit advisory role charged with the collection and dissemination of knowledge and the gathering together of networks of people uniquely illustrates the generative nature of repetition. The agency's work does not so much require iteration at regional, national, and community levels, as the iterative nature of the work itself generates the regional, the national, and the subject as scales of action. The WHO itself only becomes meaningfully global if it succeeds in producing articulate and agentive regions, nations, and subjects. The nested administrative structure is, in other words, what makes the WHO and its work global.

Tracing how global health governance renders the world as scalar through iterative bureaucratic processes illustrates that the nation, as well as global subjects with national ties, remain emergent within global relations. The argument in this chapter illustrates that unidirectional critiques of transnational development organizations, as mediums through which the West imposes itself (its values, priorities, practices, etc.) on Africa and other parts of the Third World, are too simple. The sorts of categorizing, organizing, generalizing, and abstracting critical to the global evokes the West as well as its Others. This process is evident when examining the production of a global traditional subject. Efforts to define and train TBAs as outreach workers in health development most explicitly articulate the West as the area without "traditional" actors.

Central to the world-making work of the WHO is the management of mobility. This chapter has striven to account for the kinds of mobility (and fixity) that facilitate a particular notion of globality and produce the subjects critical to it. Attention to who moves, where, and at what times reveals the forms of mobility that are productive of the universal logics justifying (and bureaucratically useful to) global health governance. I have argued that the carefully choreographed movements of paper and people organize the global, regional, national, and the subject into scales of action. The nested administrative structure is an effect of deferring all variation to the "lower" level. At the global level, variation defines the level of the region, at the regional level variation defines the level of the nation, at the national level variation defines the level of the province or community, and at the provincial level variation defines the level of the subject.

Acknowledgments

I thank both the University of Florida and the Max Planck Institute for funding the archival research on which this chapter draws, in 2005 and 2007 respectively. I am also very grateful to the archivists and the librarians at the World Health Organization who were extremely generous with their knowledge and time. In particular, Marie Villemin and Avril Reid went above and beyond the call of duty.

Notes

1. For more on the history of world health, see Bashford (2006, 2007).

2. Critiques of TBA programs and skepticism of their value in achieving biomedical goals are summarized in the 2005 World Health Report (WHO 2005).

3. This referencing system is that used by the WHO in their archive. My argument in this chapter emerged from a close reading of the WHO archive on work with TBAs. The primary file on this topic was N2/180/3. This is a large file that includes numbered jackets for material from HQ and regionally labeled jackets from material collected from the regions (example N2/180/3 EMO). I also drew on file N2/445/16. Each of these files is a collection of internal memos, travel reports, correspondence, drafts of projects, and all other documents that the departments kept relating to TBA projects. Some of these pages are numbered, some are not. I have included as much information as possible in my references to enable others to find these documents if they wish.

4. See the WHO web page for more specifics on the public face of the organization. http://www.who.int/about/en/.

5. For more on this interaction see Langwick (2010).

6. For a more detailed account of debates about native midwives in western Tanzania, see chapter 2 of Allen's (2004) *Managing Motherhood, Managing Risk*. In this book Allen carefully examines the joint efforts of international organizations, including the WHO, in designing and implementing the Safe Motherhood Initiative as well as the effects of this work in western Tanzania.

7. I refer to this individual as Dr. Maglacas in the text, as this is the name that usually appears in professional documents and minutes. However, she authored her publications under the name Mangay-Maglacas.

8. File entitled "Agenda for the Meeting of the Planning Committee for the Study of the Activities of the Traditional Birth Attendants."

9. On the politics of naming target populations in health development work, see Cohen (2005).

10. For thoughtful and sensitive examples of how global health policy shapes clinics in East Africa, see Booth (2004) and Richey (2008). In this volume, chapters 4 and 5 also illustrate the effects of international agendas and how the movement of international experts shapes local conditions and options.

11. This paper, published in March 1979, was the first in a series of AID Program Evaluation Discussion Papers out of the USAID Office of Evaluation, Bureau for Program and Policy Coordination (N2/180/3).

12. An exceptional example of such work is Riles (2000). George Marcus and a team of his students have also begun important research on such global bureaucratic practice in their ethnographic investigation of the work of the WTO (see 2008 AAA panel entitled "Collaborative Ethnography Inside the World Trade Organization" held November 22 in San Francisco, Calif.).

13. A memo from the director of Health Manpower Division to the Acting Director General on April 3, 1979, noted that the interest in and work related to TBAs warranted assigning one person as the focal point for communication.

> As we agreed [in our discussion yesterday] there is now in HQ wide interest in the subject of traditional birth attendants. It is expected that more and more activities will be envisaged since TBAs in several countries of the developing world represent a good resource pool for work linked to primary health care in the community, i.e., MCH, diarrhoeal diseases, family planning, hygiene and sanitation, etc.. Known programme areas in HQ presently interested in this subject are: CDS (diarrhoeal diseases), EPI, PHE, HMD, and TRM.
>
> In order to effectively coordinate, minimize duplications, monitor activities, as well as generate more extrabudgetary resources efficiently for this programme, it is recommended and advisable to have a focal point in HQ on all activities that have to do with TBAs. As I said I would suggest Dr. A. Mangay Maglacas, Senior Scientist for Nursing, to be designated with the understanding that she would carry out this assignment in closest cooperation with TRM (N2/180/3 Jkt 4).

14. My thinking about the temporal and spatial characteristics of bureaucratic practice is influenced by Guyer (2007).

15. In preparation for the Mexico City consultation on TBAs in December 1979, for example, the WHO designed and circulated a questionnaire to update the information in the 1973 background document entitled "Report of Review and Analysis of Information and Data on TBAs" by Miss Verdersese (N2/180/3).

16. She also suggested bringing the results of this proposed meeting to the 26th Regional Committee in Kampala in 1976, for which the subject of the technical discussions was "Traditional Medicine."

17. Other regional offices also passed WHO primary documents and reports, as well as regional variations, on to field staff in the country to guide community-level training. At the end of the PAHO seminar, participants explicitly recommended "[t]hat countries should take the results of this Seminar as a basic working document. It can be used to guide the preparation of programs for the training and utilization of the traditional birth attendant, adapted to the resources and specific situation of each country" (N2/180/3).

18. Yet not all repetition is considered productive, and not all requests of desiring nations justify repetition. Dr. Maglacas expressed frustration when she saw others as "repeating" work already accomplished after a visit from Bonnie Pederson, the Project Director of the International Project for TBAs at the American College of Nurse-Midwives, in July 1982. A contract from the International Training Programs in Health (INTRAH) at the University of North Carolina at Chapel Iill funded by the United States Agency for International Development (USAID) was sending Pedersen to work in TBA trainings in five African countries (Tanzania, Zambia, Liberia, Upper Volta, and Zaire). Dr. Maglacas wrote a note for the file, copied to the African Regional Office, detailing the information on TBAs she and her staff gave to Pederson during the latter's visit to Geneva. In the end, however, Maglacas concluded: "It is likely that Mrs. Pedersen will repeat (and I hope I am wrong) what is already known and documented and in the process she and staff working with her will really be getting educated about TBAs and about African conditions" (N2/180/3 dated July 22, 1982).

Although earlier WHO work had not focused on the five countries to which Pedersen would be traveling, and although Maglacas commented that Pedersen "claims that all these countries made requests for their assistance," she saw Pederson's efforts in Africa as out of step with the phases of WHO work and therefore redundant, arguing that "[t]here is no need to further make a means assessment for TBAs since all of this has already been documented." With this language, she rendered knowledge of any additional variation in the characteristics of TBAs and their categories of practice useless. In fact, she and her staff emphasized to Pederson that "isolated projects on TBAs will only make matters worse if not part of the totals [sic] development for MCH in a country."

References

Allen, Denise Roth. 2004. *Managing Motherhood, Managing Risk: Fertility and Danger in West Central Tanzania.* Ann Arbor: University of Michigan Press.

Bashford, Alison. 2006. "Global Biopolitics and the History of World Health." *History of the Human Sciences* 19 (1): 67–88.

———. 2007. "Nation, Empire, Globe: The Spaces of Population Debate in the Interwar Years." *Comparative Studies in Society and History* 49 (1): 170–201.

Booth, Karen. 2004. *Local Women, Global Science: Fighting AIDS in Kenya.* Bloomington: Indiana University Press.

Brew-Graves, S. H. 1977. "Pilot Project for Establishing the Training and Roles of Traditional Birth Attendants (TBAs) in the Kabwe Health Demonstration Zone." Prepared by WHO MO/MCH and presented at the Provincial Health Staff Seminar, Jan.

Cohen, Lawrence. 2005. "The Kothi Wars: AIDS Cosmopolitanism and the Morality of Classification." In *Sex in Development: Science, Sexuality, and Morality in Global Perspective,* ed. Vincanne Adams and Stacy Leigh Pigg, 269–304. Durham, N.C.: Duke University Press.

Collier, Stephen J., and Aihwa Ong. 2005. "Global Assemblages, Anthropological Problems." In *Global Assemblages: Technology, Politics, and Ethics as Anthropological Problems,* ed. Aihwa Ong and Stephen J. Collier, 3–21. Malden, Mass.: Blackwell Publishing.

du Gas, Beverley, Amelia Mangay-Maglacas, and John Simons. 1979. *Traditional Birth Attendants: A Field Guide to Their Training, Evaluation, and Articulation with Health Services*. WHO Offset Publication No. 44. Geneva: World Health Organization.

Fassin, Didier. 2008. "The Humanitarian Politics of Testimony: Subjectification through Trauma in the Israeli–Palestinian Conflict." *Cultural Anthropology* 23 (3): 531–558.

Feierman, Steven. 1990. *Peasant Intellectuals: Anthropology and History in Tanzania*. Madison: University of Wisconsin Press.

Ferguson, James. 1990. *The Anti-Politics Machine: "Development," Depoliticization, and the Bureaucratic Power in Lesotho*. Minneapolis: University of Minnesota Press.

Guyer, Jane. 2007. "Prophecy and the Near Future: Thoughts on Macroeconomic, Evangelical, and Punctuated Time." *American Ethnologist* 34 (3): 409–421.

Hunt, Nancy Rose. 1999. "STDs, Suffering, and Their Derivatives in Congo-Zaire: Notes Toward an Historical Ethnography of Disease." In *Vivre et penser le sida en Afrique/ Experiencing and Understanding AIDS in Africa*, ed. Charles Becker, Jean-Pierre Dozon, Christine Obbo and Moriba Touré, 111–131. Paris: Codesria, IRD, Karthala.

Langwick, Stacey. 2011. "Traditional Birth Attendants as Institutional Evocations." In *Bodies, Politics, and African Healing: The Matter of Maladies in Tanzania*, by Stacey Langwick. Bloomington: Indiana University Press.

Mangay-Maglacas, Amelia, and Helena Pizurki, eds. 1981. *The Traditional Birth Attendant in Seven Countries: Case Studies in Utilization and Training*. Public Health Papers No. 75. Geneva: World Health Organization.

Mohanty, Chandra Talpade. 1986. "Under Western Eyes: Feminist Scholarship and Colonial Discourses." *Boundary 2* 12 (3): 338–358.

Nguyen, Vinh-Kim. 2005. "Antiretroviral Globalism, Biopolitics, and Therapeutic Citizenship." In *Global Assemblages: Technology, Politics, and Ethics as Anthropological Problems*, ed. Aihwa Ong and Stephen J. Collier, 124–144. Malden, Mass.: Blackwell Publishing.

Peterson, Kristin. Forthcoming. "AIDS Policies for Markets and Warriors: Dispossession, Capital, and Pharmaceuticals in Nigeria." In *Lively Capital*, ed. Kaushik Sunder Rajan. Durham, N.C.: Duke University Press.

Pigg, Stacy Leigh. 1997a. "Authority in Translation: Finding, Knowing, Naming, and Training 'Traditional Birth Attendants' in Nepal." In *Childbirth and Authoritative Knowledge: Cross-Cultural Perspectives*, ed. Robbie Davis-Floyd and Carolyn Fishel Sargent, 233–262. Berkeley: University of California.

———. 1997b. "'Found in Most Traditional Societies': Traditional Medical Practitioners between Culture and Development." In *International Development and the Social Sciences*, ed. Fredrick Cooper and Randall Packard, 259–290. Berkeley: University of California Press.

Redfield, Peter. 2005. "Doctors, Borders, and Life in Crisis." *Cultural Anthropology* 20 (3): 328–361.

———. 2006. "A Less Modest Witness: Collective Advocacy and Motivated Truth in a Medical Humanitarian Movement." *American Ethnologist* 33 (1): 3–26.

———. 2008. "Sacrifice, Triage and Global Humanitarianism." In *Humanitarianism in Question: Politics, Power, Ethics*, ed. Michael Barnett and Thomas G. Weiss, 196–214. Ithaca, N.Y.: Cornell University Press.

Richey, Lisa. 2008. *Population Politics and Development: From the Polities to the Clinics*. New York, N.Y.: Palgrave Macmillan.

Riles, Annelise. 2000. *The Network Inside Out.* Ann Arbor: University of Michigan Press.

Tsing, Anna Lowenhaupt. 2005. *Friction: An Ethnography of Global Connection.* Princeton, N.J.: Princeton University Press.

Verdersese, Maria de Lourdes, and Lily M. Turnbull. 1975. *The Traditional Birth Attendant in Maternal and Child Health and Family Planning: A Guide to Her Training and Utilization.* WHO Offset Publication No. 18. Geneva: World Health Organization.

Whyte, Susan Reynolds. 2011. "Writing Knowledge and Acknowledgement: Possibilities in Medical Research." In *Evidence, Ethos, and Ethnography: The Anthropology and History of Medical Research in Africa,* ed. Paul Wenzel Geissler and Sassy Molyneux. New York: Berghahn Books.

World Health Organization. 1973. *Consultation on the Role of the Traditional Birth Attendant in Family Planning.* 12–19 March. Available in WHO HQ archive N2–180–3 Jacket 2.

———. 1978a. *Alma Ata 1978: Primary Health Care, HFA Sr. No. 1.* Electronic document: http://www.paho.org/English/DD/PIN/alma-ata_declaration.htm.

———. 1978b. *Primary Health Care: Report of the International Conference on Primary Health Care Alma-Ata, USSR, 6–12 September.* Jointly sponsored by the World Health Organization and the United Nations Children's Fund. Geneva: World Health Organization.

———. 1992. *Traditional Birth Attendants: A Joint WHO/UNFPA/UNICEF Statement.* Geneva: World Health Organization.

———. 2005. *World Health Report.* Geneva: World Health Organization.

TWO

Targeting the Empowered Individual: Transnational Policy Making, the Global Economy of Aid, and the Limitations of Biopower in Tanzania

Hansjörg Dilger

In October 2001, Amelia Jacob from Tanzania was among the four awardees of the prestigious Africa Prize for Leadership, an award presented on an annual to biannual basis to outstanding African leaders whose "accomplishments have improved the lives of tens of millions of people."[1] The award—among whose previous recipients were the former South African President Nelson Mandela (1994) and the founder of the Green Belt Movement in Kenya, Wangara Muta Maathai (1991)—acknowledged Jacob's long-term engagement in the fight against HIV/AIDS in Tanzania. According to the award-giving institution, the New York–based Hunger Project, the example set by Jacob, who has lived openly with her illness since she was diagnosed as being HIV-positive in 1993, "has empowered people living with HIV/AIDS to come forth and become spokespersons. [Jacob] has demanded that the public treat people with HIV/AIDS with dignity and compassion while advocating that any effective treatment must include warmth and respect to those living with HIV/AIDS."[2]

The Africa Prize for Leadership—which in 2001 included a grant of 50,000 USD—helped to change the work and face of the Tanzanian self-help organization SHDEPHA+ (Service, Health, and Development for People Living Positively with HIV/AIDS) of which Jacob was one of the co-founders. While the award was probably not exclusively responsible for the subsequent developments, it certainly contributed to the organization's steep rise in membership, which according to SHDEPHA+ had grown to 50,000 by 2003. In the same year, the NGO opened its membership to people who are not infected with HIV but "who show solidarity with those who are." Furthermore, SHDEPHA+ expanded its services in counseling, care, and advocacy and started to implement a wide range of programs targeting the capacity-building of community groups as well as "the elimination of stigma" in Tanzanian communities. When I returned to the organization in 2003, three years after I had completed the bulk of my fieldwork, approximately 40 branches had been, or were in the process of being, established all over the country; the new building in Dar es Salaam into which the NGO headquarters had moved was buzzing with new and old members. An external consultant had been contracted in order to help the organization to come to grips with the challenges that the growing membership presented (in addition to problems stemming from claims of embezzlement of funds that were circulating inside and outside the donor community). Finally, there were signs of a growing political consciousness within the organization itself: in 2003, the tenth anniversary of SHDEPHA+, a group of about 80 to 100 men and women, many of them living openly with HIV, marched through the streets of downtown Dar es Salaam demanding from the government the provision of free access to antiretroviral medications (ARVs).

The developments within the Tanzanian self-help organization SHDEPHA+ at the turn of the century are emblematic of the HIV/AIDS response as it evolved across wide parts of southern and eastern Africa from the early 2000s onwards. Not only was the organization among the many NGOs in the region that became involved in the fight against the epidemic during the 1990s and that received a significant boost in funding after the establishment of the Global Fund for the Fight Against AIDS, Tuberculosis, and Malaria in 2001, and the U.S. Presidential Emergency Plan for AIDS Relief (PEPFAR) in 2003. The work of SHDEPHA+ also reflects an internal shift in the world of HIV/AIDS work, which has increasingly come to integrate people living with HIV/AIDS into a holistic approach to the fight against the epidemic and which relies heavily on an internationally compatible language of empowerment, dignity, and human rights (see, e.g., UNAIDS 1999). Finally, the example of SHDEPHA+ has become emblematic of the positioning of civil society actors in a country where the formerly socialist government has had difficulties in coming to terms with the political engagement of non-governmental organizations (NGOs) (Mercer 1999), and where the face of the civil society response to HIV/AIDS has been increasingly shaped by neoliberal market forces and by the increased privatization of the health field and its dependency on international funding priorities.

Introduction: The Anthropology of Policy Making in the Era of AIDS

This chapter is concerned with the field of transnational policy and program making and the implementation of health interventions in the wake of structural adjustment, the increasing transnationalization and NGO-ization of the health sector, and the HIV/AIDS epidemic in Tanzania. As in other parts of sub-Saharan Africa, HIV/AIDS policies in Tanzania over the last three decades have been molded by country-specific epidemiological developments and the growth in mortality and morbidity rates that has entailed programmatic shifts from prevention to care and counseling to treatment—and ultimately toward a combination of these different components. Furthermore, HIV/AIDS work has been characterized by the way in which the various governmental and non-governmental authorities and organizations involved in the fight against the epidemic in Tanzania have been incorporated into a transnationalized system of health governance and funding, which in turn has affected the shape, contents, and language of specific programs. Finally, HIV/AIDS policy making in the country has been characterized by the repeated and often failed attempts of internationally funded interventions to connect to the social, economic, and moral configurations which have come to shape the ways in which people in the region are dealing with the complex challenges arising from the epidemic (for a related critique in other African regions see Heald 2003; Allen and Heald 2004; Campbell 2003; Dilger and Luig 2010).

In her book *Just One Child: Science and Policy in Deng's China,* Susan Greenhalgh (2008) draws our attention to the processes and modes of policy making as a new subject of anthropological inquiry. In the context of modern governance, Greenhalgh argues, the governance of human life is no longer an object of the state, but has shifted to a triad of governing authorities: the state bureaucracies, professional (knowledge-based) disciplines, and self-governing individuals. The forms of governance emerging in the interplay between these different levels are intimately intertwined with the formulation of policies which are regulating "virtually every domain of modern life" (Greenhalgh 2008: 7): from birth to death, school to work, and the lives and developments of populations as a whole. However, while policy can thus be understood "as the crystallization of authoritative norms" in modern systems of governance, an understanding of *the politics of these policies*—"who makes them, with what techniques and logics, through what negotiations and contests, and with what intended and unintended effects" (Greenhalgh 2008: 7f)—has hardly been achieved.

In her book, Greenhalgh continues to analyze the ways in which scientific experts in China have come to frame and interpret the growth of the Chinese population since the late 1970s and how the scientific knowledge that has been produced in this process has been translated into specific policies aimed at controlling the size and form of the population. Given the fact that HIV/AIDS is probably the best-explored epidemic in human history, in that an immense amount of data has been accumulated about the disease by a wide range of academic as well as non-academic disciplines and authorities (Treichler 1999), an epistemic approach to the analysis of HIV/AIDS-related policy making would certainly make for an excellent challenge. In this chapter, however, I choose a different approach, focusing less on the scientific knowledge and procedures which have prepared the ground for the formulation of policy responses to HIV/AIDS, and instead on the political and economic *contexts* in which HIV/AIDS-related policies in Tanzania have been produced, as well as on the way these policies have been translated into programs and projects, and finally on how these programs and projects in turn have come to relate to the lives of people in Tanzania in the era of neoliberal reform processes and HIV/AIDS. I will argue that the transnationally embedded health responses to HIV/AIDS have led to the formulation of specific subject formations and ways of relating to one's body which are promoted by NGOs and the media, as well as by a conglomerate of peer educators, health staff, and other actors who have become incorporated into the globalized AIDS response. Ideas about the subject, gender, and the person that are implicated in these formulations are in turn appropriated by people in rural and urban Tanzania to varying degrees, and are becoming intertwined with alternative ways of thinking and acting upon health, illness, and the body in a variety of (often overlapping) situations and social constellations.

In the following I will first discuss the globalizing political and economic conditions under which policies and health care interventions in Tanzania have been designed and implemented over the last two to three decades in the context of structural adjustment, the transnationalization of the country's health sector, and HIV/AIDS. I will then describe how transnational policies and funding structures have translated into a myriad of activities in the fields of prevention, care, and treatment, which have been molded by both market-driven forces and a growing focus on human rights and empowerment. Third, I will look beyond the policy-making context and describe how the various ways in which people in Tanzania have responded to HIV/AIDS, rather than being congruent with the messages and the knowledge produced and mediated by biomedically driven health campaigns, are to be understood as part and parcel of a "moral practice and experience" that emphasizes the *social relatedness* of illness, that is, the connectedness between individual bodies and the social and moral state of kinship, community networks, and society at large.

In the formulation of my argument, I will draw strongly on my fieldwork in Tanzania, which from 1995 to 2006 has explored different aspects of the interconnection between HIV/AIDS and social relationships in the context of globalization and modernity—including issues surrounding sexuality and gender relations; relationships of care and support; the moral management of AIDS-related illnesses and deaths; and, recently, the introduction of the antiretroviral treatment which has shaped health policy in Tanzania since the end of 2004. What struck me during all the phases of my research was that while people in Tanzania were often well aware of how HIV is transmitted, how to protect oneself from infection, or how one should *supposedly* behave toward people with HIV / AIDS, their actual behaviors concerning sexuality or HIV / AIDS-related illnesses and deaths were often not congruent with this information—indeed, were often starkly opposed to it. Thus, while health messages about HIV / AIDS were acknowledged among wide segments of Tanzania's population even before the introduction of antiretroviral treatment, the ideas, practices, and experiences surrounding sexuality or episodes of HIV / AIDS-related illnesses and deaths were less shaped by information and knowledge drawn from governmental and / or non-governmental HIV / AIDS programs. Responses have become intimately intertwined with people's experiences of and concerns about familial, social, and economic developments in the context of modernity and globalization, and the moral and reproductive order at large (see Dilger 2005, 2008; Dilger and Luig 2010).

Governing Health in Tanzania in the Wake of Structural Adjustment and HIV / AIDS

At the end of the 1970s, most countries in the eastern and southern African regions stood on the verge of economic and political collapse. Governments were not only confronted with the growing external debts and costs of heavily subsidized economies and overfunded welfare systems; they were also struggling with the consequences of the international oil crisis and the global economic depression. These combined factors drove many African governments to turn to the World Bank and the International Monetary Fund (IMF) for assistance. The loans that were granted to African states by the World Bank and the IMF were intended primarily for use in stabilizing economies and paying off national debts. However, they were also made contingent upon the implementation of a series of structural reforms which entailed, among other things, currency devaluation, reduction of trade barriers, and the privatization of state-owned enterprises. Structural adjustment policies (SAPs), furthermore, implied a steep reduction in governmental expenditure for health care, education, and housing programs, including a significant reduction of salary expenses for public sector employees (for Tanzania specifically, see Rösch 1995; Tripp 1997).

The effects of structural adjustment on Tanzania's heath care sector were manifold. The formerly socialist country, which had banned private medical practice in 1977 in order to eliminate "profit thinking in the face of human

suffering" (Iliffe 1998: 209), reopened its health care system to private practitioners and health institutions in 1992 (Iliffe 1998: 217). In 1999, there were
already more than 500 private clinics and hospitals in Dar es Salaam alone
(Boller et al. 2003: 117); in the year 2000 the government counted more than
1,270 private and/or religious dispensaries and 76 non-governmental hospitals throughout the country.[3] Cost-sharing programs—which were initially
opposed by the former President Nyerere and his "socialist supporters" (see
Iliffe 1998: 208)—were introduced in 1993 (Iliffe 1998: 219). These measures
placed heavy burdens on patients and their families, who, in addition to hospital and clinic charges, had to cover costs for transport, food, (admission) bribes,
drugs, and other medical supplies. In 2004, a report by the Women's Dignity
Project stated that "health care charges [in the country] have placed an impossible financial burden on the poorest households," saying that many people
were failing to access primary care when they needed it most and that many
more failed to obtain the necessary referral for more skilled care (Mamdani
and Bangser 2004: 151). Finally, the introduction of SAPs led to drastic cuts in
state expenditures for the health care sector, and to the ever-growing reliance
of Tanzania's health care system on international and private funding to make
up for the growing deficit: in 1990–1991, the national budget allocation for
health care in Tanzania had fallen to 5 percent from its 1970s average of 9.4
percent (Harrington 1998: 149). In 2007, 49.9 percent of capital expenditure for
the health care sector was coming from external sources; private expenditure
on health amounted to 34.2 percent, of which 75 percent was out-of-pocket
expenditures by patients and households (World Health Statistics 2007).[4]

The growing fragmentation and privatization of Tanzania's health
care system—and the concurring influx of external funding—have become
especially pervasive in the field of HIV/AIDS. Since the UN Declaration of
Commitment on HIV/AIDS in 2001—and the subsequent launching first of
the Global Fund for the Fight Against AIDS, Tuberculosis, and Malaria (2001),
and then of PEPFAR (2003)—international funding for the epidemic has
mushroomed. In 2005, it amounted to more than 8 billion USD on the global
level (UNAIDS 2006). In Tanzania, financial resources for the fight against
the epidemic increased steeply after the country was selected as one of the
PEPFAR's 15 focus countries:[5] under the Emergency Plan, Tanzania received
more than 70.7 million USD in Fiscal Year (FY) 2004, nearly 108.8 million USD
in FY 2005, and approximately 130 million USD in FY 2006 to support comprehensive HIV/AIDS prevention, treatment, and care programs. In the year
2007 donor funding comprised 94.6 percent of the total public expenditure for
HIV/AIDS and amounted to 377.8 billion TSH (Tanzanian shillings—approximately 219.6 million USD) (TACAIDS 2008).

As in other countries in the sub-Saharan African region, the international funding for HIV/AIDS in Tanzania is channeled partly through governmental as well as non-governmental hospitals and clinics (in the case of treatment), and partly through the programs of NGOs and, increasingly, of FBOs (faith-based organizations) that have the reputation of providing transparent and accountable entry points for community-based prevention and care initiatives (Dilger 2009). In 2003, one NGO consultant in Dar es Salaam told me that HIV/AIDS had become a "hot topic" in the country: organizations that had not been involved in the topic previously were then engaging in the fight against HIV/AIDS in order to attract additional funding; new NGOs were founded on a daily basis, existing sometimes only as "briefcase NGOs" (i.e., on paper only); and, finally, there was growing competition between individual organizations aiming to develop new and innovative strategies of prevention, care, and treatment in their constant struggles to attract donor money.

While the field of HIV/AIDS work has become increasingly fragmented and also short-lived—with many AIDS organizations attracting one- or two-year funding commitments from a variety of mostly European and North American donors[6]—HIV/AIDS-related programs have gradually subscribed to a focus on human rights and empowerment. This type of programming has placed the self-reflexive individual at the center stage of HIV/AIDS-related policies and has granted the empowered actor the capacity to deal responsibly and circumspectly with the risks associated with HIV infection and AIDS illness. To phrase it in the words of Michel Foucault (1988: 18), the empowerment approach expects people to successfully apply "technologies of the self, which permit individuals to effect by their own means or with the help of others a certain number of operations on their own bodies and souls, thoughts, conduct, and way of being, so as to transform themselves in order to attain a certain state of happiness, purity, wisdom, perfection, or immortality."

To be sure, such an approach is not entirely new in the history of health care and healing in the wider eastern and southern African region; however, it has in the past years gained unprecedented prominence. Subject formation was never the focus of the predominantly repressive power regime of the colonial state, which was only marginally interested in the wider transformation of its citizens' life worlds and individual and collective consciousness (Vaughan 1991), and the promotion of self-governing individuals in the immediate postcolonial setting was constrained mostly to the level of health experts (see Langwick, this volume) and did not rely on media and market forces to the extent that it has in more recent decades. Furthermore, the more recent empowerment approaches are also different from earlier, information-based

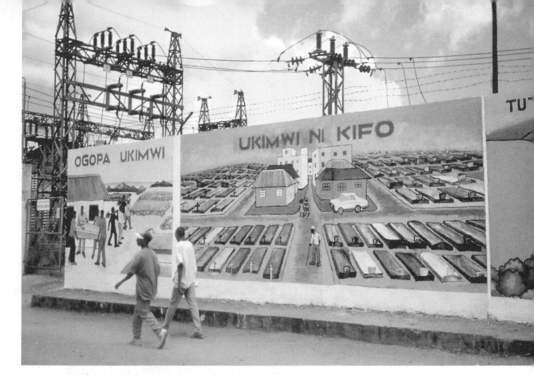

Fig. 2.1. Mural painting in Tanzania. Reads "Fear AIDS" and "AIDS is Death," 1999.
PHOTO: DILGER

approaches in HIV prevention that were directed at an undifferentiated collectivity and often tried to make people fearful of possible infection with the deadly virus. This "approach of deterrence," as I would like to call it, is exemplified by a mural painting in Dar es Salaam (figure 2.1) which simply states "AIDS is Death" (*Ukimwi ni kifo*) and, on the left, "Fear AIDS" (*Ogopa ukimwi*). Today, such generalized messages of deterrence have largely given way to empowering and participatory approaches which have also gained ground in other areas of development work (see Green 2000).[7] In contrast to the earlier information-based approaches (including the "ABC approach" which relies on the tripartite message "Abstain, Be Faithful, or Use Condoms"[8]), the empowerment approach is relying on a multiplicity of media and no longer simply tells people what to do or what not to do, how HIV is transmitted, and what the consequences of risky behavior are in terms of infection and death. While such knowledge is *implicitly* contained in the "new" type of interventions, current prevention efforts are becoming increasingly pervasive with regard to *every* aspect of individual and collective life worlds and are creating differentiated positions that *may* be assumed in relation to HIV/AIDS—based on differences in age, gender, living environment, and also with regard to the professional and educational backgrounds of the respective target groups.

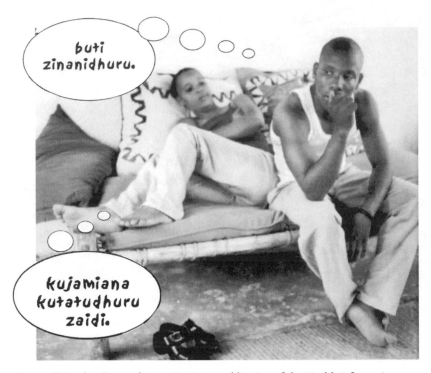

Fig. 2.2. "True love" according to Femina, a publication of the Health Information Project (HIP). FEMINA HIP, TANZANIA.

Technologies of the Self in "New" Approaches to Prevention, Care, and Treatment

In Tanzania, "technologies of the self" in relation to HIV/AIDS are to be found most explicitly in prevention programs that focus on the growing urban middle class and that promote a discourse on "romantic" and "true" love among the young generation according to which partners talk openly about sexual and reproductive health, and in particular about protection from sexually transmitted diseases. This group of young people is sometimes called the "condom generation" by health planners—and in a broader sense it can indeed be understood as a reaction to the HIV/AIDS epidemic: the young men and women addressed by these interventions have become the target of a growing market of internationally funded campaigns which use different types of media interventions, including talk shows, glossy magazines, counseling sections in newspapers, call-in radio shows, etc., and which promote a view of sexuality that has become increasingly individualized and detached from family relations. All these interventions are responding to the questions individual women and men *may* have about sexuality and HIV/AIDS. They are giving advice with regard to specific life situations that represent a risk in terms of HIV infection—and, most importantly, they talk about the pleasures and uses of sexuality. Thus, whereas earlier campaigns assumed that people know how to have sex and how to manage sexual relationships, this knowledge is no longer taken for granted and now has to be negotiated (cf. Parikh 2005). "True love," as discussed and promoted by advice columns and picture stories run by fashionable lifestyle magazines, is based not solely on sexual attraction or satisfaction—but rather on values like friendship, loyalty, trust, respect, and finally tenderness.

Such an approach is exemplified by a picture story in the lifestyle magazine *Femina*,[9] which offers a role model to young men and women who are confronted with dilemmas surrounding ideas of "true" and "romantic love"

Fig. 2.3. Femina HIP, Tanzania.

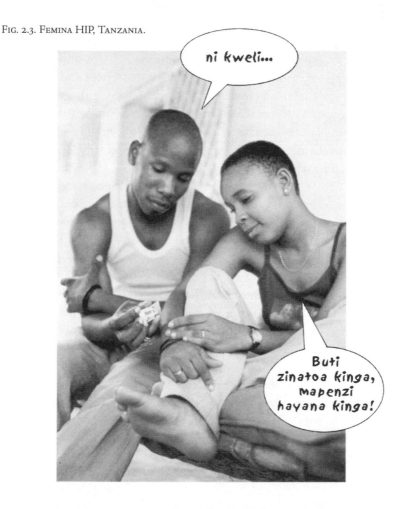

as well as prevention of HIV. A picture (figure 2.2) shows a young couple that is experiencing these dilemmas of (non)communication about sex and the associated health risks. The young man on the right, who is turning his back on his partner, expects that the use of a condom is going to "harm" him (-dhuru) in that it will decrease his pleasure in the (obviously already agreed-upon) sexual encounter. The young woman, on the other hand, is (silently) convinced that mere "trust" (in love? in the health of one's partner?) will be even *more* harmful. The story evolves over the next few pictures, showing how the couple is starting to communicate and how they finally resolve the dilemma, until the final picture (figure 2.3) shows how they have arrived at a solution that is satisfying to both of them (iconographically represented by the physical closeness between the couple). The use of condoms in this context is seen by both partners not as a sign of "lack of trust" but as an expression of mutual esteem and of acknowledging responsibility for one's partner's health (cf. Dilger 2003).

On another level, technologies of the self have come to play a crucial role in the politics of "Living Positively" that have shaped HIV-positive identities all over southern and eastern Africa during the last 10–15 years. Originating in Uganda in the early 1990s and traveling to other countries in the region from there (see Dilger 2001), this model provides a way for people with HIV/AIDS "to take care of their mind and body" and to enter into a "healthy relationship" with the life-threatening disease through a number of regulative practices and devices. At the time of my research in Dar es Salaam (i.e., before the introduction of ARVs), these practices included adherence to dietary requirements, regular medical checkups, consistent treatment of opportunistic infections, and, finally, maintenance of social activities and regular exchanges with others on dilemmas and problems associated with an HIV infection. At the turn of the century, this open communication aspect of living positively had materialized in the form of numerous NGO support groups for people with HIV/AIDS which represented fora in which to discuss, negotiate, and form opinions about various issues related to their illness. Topics discussed in the weekly or monthly support group meetings that took place under the aegis of different NGOs in Dar es Salaam in 1999–2000 included: disclosure and stigma; the challenge of balanced nutrition; "safe sexuality" in short- and long-term relationships; the lack of material support in times of illness; the writing of a will; and the benefits and disadvantages of traditional medicine. The information and advice given with regard to problems in partnerships, families, or at the workplace was specific as well as generic and was becoming an essential part of the process of building a "positive identity" despite experiences of grief,

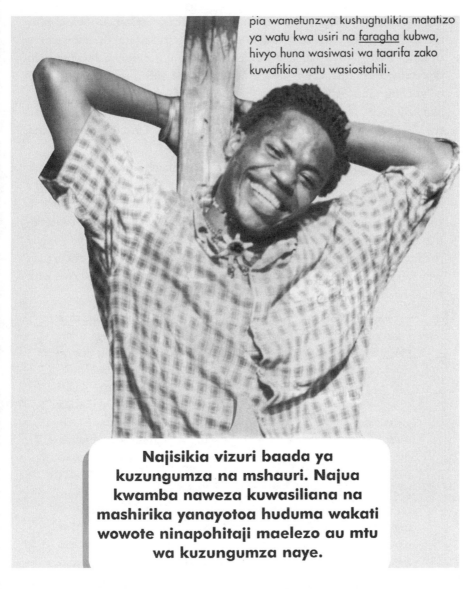

pia wametunzwa kushughulikia matatizo ya watu kwa usiri na <u>faragha</u> kubwa, hivyo huna wasiwasi wa taarifa zako kuwafikia watu wasiostahili.

Najisikia vizuri baada ya kuzungumza na mshauri. Najua kwamba naweza kuwasiliana na mashirika yanayotoa huduma wakati wowote ninapohitaji maelezo au mtu wa kuzungumza naye.

Fig. 2.4. "Living Positively" booklet published by HIP, a good example of the way in which public health responses have become embedded in transnational channels of funding and knowledge production. Adopted from the Soul City Institute for Health and Development Communication in South Africa, it was translated into Kiswahili and "culturally adapted to the Tanzanian setting" by HIP. The main character is confronted with an HIV-positive diagnosis and—after going through a period of internal struggling and despair—has accepted his HIV+ status. He says: "After I have talked to the counselor, I feel good. I know that I can talk to these organizations. They offer services whenever I am in need of advice or when I need a person to talk to." Femina, HIP, Tanzania.

stigmatization, or despair about one's material life circumstances. For most of the support group members I interviewed in Dar es Salaam, the experiences of other HIV-positive men and women had become an essential reference in describing and initiating this healing process. It was only through the repeated counseling and identification with the suffering of others that people (ideally) adopted a self-image of being HIV-positive and translated this self-image into the context of marital and non-marital relationships, kinship networks, and the wider community.

Mama Frank[10] (f, 58) stands out as an example here. After the death of her husband in 1988, she found employment as a cleaner in one of Dar es Salaam's oldest AIDS NGOs. During the monthly group counseling sessions, she had come to function as a source of experience and knowledge for others in dealing "properly" with their illness by emphasizing how important the NGOs had become in finding one's "true [HIV-positive] self." She contrasted this in turn with the experience that her late son Frank—who had been also infected with HIV—had created for himself:

> I am living a life with hope. I got tested in 1986 and they found that I carry the virus. [My husband and I] were tested at the Aga Khan Hospital [in Dar es Salaam]. When we received the results, the doctor was hesitant, but I told him: "Just tell me, don't be worried about me." The doctor told me that there is a hint of the AIDS virus in my blood. [. . .] I went to my sister-in-law[11] and told her that I have the AIDS virus and that I may die any time. Later the counselors of these NGOs came and brought me to one of these organizations. There I found that we are many. They taught us to live with hope. I also received treatment at one of the NGOs. Today I live by praying to God. I live because of the blessing of God. I don't know if it is because of these medications[12] or because of God. What also helps is that since the time of my husband's death in 1988, I haven't known any other man. My son Frank tested HIV-positive. I told him: "Don't worry, just follow the counselors' advice." But he died five years after the test.

The "open" and "positive" approach of NGO clients to their illness was ultimately supported through programs of material and legal empowerment which predominantly represented the social and economic backgrounds of the NGO clientele. At the turn of the century the NGOs were most frequently visited by middle-aged women who had come from rural regions with relatively low education. Many of them (including Mama Frank, who had been fortunate to find employment with one of the NGOs) were widows who lived alone or with their children and earned their living on a piecemeal basis. At the time of my research, NGOs in Dar es Salaam were offering legal assistance to widows whose hereditary entitlement was being contested by their in-laws. Others offered "home-based care," which is a service for providing care to sick family members in the home. Finally, NGOs aimed at providing financial security through granting small loans for the development of small-scale businesses, issuing food rations, or covering children's school fees.

A final issue that has shaped the politics of HIV-positive identities in more recent years is the introduction of the ARVs, which have become available in Tanzania since the end of 2004. In collaboration with the U.S.-funded PEPFAR program and the Global Fund for the Fight Against AIDS, Tuberculosis, and Malaria, newly created treatment centers have been established all over the country that connect counseling and testing procedures to the patients' enrollment in specific ARV treatment programs. Depending on the test results of their CD4 counts, patients undergo specific "adherence classes" in hospitals and clinics, where they are trained to observe their bodies carefully and to report unusual changes, symptoms, and side effects to their physicians and the health staff. The knowledge acquired in these adherence classes is carefully tested in individual "adherence panels," and patients are returned to further training if the desired effect hasn't been achieved yet (Mattes 2011).

This refined treatment apparatus that has been established around ARV provision in Tanzania and other African countries over the last years can be said to have become one of the largest public health intervention in the history of health care in Africa. ARV treatment programs now try scrutinously to regulate ARV patients' life worlds in addition to the possibility of emerging drug-resistant viral strains; and this has led to the further diversification of funding arrangements and institutional setups (Hardon and Dilger 2011). In Tanzania, ARVs are prescribed on a monthly basis and the dates of the last health clinic visit as well as of the recommended return for checkup are marked on a blue card that is used specifically for the prescription of ARVs and that allows people to visit other treatment centers around the country while traveling. A number of booklets and handouts stress the necessity of taking ARVs according to a fixed schedule and being aware of the importance of sticking to these drugs—forever: "These expensive medicines," reads one booklet which was adopted from the Soul City project in South Africa, "have to be taken every day, every month, your whole life." Finally, the health planners see it as crucial for the success of ARV treatment that families and friends establish an open dialogue about these drugs in order to create a supportive environment for consistent and continuous drug regimens: "It is good to be with someone you trust," reads one leaflet, "be it a relative or a friend—he will help you to remind you to take your medicine [as prescribed]." Thus, while people have been urged "to live positively with HIV" for more than a decade

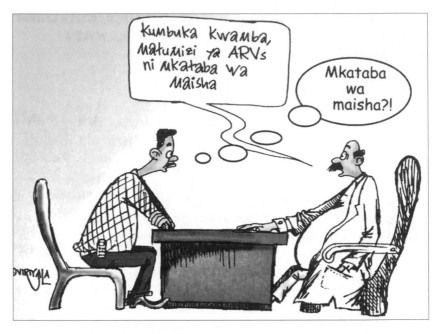

Fig. 2.5. Leaflet emphasizing the long-term aspect of ARV treatment. Doctor: "The taking of ARVs is a life-long contract." Patient: "A life-long contract?" NATIONAL AIDS CONTROL PROGRAM, TANZANIA.

now, today they are required to "make a life-long contract" with medications that have transformed the life-threatening disease into a chronic condition (see fig. 2.5).

Beyond NGOs and Biological Citizenship: Local Moral Worlds and the Limitations of Biopower in Tanzania

Looking at the numerous interventions that have been established in the field of HIV/AIDS over the last decades, one may wonder which particular "truths" about the disease (in the sense of Paula Treichler [1999]), or, alternatively, which type of "moral regimes and knowledge" (in the Foucauldian sense) are being promoted by health programs in Tanzania that have evolved in the context of a market-driven, mostly non-governmental and transnationalized response to the epidemic. I want to argue that the empowerment approach—and the social, cultural, and economic practices that are implied in it—are confined to specific settings; these settings can be described as *islands of biopower and self-care* that are sustained by the international AIDS industry, which has increasingly based its activities on notions of human rights and self-responsibility and in recent years has aimed to involve "affected communities" into its manifold activities.

In medical anthropology, practices, ideals, and technologies of the self originating in the context of illness, health, and well-being have in recent years become closely related to discussions of biological citizenship, a form of citizenship that refers to the biological dimension of human life and "embodies a demand for particular protections, for the enactment or cessation of particular policies and actions [and for] access to special resources" (Rose and Novas 2005: 441). In the context of HIV/AIDS, Vinh-Kim Nguyen (2005: 126) has subsumed the various practices, values, and ideas that have emerged in the context of a globalized health response under the concept of therapeutic citizenship—a transnationalized form of biological citizenship which makes claims on the global economic and social order based on a "shared therapeutic predicament." According to Nguyen (2005: 125f), the social and cultural practices that have evolved in this context over the last 10–15 years have been organized around a complex set of confessional technologies and processes of self-fashioning which are closely interwoven with internationally acclaimed forms of HIV/AIDS activism and essentially draw their legitimacy from the economic, political, and biological inequalities existing in a globalizing world.

The practices and technologies of the self which are evolving under these circumstances can now be described with the concept of "biopower," which, according to Foucault (1977), involves the exercise of power on two mutually intertwined levels and at the center of which lies the control—and the proper conduct—of sexuality and life itself. On the individual level, the exercise of biopower presupposes a specific type of relationship with one's body, as well as a specific type of subjectivity. Thus, while the exercise of state power aims at the regulation and control of the population as a whole, the exercise of individual power aims at the disciplining of one's own body, the regulation of desire, and the refashioning of the responsible (sexual) self. In this context, the care of one's own health and body are intimately intertwined in that both are protected, cultivated, and isolated from anything that is considered undesirable and dangerous. This creation of the "healthy self" through the application of technologies of truth and knowledge seems not dissimilar to the way in which the interventions of the mostly transnationally funded AIDS NGOs in southern and eastern Africa have come to present sexuality and health. According to Deborah Posel (2005: 134), for AIDS NGOs in South Africa—and certainly to some of their clients and target groups—sexuality has become a "site of rational, individual choice and agency—an opportunity for empowerment and 'healthy positive living.'"

If we look now at rural areas of Tanzania—and also beyond NGOs and clinical settings in urban centers[13]—we find that the ways people deal with HIV/AIDS are not based *exclusively* on knowledge, discursive processes, and technologies of the self that are derived from governmental and non-governmental AIDS campaigns. While public health information has become important for how people think about and act upon health and illness in the context of HIV/AIDS, the ways they are responding to health challenges and suffering bodies have become embedded simultaneously in the wider political economies of health care in Tanzania, as well as in the social and moral priorities formulated by communities and families in relation to the disease. I want to illustrate this aspect with regard to the ways families and communities in the rural Mara Region in northwestern Tanzania—as well as in a Pentecostal congregation in Dar es Salaam—have come to deal with HIV/AIDS-related illnesses and deaths. However, while I focus on the ways in which people's responses to HIV/AIDS have been shaped in specific settings in Tanzania beyond the NGO context, it should become clear that the processes and practices I describe here are not situated *outside* the globalized AIDS response and the health sector in Tanzania. They have become inseparably intertwined with the processes described above in that they evolve *in relation to* the needs and challenges experienced in the wake of structural adjustment, privatization, and the implication of Tanzania's health system in transnationalized forms of governance. Furthermore, it has to be kept in mind that many of the HIV-positive women and men I encountered in Tanzania belong not to one neatly bounded social entity or group, but, rather, identify themselves (sometimes only temporarily) as NGO clients and/or church members in addition to emphasizing their identities as part of one or more kinship networks.

KINSHIP, CARE, AND RELATEDNESS IN RURAL MARA

At the time of my research in the rural Mara Region in 1999–2000, governmental and non-governmental care programs were only established in rudimentary ways.[14] The expensive care and treatment provided by local private hospitals were affordable to only a few rural families, who lived primarily from agriculture and petty trade—in part from fishing and through the support of family members who were living and working in the cities. Relationships of care and welfare in this context were shifted out of necessity to the families with members with HIV/AIDS and were embedded in, among other things, family conflicts that had often begun long before the outbreak of illness. Especially with regard to sick relatives from cities like Dar es Salaam, Mwanza, or Arusha, family tensions had an effect on situations of care provision, as sick relatives who had been living in the city often returned to their home villages unwillingly and under pressure from their (urban) relatives. On the other hand, the return of these relatives, who in some cases had paid little attention to the well-being of their rural families during preceding years, presented a significant economic, social, and emotional strain for their rural family members (Dilger 2005, 2006, 2008). This aspect was expressed in the following interview with a male farmer:

> Samson Mrungu (m, 38): Some fear [people with HIV/AIDS] because they think: "If I eat with him or touch him, I will get his disease." It has also occurred that families have chased away their sick relatives. If somebody became sick in Dar es Salaam or Mwanza and returns home people will say: "Go back to where you came from! Don't bother us with your disease! You got your disease from the town and now you bring it to us." This happens.

> HD: Do these sick people return to town then?

> SM: No, they won't return, they say: "Where shall I go while my home is here in the village?"

In addition to the internal family conflicts and significant social and economic difficulties that the care of family members sick with AIDS implied in this rural setting, the differences in the quality of care and the availability of the care provided was determined above all by gender-specific dynamics. The latter played a particularly important role with regard to the care situations of young women. In the patrilineal family structures of the research region, women and their children were considered part of the husband's family following marriage. As such, their care in times of sickness or in the case of the death of their husbands was considered the responsibility of their husbands' relatives. In reality, however, these rules and expectations often represented the basis for tensions and discussion across family networks: in particular, questions would be raised with regard to young wives who became ill with HIV/AIDS about whether they were "properly" married and if the marriage had been "correctly" confirmed through a dowry. Discussions concerning proper marriages—and thus about the recognition of the woman's status as a wife—were especially common in regard to childless women, as well as to widows, in whose case claims on their husbands' inheritance would be shared not only with their children but with their in-laws (see Dilger 2005, 2006).

On another level, relationships of care and support were shaped by the kinship-based politics of burial and belonging, which forced people who had worked and lived outside of their villages for extended periods to return to their rural homes when death was approaching. Questions concerning care and the subsequent burial—and especially about the place of burial—were thereby potentially conflictive and reflected again on the dynamics of age, gender, and belonging within patrilineal kinship networks (cf. Cohen and Odhiambo 1992). Thus, while the need to care for and bury male relatives raised questions concerning (unfulfilled) solidarity and kinship obligations in some cases, the situation of women routinely became more troubling to the involved families. Especially in the case of younger women who had been married to their husbands only recently and who had no or only a few children at the time of their death, the question posed was: to which family did they actually belong, and who was responsible for their care and their burial— their husband's or their father's family? Unmarried (or not formally married) women, on the other hand, were cared for mostly by their family of origin and buried on the compound of their brother-in-law, who thus provided the deceased with the status of a co-wife.[15]

Finally, the way families in rural Mara dealt with HIV / AIDS illnesses prior to the arrival of ARVs consisted of a persistent silence that surrounded the infections and deaths of family members. Prior to the arrival of ARVs, only a very few HIV-infected men and women among my informants knew about their diagnosis and almost none of them talked openly about it. Testing and counseling were carried out in the local hospitals only for those patients who were suspected by the health staff to be infected with HIV. Those patients who were found to be HIV-positive were often not informed about their diagnoses—and those who were, were sent home due to the high costs of nursing AIDS patients and as beds in the local hospitals became increasingly over-occupied. However, while for people in Mara at the turn of the century the silence on the *biological* dimensions of the disease had become an integral part of referring to illnesses and deaths in the time of AIDS, this didn't mean that there was no talk *at all* about the illnesses of dying community members or relatives. On the one hand, HIV / AIDS-related illnesses and deaths were the subject of multiple rumors that were circulating in the villages and that discussed the nature and origin of suffering—as well as the sexual relationships and networks that were its alleged root cause—in detail. As figure 2.6 shows, the targets of this talk were carefully trying to prevent these rumors from spreading—sometimes even beyond their deaths—and many people were hesitant to discuss their claims openly, especially if the person who was suspected of an HIV infection was a powerful and influential member of the community. On the other hand, many individuals and families in Mara referred to HIV / AIDS in terms of other diseases such as tuberculosis or *herpes zooster*, or associated it with witchcraft or the disease *chira,* said to be caused by the non-observance of ritual prescriptions, the symptoms of which were

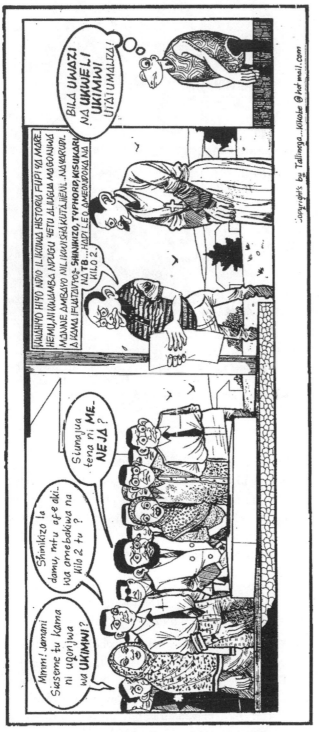

Fig. 2.6. Cartoon discussing the silences—and the multiple rumors—around HIV/AIDS at funerals. From left to right: "Mmm! Why doesn't he say that it was AIDS?" "Can a person die of high blood pressure when he only weighed 2 kilos at his death?" "Don't you know that he was a MANAGER?" "This was the story of the deceased. Our relative died of the four diseases, which I have already mentioned and will now repeat: HIGH BLOOD PRESSURE, TYPHUS, DIABETES, and TB . . . In the end, he only weighed 2 kilos." "Without openness and sincerity AIDS will kill us all." MSEMAKWELI, 16—JAN. 22, 2000.

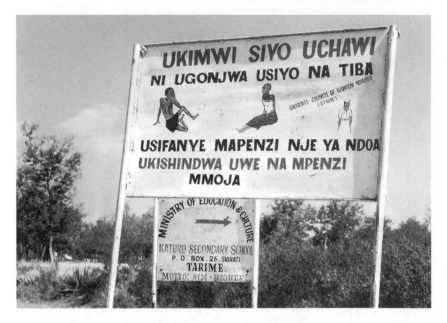

Fig. 2.7. Associations of HIV/AIDS with witchcraft have been integrated into community-based health campaigns in Mara, as is exemplified by this billboard—which, however, takes an explicitly negative approach to such interpretations of disease: "AIDS is not witchcraft," it says, "it is a disease which can not be treated / which doesn't have a cure." And below it reads: "Don't make love outside marriage. If you fail, stay with one partner." PHOTO: DILGER

described as being very similar to AIDS (Dilger 2006, 2008). While at the time of my research not all people in Mara would have argued that *all* cases of HIV/AIDS were related to *chira,* in those cases where the connection was established this had immediate effects on the way treatment was sought for patients and how care and support were being organized within family networks (this being related essentially to the fact that *chira* was said to be curable with the help of local herbs).

HEALING, COMMUNITY, AND CARE IN A NEO-PENTECOSTAL CONGREGATION IN DAR ES SALAAM

In rural areas as in urban centers of Tanzania the daily lives of people living with HIV/AIDS are often more complex than public health programs suggest. In particular, in Dar es Salaam, Neo-Pentecostal churches, which have seen drastic increases in the number of members in large sections of sub-Saharan Africa in recent years, have played an important role in the social, economic, and religious life situations of people with HIV/AIDS (see also the quotation above by Mama Frank). The Full Gospel Bible Fellowship Church

(FGBFC) in Dar es Salaam in which I conducted fieldwork in 1999–2000 was founded in 1989 by Zachariah Kakobe, a charismatic bishop from southern Tanzania who had earned his living as a musician and meteorologist before receiving his calling in 1980. Over the last 20 years, the church has established branches in almost all regions and districts of the country and counted more than 120,000 members nationwide in the year 2000. In 1999, the FGBFC caused a stir through its public AIDS healings, which attracted 300–400 people a week and were hotly debated in the print media and among the public (see Dilger 2007).

For the members of the FGBFC I encountered during my fieldwork, the church became a source of hope mainly through its Gospel of Prosperity and, intimately related to it, the concepts of "awakening" and "salvation." According to Corten and Marshall-Fratani (2001), salvation in a Pentecostal church is "an ongoing existential project" that requires engagement in church activities and healing prayers in order to ward off attacks by diabolic forces, as well as a break with many of the obligations church followers have toward their families (especially the "cultural" and "ritual" obligations which are associated with the central phases of life, i.e., birth, marriage, and death; see also Meyer 1998). In the case of the FGBFC, the church teachings required furthermore the abandonment of sinful lifestyles such as consumption of alcohol or engagement in extramarital sexual relationships. It was only if these (admittedly difficult) conditions were fulfilled that the manifold promises of salvation began to work in multiple directions. Thus, the gospel of health and wealth in the FGBFC promised not only material success and progress for those living in poverty: salvation also meant relief from all kinds of distress, from trouble at work or with the Tanzanian bureaucratic system to diseases such as infertility, cancer, high blood pressure, or AIDS (see Dilger 2007). These promises of healing were backed up by the testimonies of members who claimed that the healings had been "proved" by scientific tests in a hospital or clinic, and these testimonies were also circulated in leaflet form. One of my interviewees recounted:

> Consolata Msemo: Before I got tested in 1998, I felt a strong heat (*moto*) in my body—as if you get burnt. Then I felt something like paralysis (*ganzi*)—I was freezing. And my head was aching. Every time I had a cold, I became critically ill. [. . .] At [the NGO] CCBRT[16] they found out that I am [HIV] positive. They told me to return for another test after three months. I told them that I am not worried because God has the power to do everything. Humans cannot heal AIDS, but if you believe in God—He can. I returned to Kakobe[17] and showed him the certificate (*cheti*). This was when we started officially (*rasmi*) with the healing prayers.

Apart from the AIDS healings—which, according to the church's bishop and his followers, have been confirmed by biomedical tests in some cases—the church has established a network of mutual solidarity that provides help and support for members in times of need and crisis. At the time of my research, the church had established a dense network of small neighborhood churches comprised of 20–30 members each, in which the idea of a "spiritual family"— defined in opposition to the worldly family—was promoted. This concept of spiritual family aimed to build a new moral community that was to disperse any doubts the church members might have about the righteousness of their path. This path to relation- and community-building was an ambiguous process that implied a high potential for intra-familial conflict, stemming both from unsaved relatives who tried to make church members depart from the path of salvation *and* from the church followers who persistently urged their families to give up their "dark" and "sinful" ways. However, the FGBFC was described to me by its members not only as a source of conflict, but also as a beneficial network of care and support that flexibly reacted to the needs of its individual followers. Especially in cases of serious illness, the charitable behaviors of other church followers went far beyond immediate acts of caring or nursing and often included arranging funerals, etc. The provision of such acts of solidarity had become particularly beneficial for the mostly female members of the church, mainly young to middle-aged women with low educational status who had migrated to Dar es Salaam in search of employment or business opportunities during the 1980s or 1990s. To these women—as well as to the fewer male members of the church, most of whom had a similar social background—the FGBFC was appealing essentially because it offered a space of hope, stability, and moral orientation in an urban context that was experienced as increasingly risky and ambivalent.

What can be drawn now from these two case studies on the FGBFC and on kinship networks in rural Mara? As I hope to have shown, there may be significant gaps between the ways in which the "empowered individuals" of transnationally designed health programs (as well as the subjects formulated predominantly on the ground of NGOs), on the one hand, and people who perceive of themselves mainly as members of kinship- and other community-based networks, on the other, conceive of illness and well-being in the time of AIDS. People in Tanzania—who may have a range of resources at their disposal and who may depend in their decisions on a variety of social and cultural settings and relationships—act not always in accordance with public health messages or with regard to the greatest benefits to their own (or others') biologically defined health. At the turn of the century, individual and

collective behaviors in the era of AIDS were constrained by the growing economic pressures and the lack of access to health care services that have been
triggered by neoliberal economics and political reforms in the health sector
over the last two decades. They were also rooted in the logics of community
and kinship politics and in the moral, cultural, and religious priorities that
people had with regard to the persistence of social relationships in and beyond
the context of death and suffering. The *exclusive* focus on life worlds that are
promoted and represented by state actors, non-governmental organizations,
and humanitarian interventions would have revealed only a partial view of
the complex social and cultural processes that have come to shape the lived
experience and practice surrounding HIV/AIDS in Tanzania and other parts
of sub-Saharan Africa. Consequently, I would argue that if we are to think
critically about notions of citizenship and self-care in relation to HIV/AIDS,
we need to take account of the complex relationships between power, experience, and practice that have shaped people's identities and subjectivities in the
wake of globalization and the emerging epidemic.

Knowledge, Experience, Power: The Making of Subjectivities in the Era of Globalization and HIV/AIDS

In contrasting the different ways in which individuals, families, communities, and a wide range of governmental and non-governmental institutions
have come to deal with HIV/AIDS in rural and urban Tanzania, three things
should be emphasized. All of them shed light on the way in which the relations
between knowledge, practice, experience, and (bio)power have been shaped
and reconfigured in the context of globalization and neoliberal reform processes over the last few decades.

First, the analysis above has made clear that the various contexts in which
people have come to act on HIV/AIDS in Tanzania imply shifting understandings of the (causal) connection between knowledge and practice and the larger
social contexts in which they are embedded. While earlier approaches in HIV/
AIDS prevention were based on the "rational actor model" and assumed that
the accessibility of knowledge (in the sense of information) translates inevi-
tably into practice (in the sense of behavior), more recent approaches have
adopted a more complex view of this relation. Thus, NGO approaches that are
based on the notion of empowerment acknowledge that biomedical and public health knowledge acquire meaning only in relation to the larger contexts
in which individual behavior and practice materialize. This understanding has
enabled approaches to issues of the (gendered) relationships between sexual

partners; emotional states like fear, love, or hope; the challenges of disclosure, stigma, and care, and, related to this, the dynamics in (nuclear) families; and finally, albeit to a minor extent, the socioeconomic and legal conditions that shape the lives of individual actors in contemporary Tanzania. Issues that remain excluded, however, are the larger transformations in politics and health care in the country (including the issue of access to health services); alternative notions of illness, healing, and trust; and the dynamics of relatedness and belonging in relation to extended family networks and religious communities in urban and rural settings. As argued above, these latter aspects may play a crucial role in shaping individual and collective practice, knowledge, and experience in relation to HIV/AIDS in rural and urban areas.

Second, the different types of knowledge, practice, and experience that have emerged in the context of globalization and HIV/AIDS in Tanzania are inseparably intertwined with different types of subjectivities and reflexive selves, which are in turn built around shifting concepts of person and gender. Thus, in their approaches and interventions NGOs perceive their target groups and clients largely as autonomously acting individuals who, in the case of women, need to be empowered socially, economically, and legally in order to be able to make healthy and responsible decisions. Men, on the other hand, are seen as economically, socially, and legally privileged and as being largely in charge of most decisions that relate to their partnerships and families. Only in recent years have NGOs and local interest groups come to reflect critically on socially constructed modes of masculinity and male sexuality and to emphasize the need for men's "cultural empowerment" which might enable them to assume a "positive" gender role as responsible husband, son, father, and sexual partner (for the discourse on the "new men" in South Africa, see Morell 2001).

Such discourses and images contrast with the expectations, roles, and responsibilities that are formulated for the behaviors of men and women in other areas of life in Tanzania. In the patrilineal kinship networks in rural areas, the well-being of individual men and women is often closely interwoven with the fate of their—and, in the case of women, their husbands'—nuclear and extended families. Illness and suffering are often understood here as a reflection of the wider state of (gender- and age-specific) social relations which are perceived as being disturbed by globalization and migratory processes and which need to be worked upon in order to ensure individual and collective well-being. In contrast, Neo-Pentecostal churches like the FGBFC in Dar es Salaam offer new spaces of solidarity and attachment, especially for women, and thus provide an alternative to the male-centered kinship networks of rural and urban areas. Such churches often pursue a highly conservative gender ideology, however, which is centered on the nuclear family and which expects decency and submissiveness from women toward their husbands. It is important to emphasize that these different types of gendered subjectivities and concepts of the person as sketched out here are not mutually exclusive. People's lives are often shaped in relation to different urban as well as rural localities and social settings through which they are exposed to shifting, and often conflicting, types of expectations, knowledge, and values.

Finally, the way knowledge, truth, and meaning are produced and reproduced in relation to HIV/AIDS in various settings in Tanzania has been shaped by the context of global development and health restructuring over the last two to three decades—as well as by the multiple iconographies and textual representations that have become part and parcel of the process of producing meaning and truth in the era of globalization. On the one hand, globally driven development precludes the integration of certain types of truth and knowledge into health interventions, a fact that is amply illustrated by the various images, texts, and statistics produced by governmental as well as nongovernmental actors in the form of flyers, booklets, and reports. In particular, the multiple moral conflicts relating to decisions concerning health and sexuality—but also people's alternative knowledges and experiences concerning illness, healing, death, and mourning—are seldom addressed by internationally funded interventions and programs. Thus, while "local knowledge" and experience are highly valued in other areas of development work in Tanzania (especially in agriculture and more recently, again, in the field of traditional medicine), HIV/AIDS interventions in the country have often engaged a modernizing approach that reproduces established dichotomies like "tradition vs. modernity," "belief vs. knowledge," and "religion vs. medicine and science." In this context, local knowledge, experience, and practice, as partially represented in local Kiswahili publications and cartoons, are often branded as "superstitious," "harmful," and "backwards."

On another level, and related to this, the production and dissemination of knowledge, meaning, and truth in the neoliberal era have been shaped by the growing disjuncture between the practices, experiences, and ideas of (internally further differentiated) families and communities, on the one hand, and the expectations and values that are promoted by the (equally differentiated) HIV/AIDS industry, on the other. Thus, this text has shown that the promises and services of NGOs have had an impact on the lives of many individuals, some of whom have benefited from the new funding arrangements that have also opened up new avenues into the globalized health order on a personal level (as exemplified by the case study of Mama Frank and the introductory case of Amelia Jacob). Furthermore, the privatization and NGO-ization of the health care sector in Tanzania have also led to shifting understandings of rights and citizenship. While colonial and post-independent understandings of law in the country regarded the existence of legal frameworks predominantly as "constitutive of state power, not as a limitation upon it" (Harrington 1998: 151), the transition to a multi-party system and the growing influence of the international development community from the mid-1990s onwards have defined law as a code for which the state can be made liable; thus opening a space for the perception that health is a right individuals are entitled to (Harrington 1998). In Tanzanian society, such shifting perspectives have not resulted, however, in an open challenging of the state in relation to its alleged responsibility toward people with HIV/AIDS—as for instance in South Africa, where the demonstrations and activities of the Treatment Action Campaign have become symbolic for practices of health citizenship in the post-Apartheid state (Robins 2004). In Dar es Salaam, it was almost exclusively on the safe ground of the NGOs that members of the HIV/AIDS support groups expressed their critique of governmental authorities which, according to them, have failed to take care of their HIV-positive and AIDS-sick citizens (Dilger 2005). This seems understandable given the fact that during the 1990s the work of NGOs depended largely on the benevolence of the government, which often conceived of them as a threat to the social order (Mercer 1999: 250ff.).

Under these circumstance, many people in rural and urban Tanzania are relying on knowledge and relationships beyond the biomedically defined health settings, and are trying to act on their bodies and illnesses by drawing on a wide range of resources that have emerged, and have been transformed, in response to HIV/AIDS and shifting social and political-economic conditions. In conclusion, I would therefore like to argue that this disjuncture has become reflective of how the circulation of medicine and biopower in the neoliberal era has been shaped by the way global capital and development are "hopping" over sub-Saharan Africa (Ferguson 2006), thereby reconfiguring social, economic, and cultural constellations on the continent in only fragmentary ways. Thus, while the production and spreading of biopower in Tanzania have become embedded in globalized channels of funding which govern "regimes of truth and knowledge" in the context of HIV/AIDS and structural adjustment in often contradictory ways, the state and its institutions—as well as the non-governmental actors that have become complementary to them—have only a limited ability to establish and exercise biopolitical authority (also in its more beneficial form) in a *pervasive* way. Under these conditions, many Tanzanians have developed a critical sense of their government's ability to control the living conditions of its citizens on a daily basis and turned to looking for "collective solidarity" and "moral beneficence" outside of the state altogether (Ferguson 2006: 85). In this regard, moral knowledge, practice, and experience—and the various forms of sociality and belonging that have been built around them—have remained of crucial importance to individuals, communities, and families in making sense of the transformations and challenges related to globalization and in responding actively to the suffering associated with HIV/AIDS.

Notes

1. http://www.thp.org/what_we_do/key_initiatives/honoring_africa_leadership/laureate_list (accessed Aug. 30, 2010).

2. http://www.thp.org/what_we_do/key_initiatives/honoring_africa_leadership/laureate_list/amelia_jacob (accessed Aug. 30, 2010).

3. http://www.tanzania.go.tz/health.html (accessed Aug. 30, 2010).

4. http://apps.who.int/ghodata/?vid=20700 (accessed Sept. 14, 2010).

5. Among PEPFAR's 15 focus countries—which represent collectively approximately 50 percent of HIV infections worldwide—are five East African countries: Ethiopia, Kenya, Rwanda, Tanzania, and Uganda.

6. During my research in 1999–2000, some of the donors to AIDS NGOs in Dar es Salaam were: NORAD (Norwegian Agency for Development Cooperation), DANIDA (Danish International Development Agency), HIVOS (Humanist Institute for Co-operation with Developing Countries), UNDP (United Nations Development Programme), and UNAIDS (Joint United Nations Programme on HIV/AIDS) (see Dilger 2005).

7. "Participatory approaches" and "partnership" in development, as defined by representatives of the development complex, imply the planning and implementation of development projects as the result of a process of mutual learning and interaction that is targeted first and foremost at the "empowerment" of local populations. As Green (2000: 69) has put it,

> "Development" is not [then] simply a process of directed change leading to certain kinds of economic and social transformation, but depends on the accomplishment of a series of corresponding moral transformations in the consciousness of people participating, as change agents and changed, in the development process. Consequently, the proper task of development organizations and their personnel is to facilitate the necessary transformations in consciousness which can *empower* the poor as social actors to embark on locally managed change.

While this is not the focus of my chapter, it should be mentioned here that the ideals of "partnership" and "empowerment" are seldom translated into actual practice and that attempts at their realization have led to paradoxical relations between actors in the field who, while often being critical or even cynical about the contradictions contained in development, ultimately affirm and reproduce the overall system (Green 2000; Rottenburg 2002; Marsland 2006).

8. For a critical analysis of the ABC approach, see Heald (2002).

9. *Femina* is a publication of the Health Information Project (HIP). The HIP is a multimedia initiative which is funded by a multitude of international donors, including the German Society for Technical Cooperation (GTZ), NORAD, and SIDA. The HIP has developed a broad range of publications and activities that help young people to "get the facts and make better decisions about how to stay safe, improve [their] relationships and learn more about job opportunities." (http://www.chezasalama.com/G-Behind/view.partner.php?id=384, accessed Nov. 10, 2007).

10. All interviewees' names are pseudonyms.

11. Sister of Mama Frank's late husband.

12. During the time of our interview (2000), Mama Frank received basic treatment for opportunistic infections.

13. While my critique of concepts like "biological" or "therapeutic citizenship" in this section focuses mostly on settings and relationships situated *outside* of NGOs and biomedical institutions, the validity of these concepts has also to be questioned for the context of NGOs themselves and of the biomedical sector in general. Thus, as Whyte, Whyte, and Kyaddondo (2010) and Whyte (2009) have argued, the rollout of ARVs raises challenging questions for anthropological debates on ethics, subject formation, and understandings of biological and/or therapeutic citizenship. These questions may become even more pertinent with the current cutbacks in global funding for antiretroviral treatment and the impact this may have on the accessibility of local and national treatment programs (Médecins Sans Frontières 2010). Furthermore, the confines of this article do not allow me to elaborate on the manifold social and cultural processes influencing not only the domains of care and illness experience but also sexuality in rural Tanzania. Thus, while a discourse on "true love" is taking place even in rural areas, there are many other aspects (such as inequality between the sexes, the significance of gifts and money for sexuality, and concepts of moral integrity and sexual pleasure) that are just as essential for the shaping of sexual relationships between young men and women as the knowledge being conveyed by national and international campaigns (see Dilger 2003).

14. In the year 2001 around 9% of the region's adult population was infected with HIV. However, there was no continuous HIV/AIDS response in the villages until 2005, when an ARV treatment center was put in place by the government in collaboration with one of the private, mission-based hospitals in the area.

15. On the liminal situation of (young) women in patrilineal kinship networks in Uganda, and the challenges this liminality entails for their burials in the time of AIDS, see Whyte (2005). In western Mara, conflicts and discussions concerning the burials of men and women in the context of HIV/AIDS were also driven by the concern that the spirit of a deceased person might seek revenge if ritual prescriptions were not observed. The danger was considered especially high from women or young girls who were not married at the time of their death. If they were buried within their father's compound they were said to attract evil spirits and unleash infertility among their female relatives.

16. Comprehensive Community Based Rehabilitation, Tanzania.

17. The Bishop of the Full Gospel Bible Fellowship Church.

References

Allen, Tim, and Suzette Heald. 2004. "What Has Worked in Uganda and What Has Failed in Botswana?" *Journal of International Development* 16 (8): 1141–1154.

Boller, Christoph, Kaspar Wyss, Deo Mtasiwa, and Marcel Tanner. 2003. "Quality and Comparison of Antenatal Care in Public and Private Providers in the United Republic of Tanzania." *Bulletin of the World Health Organization* 81 (2): 116–122.

Campbell, Catherine. 2003. *Letting Them Die: Why HIV/AIDS Prevention Programmes Fail.* Bloomington: Indiana University Press.

Cohen, David William, and E. S. Atieno Odhiambo. 1992. *Burying SM; The Politics of Knowledge and the Sociology of Power in Africa.* Portsmouth, N.H.: Heinemann.

Corten, André, and Ruth Marshall-Fratani. 2001. "Introduction." In *Between Babel and Pentecost; Transnational Pentecostalism in Africa and Latin America,* ed. André Corten and Ruth Marshall-Fratani, 1–21. Bloomington: Indiana University Press.

Dilger, Hansjörg. 2001. "Living PositHIVely in Tanzania: The Global Dynamics of AIDS and the Meaning of Religion for International and Local AIDS Work." *afrika spectrum* 36 (1): 73–90.

———. 2003. "Sexuality, AIDS, and the Lures of Modernity: Reflexivity and Morality among Young People in Rural Tanzania." *Medical Anthropology* 22 (1): 23–52.

———. 2005. *Leben mit Aids. Krankheit, Tod und soziale Beziehungen in Afrika. Eine Ethnographie.* Frankfurt am Main: Campus.

———. 2006. "The Power of AIDS: Kinship, Mobility, and the Valuing of Social and Ritual Relationships in Tanzania." *African Journal of AIDS Research* 5 (2): 109–121.

———. 2007. "Healing the Wounds of Modernity: Community, Salvation, and Care in a Neo-Pentecostal Church in Dar es Salaam, Tanzania." *Journal of Religion in Africa* 37 (1): 59–83.

———. 2008. "'We are all going to die': Kinship, Belonging, and the Morality of HIV/AIDS-Related Illnesses and Deaths in Rural Tanzania." *Anthropological Quarterly* 81 (1): 207–232.

———. 2009 "Doing Better? Religion, the Virtue-Ethics of Development and the Fragmentation of Health Politics in Tanzania." *Africa Today* 56 (1): 89–110.

Dilger, Hansjörg, and Ute Luig, eds. 2010. *Morality, Hope, and Grief: Anthropologies of AIDS in Africa.* Oxford: Berghahn Books.

Ferguson, James. 2006. *Global Shadows: Africa in the Neoliberal World Order.* Durham, N.C.: Duke University Press.

Foucault, Michel. 1977. *Der Wille zum Wissen. Sexualität und Wahrheit.* Frankfurt am Main: Suhrkamp.

———. 1988. "Technologies of the Self." In *Technologies of the Self: A Seminar with Michel Foucault,* ed. Luther H. Martin, Huck Gutman, and Patrick H. Hutton, 16–49. Amherst: University of Massachusetts Press.

Green, Maia. 2000. "Participatory Development and the Appropriation of Agency in Southern Tanzania." *Critique of Anthropology* 20 (1): 67–89.

Greenhalgh, Susan. 2008. "An Anthropology of Science and Policy-Making." In *Just One Child: Science and Policy in Deng's China,* by Susan Greenhalgh. Berkeley: University of California Press.

Hardon, Anita, and Hansjörg Dilger. Forthcoming. "Global AIDS Medicines in East African Health Institutions. Introduction." *Medical Anthropology* 30 (2): 136–157.

Harrington, John A. 1998. "Privatizing Scarcity: Civil Liability and Health Care in Tanzania." *Journal of African Law* 42 (2): 147–171.

Heald, Suzette. 2002. "It's Never as Easy as ABC: Understandings of AIDS in Botswana." *African Journal of AIDS Research* 1 (1): 1–11.

———. 2003. "An Absence of Anthropology: Critical Reflections on Anthropology and AIDS Policy and Practice in Africa." In *Learning from HIV and AIDS,* ed. George Ellison, Melissa Parker, and Catherine Campbell, 191–216. Cambridge: Cambridge University Press.

Iliffe, John. 1998. *East African Doctors: A History of the Modern Profession.* Cambridge: Cambridge University Press.

Mamdani, Masuma, and Maggie Bangser. 2004. "Poor People's Experiences of Health Services in Tanzania: A Literature Review." *Reproductive Health Matters* 12 (24): 138–153.

Marsland, Rebecca. 2006. "Community Participation the Tanzanian Way: Conceptual Contiguity or Power Struggle?" *Oxford Development Studies* 34 (1): 65–79.

Mattes, Dominik. 2011. "'We Are Just Supposed to Be Quiet'—The Production of Adherence to Antiretroviral Treatment in Urban Tanzania." *Medical Anthropology* 30 (2): 158-182.

Médecins Sans Frontières. 2010. *No Time to Quit: HIV/AIDS Treatment Gap Widening in Africa.* Brussels: Médecins Sans Frontières, Brussels Operational Centre.

Mercer, Claire. 1999. "Reconceptualizing State–Society Relations in Tanzania: Are NGOs 'Making a Difference'?" *Area* 31 (3): 247–258.

Meyer, Birgit. 1998. "'Make a Complete Break with the Past': Memory and Postcolonial Modernity in Ghanaian Pentecostal Discourse." In *Memory and the Postcolony: African Anthropology and the Critique of Power,* ed. Richard Werbner, 182–208. London: Zed Books.

Morrell, Robert. 2001. "Introduction—The Times of Change: Men and Masculinity in South Africa." In *Changing Men in Southern Africa,* ed. Robert Morrell, 3–34. Pietermaritzburg, South Africa: University of Natal Press.

Nguyen, Vinh-Kim. 2005. "Antiretrovirals, Globalism, Biopolitics, and Therapeutic Citizenship." In *Global Assemblages: Technology, Politics, and Ethics as Anthropological Problems,* ed. Aihwa Ong and Stephen J. Collier, 124–145. Oxford: Blackwell Publishing.

Parikh, Shanti A. 2005. "From Auntie to Disco: The Bifurcation of Risk and Pleasure in Sex Education." In *Sex in Development: Science, Sexuality, and Morality in Global Perspective,* ed. Vincanne Adams and Stacy Leigh Pigg, 125–158. Durham, N.C.: Duke University Press.

Posel, Deborah. 2005. "Sex, Death, and the Fate of the Nation: Reflections on the Politicization of Sexuality in Post-Apartheid South Africa." *Africa* 75 (2): 125–153.

Robins, Steve. 2004. "'Long Live Zackie, Long Live': AIDS Activism, Science, and Citizenship after Apartheid." *Journal of Southern African Studies* 30 (3): 651–672.

Rösch, Paul-Gerhardt. 1995. *Der Prozess der Strukturanpassung in Tanzania.* Hamburg: Institute for African Affairs.

Rose, Nikolas, and Carlos Novas. 2004. "Biological Citizenship." In *Global Assemblages: Technology, Politics, and Ethics as Anthropological Problems,* ed. Aihwa Ong and Stephen Collier, 439–463. Oxford: Blackwell Publishing.

Rottenburg, Richard. 2002. *Weit hergeholte Fakten. Eine Parabel der Entwicklungshilfe.* Stuttgart, Germany: Lucius & Lucius.

TACAIDS. 2008. "Tanzania Public Expenditure Review. Multi-Sectoral Review: HIV-AIDS December 2007." Electronic document: http://www.tacaids.go.tz/component/content/article/13-tacaids-news/177-tz-public-expenditure-multi-sectorial-hiv-aids-2007.html.

Treichler, Paula. 1999. *How to Have Theory in an Epidemic: Cultural Chronicles of AIDS.* Durham, N.C.: Duke University Press.

Tripp, Aili Maria. 1997. *Changing the Rules: The Politics of Liberalization and the Urban Informal Economy in Tanzania.* Berkeley: University of California Press.

UNAIDS. 1999. *From Principle to Practice: Greater Involvement of People Living with or Affected by HIV/AIDS (GIPA).* Geneva: UNAIDS.

———. 2006. *Report on the Global AIDS Epidemic.* Geneva: UNAIDS.

Vaughan, Megan. 1991. *Curing Their Ills: Colonial Power and African Illness.* Cambridge: Cambridge University Press.

Whyte, Susan Reynolds. 2005. "Going Home? Belonging and Burial in the Era of AIDS." *Africa* 75 (2): 154–170.

———. 2009. "Health Identities and Subjectivities: The Ethnographic Challenge." *Medical Anthropology Quarterly* 23 (1): 6–15.

Whyte, Susan Reynolds, Michael A. Whyte, and David Kyaddondo. 2010. "Health Workers Entangled: Confidentiality and Certification." In *Morality, Hope, and Grief: Anthropologies of AIDS in Africa,* ed. Hansjörg Dilger and Ute Luig, 80–101. Oxford: Berghahn Books.

THREE

Health Security on the Move: Biobureaucracy, Solidarity, and the Transfer of Health Insurance to Senegal

Angelika Wolf

"Ce n'est pas facile!" Mr. Dembele shook his head. He was trying to understand the difference between budget and capital, as well as between budget and money. Understanding this was necessary to evaluate the financial viability of his mutual health organization in one of the quarters of Diourbel town in Senegal. As one of the many volunteers in the administration of such an organization, he had been invited to participate in a workshop on "planning, monitoring and evaluation for administrators of mutual health organizations."[1] For two days he and the other 30 participants attempted to learn how the administration of a *mutuelle de santé*—a mutual health organization—should work, in particular how its staff should organize, oversee, and assess their organization. The workshop was conducted by one of the district hospital's vice directors under the auspices of the regional office of the Health Ministry. It was, however, organized by the umbrella organization of the regional health insurance initiative Coordination Régionale des Mutuelles de Santé de Diourbel (CORMUSAD) and financed by the German Society for Technical Cooperation (Gesellschaft für technische Zusammenarbeit, GTZ), a development organization working on behalf of the German government. Such events occasionally occur in Diourbel and comprise part of development organizations' activities to set up mutual health organizations (MHOs) in Senegal.

The workshop opened with speeches by the president of CORMUSAD and the health ministry representative. Then, one of the vice presidents of the regional hospital, who is also responsible for supporting MHOs, began with the workshop program. His PowerPoint presentation mainly focused on issues such as corporate planning and objectives of MHOs, the most important goal being to raise the number of members in the MHO and to secure membership fees. The two factors of income from membership fees and an increasing number of participants in the MHO would determine its survival. Each MHO must be economically independent, economic self-sufficiency being a major goal since financial support from German development aid was to be limited to only a few years.

After this warning about the limited period of support, the vice director turned to the topics of the day. As the title of the workshop suggests, the meeting was completely dedicated to administration issues. In the technical language typical for development organizations, he tried to teach the participants how to distinguish functional viability from financial viability and how to make use of the corresponding formulas. From time to time, especially when confusion among the workshop participants arose, he was supported by a young man who sought to clarify the problems by referring to the participants' daily situations. The young man was a Senegalese sociologist employed by GTZ to coordinate the newly funded MHOs and to support them in keeping records and writing reports. He and some teachers among the participants would reassure their fellows if matters appeared too complicated.

When I spoke with the vice director during the coffee break, he stressed: "The problem is the level of administrative professionalism; only two or three organizations work on a high level, otherwise it's simply too low. In this way they have no chance to survive." However, the participants' remarks indicated a contrary attitude: they were dubious that any MHO administrator really needed to know all these intricacies of management and accounting to run their organization. Nevertheless, the workshop went on with some more bureaucratic refinement, and after two days of hard work each participant received a certificate presented by the regional representative of the Health Ministry.[2]

The account of this workshop shows some of the complications that occur in conjunction with the establishment of health insurance schemes in the informal sector of many African countries. Supported by transnational agencies, laymen are expected to develop mutual health organizations so as to assure access to health services for poor people in their communities. In order to do so, they must acquaint themselves with administrative constraints. Thus, the transfer of health insurance takes part within a certain framework of biobureaucracy.[3] Kohrmann (2005) introduced this term to describe the relationship between actors and a health-related bureaucracy. This understanding of health, however, is bound to biomedicine and the concept of biology. Increasing concerns about how to finance biomedical services accompany the global flow of biomedicine and lead to the emergence of this new form of bureaucracy in the context of biomedical funding.

Aspects of biobureaucratic institution building have rarely been discussed from an anthropological point of view. The associated problems of the transfer of health insurance have so far mainly been analyzed in a rather technical context. With some exceptions (such as Klocke-Daffa 2001; Arhinful 2003; Damen 2003; Steinwachs 2006; Schulze 2010; and Wolf et al. forthcoming) most of the literature about health insurance in Africa deals with questions of financing systems, policy options, risk protection, resource mobilization, or market mechanisms (see, among others, Drechsler and Jütting 2005; Preker et al. 2002; Atim 1998; Nolan 1995). Local strategies for providing social security and securing health have rarely been discussed (see Neubert 1986; Foley 2008).

The aim of this chapter is to depict some of the social, economic, and cultural factors that facilitate or hinder the adoption of Western ideas about financial arrangements for guaranteeing access to health care in Senegal. It describes the historical background of formal health insurance in Europe and considers how a certain concept of solidarity makes transferring the idea of social health protection interesting for agencies acting transnationally. Despite this interest, though, MHOs in Diourbel are struggling to survive. One reason for the strain is that the meaning of solidarity in informal settings differs from its meaning under formal health protection arrangements.

It is often claimed that African governments lack the administrative and management capacities to establish and run social security systems (Preker et al. 2004) and that these governments have insufficient credibility to organize and maintain social insurance schemes. Such a perspective hardly considers the negative impact of the structural adjustment programs (SAPs) that have limited the scope of African economies. The destruction of national economic spaces accompanies the construction of global ones. Global networks increasingly dominate the political sphere on the African continent, thus undermining former "vertical topographies of power" between state governments and local communities (Ferguson 2006). The establishment of social security mechanisms is occurring precisely as these vertical power topographies are vanishing.

The Idea of Social Security in Europe: Compulsory Social Health Insurance or State Health Services?

The first law to establish social insurance schemes in Europe was instituted in Germany (Sigerist 1943). In the late 1890s, due to unbearable working conditions, socialist movements had become strong in the German Empire. Chancellor Otto von Bismarck tried two methods to suppress socialist influence on workers: repression and social reforms. One idea of the emerging model of social security was to provide health insurance for workers. Thus, the first health insurance act in history was passed in June 1883 in the German Empire. It was part of what can be considered the first European labor laws.

Sigerist (1943) states that social insurance institutions result from world-wide industrialization. In feudal systems, the liege lord was supposed to bear responsibility for the poor. Later on, trade guilds would establish aid funds for mutual assistance, or mine workers would organize themselves into brotherhoods for mutual support. However, the idea of social welfare became even more important after the Industrial Revolution in the nineteenth century, since workers often died in accidents or lost their jobs due to illness or old age. They started to organize themselves into groups that could stock a kind of voluntary kitty or social cash box. Thus, the idea of social insurance was accepted in Germany long before Bismarck came up with his model; it was only having a mandatory formal system for the majority of the population that was new. In that compulsory social health insurance system both employer and employees contribute progressively based on the employee's wages. However, all those insured are supposed to receive the same medical services from their provider regardless of the premiums they pay. The basic idea of having a solidarity-based national health system in which contributions are scaled according to income still prevails in Germany.

Routinely contrasted with the Bismarck model of contribution-based social security related to formal employment is the Beveridge model, a tax-based social security system with the state as sole provider of care.[4] In Britain the National Health Service Act of 1946 established the provision of services free of charge based on the recommendations of the director of the London School of Economics, and so the National Health Service (NHS) of the United Kingdom was created (Musgrove 1996). That the state must play a substantial role in the health sector, particularly in regulating and financing it, was the dominant idea until market-based reforms were introduced into the NHS in 1989.

Nowadays both the Beveridge system of state taxation and the Bismarck model of employment-based contributions are common in Europe. Both systems have been transferred around the world and been subjected to change and adapted to local conditions. At the same time, they have been transformed in their countries of origin due to the cutbacks and financial constraints Europe has recently been facing (Mossialos et al. 2002). The ongoing discussion as to whether national tax-based health care services or social health insurance provide a better solution to health finance notwithstanding, social protection was an important achievement in Europe during the Industrial Revolution and after the Second World War. However, its regulation depends on a strong *formal* working sector for both. Since many countries in the world have a predominantly *informal* working sector with larger parts of the population living in rural areas, the worldwide introduction of health insurance schemes creates a challenge for development organizations and cooperating states alike.

Besides tax revenue and formal employment-based contributions, there are a number of other sources for financing health care, among them community-based micro-insurance, private insurance, medical saving accounts, and out-of-pocket payment including direct as well as informal payments. For people with low or mid-level incomes, direct payments are the most ineffective type of payment; they increase the risk of impoverishment (Kawabata, Xu, and Carrin 2002). Prepayment mechanisms such as health insurance not only prevent people from incurring catastrophic expenditures; they moreover offer better resource management and promise a more sustainable way of financing health services. Most countries have mixed financing mechanisms for health care (Preker et al. 2002). However, tax-financed health services as well as social health insurance offer the best options for financing health care in terms of equity and universal coverage (Weber et al. 2005; Doetinchem, Schramm, and Schmidt 2006).

Social protection has been on the agenda of development cooperation in the last decade.[5] After years of cutbacks due to structural adjustment programs (SAPs) in the social sector, both the donor community and many African governments are striving for the "rediscovery of the social" (Diop 2001 in Bührer 2006: 11). Government agencies such as USAID, along with the WHO, World Bank, and ILO (International Labour Organization), are active in setting up health financing systems. The transfer of *social* health insurance, however, seems to be a specific European effort. Organizations such as the Belgian health insurance fund ANMC (Alliance Nationale des Mutualistes Chrétiennes) and the Belgian NGO World Solidarity, as well as the German GTZ, claim that health insurance should be a component of social protection. European experiences should be used as a pool of know-how (Huber, Hohmann, and Reinhard 2003: 11). In 2004 the members of the Executive Board of the WHO emphasized the importance of solidarity, equal opportunities, and universal access to health services. Since then the Bismarck approach has served as a role model for universal coverage in health insurance.

An important aspect of social protection is the perception of solidarity. Distinct awareness about solidarity and fairness seems crucial when establishing social insurance programs. "In Western Europe the general understanding of fairness is collective and need-based; it refers to mutual support and equity between society members. This notion is directly antithetical to the politically-fanned belief in the United States that social programs are in fact individual savings accounts" (Weber et al. 2005: 26). According to the authors, to most Americans fairness means getting out exactly what they pay in. Using one person's money to cover someone else's health expenditures would be considered unfair. From this individualist perspective, there is no difference between health care systems based on tax revenue and those financed by compulsory insurance, both of which entitle members to the use of health services based on declarations of solidarity rather than individual saving. In the understanding of the WHO and many development agencies, this distinctive perception of solidarity as well as the idea of universal access to health benefits is what qualifies European approaches to social protection for transfer to developing countries. Although social protection mechanisms vary quite a bit within the European Union, it is assumed that the widespread concept of solidarity in Europe might link with pre-existing solidarity mechanisms in developing countries in Africa (Schramm, Doetinchem, and Baak 2004; Weber et al. 2005: 26; Doetinchem, Schramm, and Schmidt 2006).

The Transfer of Health Insurance to Senegal

The more common approach to health care in developing countries had been to treat receipt of free services for everybody as a right of the people. In particular, postcolonial African governments opted for free-of-charge services in publicly financed health settings (Waelkens, Soors, and Criel 2005: 19). However, World Bank experts claim that this approach prevents the government from collecting revenues from patients who are both able and willing to pay and recommended the introduction of user fees for biomedical services (World Bank 1987). In 1980, under the pressure of the economic crisis, Senegal signed a structural adjustment loan with the World Bank. To qualify for World Bank and IMF loans, the government had to withdraw funding from the public sector, which included reducing social services, and as a result the quality of health services declined (Hemenway 1997; Foley 2010). Health care professionals lost their jobs as a consequence of these public sector cuts, and between 1980 and 1993, the number of patients per nurse in Senegal increased six-fold (Schoepf, Schoepf, and Millen 2000: 112). Moreover, total health expenditure per capita diminished from 653 FCFA in 1978–1979, to 427 FCFA in 1988–1989, which led to increased exclusion from coverage for many social groups (Ndiaye 2002).[6] Thus, user charges blatantly caused a decline in the usage of biomedical services, especially among the most socioeconomically deprived (McPake 1994), and user fees "introduced to complement the government financing deprived many of access to health services" (Waelkens,

Soors, and Criel 2005: 19). Both Senegalese and international health econo-
mists agree that community-based health insurance is an acceptable source
of finance to improve access to health care and to protect poor people from
unexpected and exceptionally high health care expenditure.

To establish a sustainable health insurance system, certain political
and economic prerequisites are important. The Republic of Senegal offers
good political and relatively good economic conditions for the introduction
of health insurance schemes. The country has a stable multi-party system,
a free press, and no systematic violations of human rights. Gross Domestic
Product (GDP) was 490 USD per capita in the year 2002, which is about 150
percent of the average in sub-Saharan Africa (Gueye et al. 2001). For people
working in the formal sector, approximately 10 percent of the population,
insurance protection is mandatory. Companies with 100 or more employees
must provide health insurance (through an Institution de Prévoyance Maladie
d'Entreprise, or IPM) based on contributions from the employees and the
enterprise alike. Companies with fewer than 100 employees are obliged to join
an authorized health insurance institution (Institution de Prévoyance Maladie
inter Entreprises, or IPM-IE). A separate fund for social security for civil servants is in place directly under the Ministry of Finance. Nevertheless, a study
by the French Ministry of Health (MAE 2000) recommends not introducing
compulsory health insurance for countries with a GDP of less than 1,000 USD
per capita. Instead, it proposes the establishment of local health insurance
schemes until better economic conditions and organizational structures have
been established.[7]

Almost 90 percent of the Senegalese population works in agriculture or
the informal sector, and no legal regulation regarding health protection exists
for them. A survey conducted by the WHO among 3,600 households with
a total of nearly 28,000 family members in Senegal in 2002 has shown that
impoverished households hardly use savings as a major financing mechanism.
They try to cover health expenses by borrowing money or selling their livestock or land.[8] On average, only 3 percent of households' health expenditures
were covered through payments or reimbursement from health insurance
plans; that average represents a spectrum from 2 percent in the poorest fifth
of the study to 7 percent in the wealthiest (Asfaw 2004: 20). The national
health development plan drafted for the period of 1998–2007 attempted to
confront this situation. Some of the goals included improving the financial
viability of public services and improving vulnerable groups' access to health
care (Asfaw 2004: 5).

Since the end of the 1990s, the Senegalese government has promoted
health insurance initiatives for the rural as well as for the informal sector and
has created two organizations intended to support local initiatives: PAMS

(Programmes d'Appui aux Mutuelles de Santé) in 1986 and CAMICS (Cellule d'Appui aux Mutuelles de Santé aux IPM et aux Comités de Santé) in 1998 (IMF 1998). Although the two organizations started numerous health insurance projects, most of these ceased to function after a short time. Problems with self-management resulted due to insufficient qualification of co-workers within the projects, and in individual cases fraud and/or misappropriation of funds cropped up. Frequently, a so-called gatekeeper system to regulate referral of patients to specialists was missing, or overconsumption arose, endangering the financial viability of the insurance (due to moral hazard or adverse selection[9]). In addition, the PAMS and CAMICS staff frequently had no experience in providing support services, but only in exercising control, and were therefore rejected by many people in the locations of the projects (Huber, Hohmann, and Reinhard 2003: 21). Nevertheless, people in Senegal have in the last decade become considerably active in founding mutual health insurance associations. In 2000, approximately 70,000 persons were organized into 30 MHOs (Evrard 2002: 4); by 2004, the number of organizations had tripled. In a comparison of 11 West African countries with a combined 366 functioning organizations, Senegal, with 90 *mutuelles de santé*, appears to be the country with the highest number of working MHOs (Concertation 2004: 12).

In 1989, the first health insurance scheme for people not covered in the formal sector was created in the region of Thiès. This initiative cooperated with the Catholic hospital St. Jean de Dieu. The nonprofit hospital offered a reduction of hospital fees of up to 50 percent for health insurance members. This positive experience encouraged the creation of other MHOs in the region, and most MHOs in Thiès cover not only some percentage of hospital services but primary care treatment as well (Bührer 2006). Moreover, in 1994, they created their own technical support structure, which was supplemented by a regional coordination in 1997.

Such a success story cannot be expected everywhere. The cooperation of MHOs in the Thiès region in Senegal counts as the most authentic MHO movement in West Africa, without much interference from outside donors (Huber, Hohmann, and Reinhard 2003: 25). In the neighboring region of Diourbel, health insurance in the informal sector is a relatively new idea. It was introduced by GTZ in the year 2000, when the regional hospital was renovated and restructured.

Mutuelles de Santé in Diourbel

Establishing *mutuelles de santé* in the district of Diourbel began in combination with the rehabilitation of its regional hospital. The Hôpital Heinrich-Lübke de Diourbel was constructed in 1966 in Senegalese-German cooperation. German support ended in 1972 and was renewed in 1999 until spring 2006. In the hierarchy of the Senegalese formal health care system, the hospital is considered a second-level hospital, which means that it is a referral hospital for the whole region. The Senegalese public biomedical health care system is structured hierarchically and consists of health posts and dispensaries (*posts de santé, dispensaires*) at the primary health care level; health centers at the first level of referral (*structures du niveau primaire de référence*); one district hospital in every region, where surgery, internal medicine, and gynecology are obligatory (*structures du niveau secondaire de référence*); and finally, national hospitals with a broad range of specialties (*structures du niveau tertiaire de référence*). Although the Diourbel hospital has maintained 11 special divisions since its rehabilitation, it is no longer the only referral hospital in the region. The department of Touba also belongs to the Diourbel region, and it opened a third-level hospital on the private initiative of the Murid brotherhood, a Sufi Muslim order, in December 2005.[10]

The rehabilitation project for the Diourbel hospital had two major objectives: a) to fulfill its role as a support and referral structure for the regional health system, and b) to achieve a viable concept for hospital financing by promoting the creation of local health insurance systems. A feasibility study was conducted surveying 810 households in the Diourbel region, which consists of the four departments—Bambey, Diourbel, Mbacke, and Touba—in order to collect reliable data on the acceptance of health insurance and to familiarize the population with the idea. Of the households surveyed, 49.5 percent have an average monthly income between 10,000 and 50,000 FCFA, and 40.4 percent of households have means between 50,000 and 100,000 FCFA (Gueye et al. 2001: 29). Most heads of household (60 to 70 percent) in the four departments had never heard about the possibility of covering health expenditures by insurance. An immense majority of people in the study confirmed that they had fears of getting ill and not having the means to pay hospital bills. Many stated that they would be willing to participate in MHOs and referred to other associations they are members of. Fees or contributions for these memberships range from 100 to 3,500 FCFA (Gueye et al. 2001).

Awakening the interest of community leaders was the next step in the introduction of the new idea to the Diourbel communities. Once the results of the feasibility study had demonstrated the interest of the population in health insurance, the project consultant started activities together with the hospital staff in January 2000. After a workshop for the promotion of MHOs in the Diourbel region, a steering committee (*comité de pilotage*) was set up consisting of one of the deputy directors of the hospital, the hospital's social worker, and two other people from NGOs involved in micro-credit programs. The committee sought expertise in the neighboring region of Thiès and received support from the government agencies PAMS and CAMICS as well as from German and Belgian development organizations. CAMICS offered special training for providers of medical services, in particular for health staff in leading positions (Huber, Hohmann, and Reinhard 2003: 51). The members of the committee particularly tried to attract existing organizations such as professional associations, *dahiras* (religiously based associations for mutual assistance), and neighborhood initiatives because of their structural advantages and experience in networking (Mossa Daff, March 18, 2006). Thus, it was not primarily the hospital that created the MHOs; rather, actors within the rehabilitation project expected community leaders to take the initiative and approach the steering committee for support. After the initial period, the committee resigned but individually continued to support the seven newly founded MHOs of the umbrella organization CORMUSAD, which since then has coordinated their activities, including the promotion of new MHOs (Fane Dieng, May 10, 2007).

Recruiting new members for MHOs depended very much on the initiative of the founding persons. It was mainly people with a good education in the formal sector—such as teachers or employees in management positions at small companies—who approached the steering committee. Other interested parties without a formal education included community leaders accepted on the basis of their family status, religious leaders, and the leader of the drivers' association in Diourbel. Some of them had health insurance coverage at their workplace; thus their motivation in establishing health insurance schemes was not only to improve living conditions for others but also to improve their own reputation and boost their standing in the communities (Wolf 2007). It was also their reputation that helped attract new members to the MHO. By 2003, eight MHOs had been created. Out of these eight mutual health organizations, three were neighborhood initiatives, two were faith-based organizations (one Catholic, one Murid), one was attached to the drivers' association, and two were affiliated with an NGO. One of them had to give up after financial support from the NGO ceased, and one neighborhood initiative could not receive their donor's last allocation due to major disagreements in the leadership which resulted in the split-up of the organization (Wolf 2007).

The MHO Musgrad (short for Mutuelle de Santé Grand Diourbel) was established in 2003 on the initiative of community leaders in the Grand Diourbel quarter of the town Diourbel. Some of them had known each other since childhood. They approached the hospital and received financial support to organize a familiarization campaign in their quarter. The initiators arranged a meeting where a member of the steering committee explained to the audience how mutual health insurance functions and why it could be a solution to their health financing problems. In addition, the initiators launched radio advertisements and also went from door to door to seek the support of their neighbors and to convince them to become members of the MHO. At a general assembly meeting, the founding members of Musgrad elected the president, the vice president, the treasurer, and the secretary general. The German development program supported the newly founded MHO with office equipment, including a computer, and provided money for three years to hire an administrator. The MHO also received advice in project management, such as how to draft membership rules and how to construct a benefit package.

The Musgrad benefit package covers 50 percent of treatment costs in health centers, health posts, or hospitals. It also meets 50 percent of the costs for x-rays, laboratory tests, and those medications that can be obtained in the hospital pharmacy. However, drugs not available in the hospital must be purchased at an outside pharmacy, where, due to the Bamako initiative, they are not covered by health insurance.[11] Delivery with surgical intervention (Caesarian) is fully paid for. Before enlisting the assistance of health services, the administrator of Musgrad entitles the patient to care by issuing a certificate of guarantee (*lettre de garantie*) at the small office which was rented within the quarter. The patient shows this certificate to the health care provider's administration. Then the provider settles 50 percent of the costs directly with the MHO. Members are entitled to insurance services after a waiting period of six months. The initial membership fee amounts to 1000 FCFA. One member may include up to ten beneficiaries and contributes 100 FCFA per beneficiary monthly. One year after its foundation, Musgrad had slightly more than 700 participants, including 100 members. Their leaders still promoted membership and tried to attract new members by selling mosquito nets for half of the usual price, along with T-shirts printed with the organization's name.

It may be asked what remains from the Bismarck model of social health insurance in the Diourbel context. There is no two-prong contribution to the insurance fund. Contributions stem from insurance members only. Thus, it rather resembles the private health insurance model. There is no coverage for medication that is not available in the hospital, even if it was prescribed by a doctor. However, as already mentioned, this compulsory payment at private or non-hospital pharmacies is due to the international agreement under the Bamako initiative. Also not in accordance with the model of social insurance but rather part of private agreements is the waiting period. Admittedly, it protects smaller associations from depletion by people who might profit from the outset but do not continue paying their membership fees.

Adopted from the Bismarck model is the idea of the autonomy and self-management of health insurance. According to the strategies of international development organizations, governments should not interfere with mutualist movements. State intervention may cause a conflict of interest, because often the state is the main provider of health services (Huber, Hohmann, and Reinhard 2003: 53). MHOs should be rooted in civil society and carry out their agenda independent of government. The state's responsibility in the Bismarck model is to develop an appropriate legislative framework. Apart from the state's accountability for the political framework, the idea of solidarity among participants in health insurance is at the center of European approaches to social protection. The meaning of solidarity in this context is to provide means for mutual support and to have a common pool to cover health expenditures. However, Musgrad's greatest problem is their members' failure to make their regular payments. "People are not used to saving money for sickness" (Lamine Kane, September 1, 2004). Sometimes people stop paying even during the waiting period and just come to hand in their contribution shortly before they need a guarantee certificate to go to the hospital. Such behavior reflects the more common approach of informal saving that predominates in the quarters of Diourbel. However, it reveals a different understanding of solidarity and reciprocity than European health insurance models have.

Social Security in Diourbel

The question remains as to how people with no involvement in larger businesses, with very limited income, and with no access to bank accounts generate savings for their needs? In Diourbel there are several strategies for gathering money and means. People approach their employer, neighbors, and friends; extended family networks provide whatever they are responsible for (or considered responsible for); and last but not least, most people belong to various saving associations that meet on a regular basis and are commonly called *tontines* in French or *natt* or *mbootaay* in Wolof. These *tontines* can be found at working places among employees in companies, or at the hospital, at the market, or even in religious organizations. The groups are of mixed gender, though men usually organize themselves in *tontines* connected with their occupation, whereas *tontines* in the quarters of Diourbel are exclusively composed of women.

In their *mbootaay,* women have a variety of possible forms of financial arrangement to meet different needs. *Tek, sanni jamra,* and *tour* seem to be the most common and most important forms of support systems under the umbrella of *mbootaay.*[12] What the different forms of meeting and saving in a group have in common are their features of formal organization: they are highly structured, with a president, a vice president, a treasurer, and a secretary. Often the president is called mother, indicating a resemblance to a family structure of support and assistance, but in the wider community. The word *mbootaay* refers to the cloth that women use to tie a baby to their back, a reference which strengthens the image of family bonds. The root of the word is the Wolof verb *boot,* to put on your back.[13] The association offers protection and security, but like a child that grows and becomes independent of the mother, the members of the groups are free to stay and continue with their membership or not once all payments due are finished. They exist for certain periods of time depending on the number of members and the amount of money that is collected. Some meet on a weekly basis, collect smaller amounts of money (i.e., 150 FCFA), and stay together for only a few months; others pay higher contributions (i.e., 2,000–30,000 FCFA), meet on a monthly basis, and remain together for two or three years.

The most common forms of meeting among women in the Diourbel quarters are *tek* and *sanni jamra.* Whereas the *sanni jamra* type of meeting serves to satisfy immediate needs in daily life and is mainly an exchange of small goods, *tek* provide savings for more expensive projects and may also be used in the case of illness, although in a rather indirect way. The money circulating in the *tek* is usually distributed by a lottery among its members. Once neighbors or colleagues decide to form a *tek,* they determine the amount of money to be saved, and the names of all participants are written on individual slips of paper. These slips are kept in a bag. When the group meets on their monthly or weekly basis, usually at the president's house, each member pays the amount agreed, which is noted in a book. When throwing the money into the bowl or calabash they often say *sama tek,* my contribution. After all payments have been made, the lottery starts. The bag with the fortunes is opened and one slip is taken out. The name on the fortune is announced and the person in question will receive all the money that was collected. The fortune drawn is thrown away, but the person is obliged to continue paying and thereby enables the other members of the *mbootaay* to receive their share. In addition to the monthly payments, a small contribution is made for the group's cash box. With that money women buy mats and chairs, or even music boxes, which members may borrow for their festivities.

Not only can money be saved, food or goods count as savings as well. When meeting for *tek,* women declare an agreement on what to distribute to a certain member. One might say, for example, that she needs a bed, and when it is her turn (*tour*) the other members will buy her a bed with the money collected. At the *sanni jamra,* women gather each week at a different member's house and bring things "they just have." The gift here circulates on a more individual basis. If one woman brings vinegar to the host of the first meeting, she will get vinegar back from that person once it is her turn to host visitors. Another will bring and later get back soap, or *jumbo* (bouillon cubes), or sugar. The name *sanni jamra* refers to the pilgrimage to Mecca. One of the important tasks during the pilgrimage is to throw stones at the two pillars symbolizing Satan. Thus the meaning of *sanni jamra* is "beating the devil." Yacine explained to me, "If a person is in need, or before she is in need you give support. That is why we say 'fight the devil!'" (Yacine Sarr, December 1, 2006).

Yacine is a trader and sells drinks and ice at the market close to her quarter. When Yacine was young, she and her friends used to collect small amounts of money just to serve their "need for fun." With that money, the young people hired a *griot* (musician) to provide them music and entertainment. Over the years, her former group has evolved and now meets each Sunday at the president's house. The group provides support for family ceremonies, for daily needs, and for cases of sickness. Explaining her membership, she said, "The problem is if you work without earning much you have to be member in a *tek*. When it's your turn and you get your money, you will prefer to buy something that you usually can't afford. In case now, you need money, you may sell it again. [. . .] If you have for example jewelry and there is an emergency, you are able to deal with the problem." When Yacine was sick and had to pay a hospital bill of 50,000 FCFA, she borrowed money from a merchant at the market. After leaving the hospital she sold her golden jewelry to pay back her debts. She needed the loan from the salesman because her group consists of 76 members, and since they meet once a week, it could take one and a half years for her share to come around. In case of sickness her *tek* forms a delegation to visit the sick member. "If you are sick and you go to the hospital, they form a delegation and you will see everyone gives you what he has. [. . .] When someone has a ceremony, when someone has a funeral or a baptism it is also like that. [. . .] Some give 500 FCFA, others 100 FCFA, and others 200 FCFA, you give what you have" (Yacine Sarr, December 1, 2006).

In addition to saving and circulating money, the *tek* assumes some health insurance functions in a veiled manner. Firstly, women use their pay-out to balance hospital bills and payments for medication; secondly, members collect money to support a sick person in their group. However, in case of serious illness, the amount of money collected might not be sufficient and only a few members of the association might contribute. Since saving money is the core concept of these groups, health protection is not an explicit goal of its members.

Besides their economic purpose, the meetings also have an important social dimension, often including music, dance, and chatting. Within the associations women establish social ties that go beyond economic support. They create bonds and relationships for emotional support and mutual assistance in daily life. Their discussions of events in the neighborhood serve as social control mechanisms as well. Due to polygamy there is competition between co-wives and their respective kin. The association brings women together for mutual support and thereby may contribute to overcoming strife in the family. Since membership is a matter of time, the relationships are flexible and can be negotiated again and again. The flexible nature of the associations enables women to join other groups that better serve their needs at certain times. However, as it is the case with Yacine, some members may stay in the same association for a lifetime.

Tontines are based on a form of contract. "Each time before starting the activity you concentrate and you determine what you are going to do" (Fatou Fall, February 12, 2006). Apart from a small contribution for the cash box, at the end of a cycle each member in a *mbootaay, tek,* or *sanni jamra* has received back the same amount of money she has spent or the equivalent of the goods she has given. A balanced reciprocity among the participants is at the core of these groups. In this respect, there is a difference between family *tontines* and *tontines* in the neighborhood. In his work on the associations in Thilonge in the northern part of Senegal, Kane (2001) mentions a form of working-*tontine* that existed before monetarism reached the village. Members in those groups used to help each other build houses, work in the fields, or perform other services of mutual aid. This type of work was organized in a collective and rotating way among the families in a certain neighborhood. Women organized their means for family ceremonies in a similar way, but without a guarantee of equilibrium between giving and receiving. The same holds true for the *tontines* at family ceremonies in Diourbel. Kane also describes *tontines* in the quarters of Dakar, the capital of Senegal. There, the contributions must be balanced out. Balance between giving and getting is the basis for the verbal contract among members of the *tontines* in the quarters and markets of the smaller town of Diourbel. This concept of balanced reciprocity is, however, contradictory to the idea of health insurance, which builds on generalized reciprocity—as we will see.

Solidarity and Reciprocity

Flexibility, reciprocity, and the public character of the distribution lead women to join the associations described above rather than a *mutuelle de santé*. "Before new mutual health institutions can be successful, they need to be grounded in local values of solidarity and reciprocity" (Sommerfeld et al. 2002: 160). MHOs in Diourbel are perceived as not being flexible about membership and payments. Contributions are fixed, but contrary to the practice in *tontines,* receiving benefits remains uncertain. Not only are monthly payments difficult for people working in their fields, since they often have funds at their disposal only when harvesting, but for many it is also not clear if the money will be properly used. The money of insurance members goes to a bank account and is not visible anymore. Only "educated people" are able to deal with the requirements of administration. In *tontines* members can observe the secretary directly putting their name and the paid amount into the book, they can see who gets the money, and the group has the ability to exert social (and juridical) pressure if one does not pay. After all turns are finished, women are free to continue in the next round, they might join another group, or they stop saving money for a time. Members in an MHO have to make payments continuously each year regardless of whether they have benefited from the membership or not. Those who do not pay fees lose their financial protection against health-related costs and there is no refunding of amounts of contributions previously paid.

Reciprocity, and whether it is balanced or unbalanced, is another important issue. As Fatou explained to me, "I take myself as an example. I was member in a mutual health organization, but I did not respect the contributions, whereas with the *tek,* I contribute regularly. I always think of the day when it will be my turn, because I know I will receive all the money and buy such or such things, you know. A material person does not think of financial precautions" (Fatou Fall, February 12, 2006). For the people in Diourbel, one obvious difference between an MHO and an organization such as *mbootaay,* apart from the social value, is the lack of money circulating and the uncertainty about whether it really pays to belong to an MHO. Health insurance reveals a profound contradiction. On the one hand, nobody wants to get sick just in order to benefit from the insurance services. On the other hand, if all members in the family have the good fortune to remain healthy, the invested money is lost. Since so many activities in the daily life of the Senegalese center on reciprocity, just to give money without knowing if it will come back is a real challenge to many in Diourbel. An advantage of the *tontine* is that the use of savings is directly linked to the needs of daily life; whereas becoming sick is something they may fear but is mostly far away from the thoughts of healthy people. Often people would say, "You cannot be sure if the investment pays off," meaning that health facilities consume much money without providing certainty that the respective activities for diagnosing and treating illness will end up producing a healthy individual. Thus, with health insurance, there is no balance between the money contributed to the organization and the outcome; whereas in the saving system of the *tontines,* people can be quite sure of having equilibrium between amounts paid in and amounts paid out. Moreover, any solidarity-based health insurance would not be able to function with balanced reciprocity, since one case of health care utilization with high costs is covered only if many other members do not claim benefits. Thus, balanced reciprocity contradicts the concept of social health insurance and its appeals to solidarity.

When I asked if and how institutions such as *mbootaay* or *tek* could contribute in the case of illness, a common answer was, "If one of us falls sick, we might join and decide a certain amount. Then one of us will go and give her the help." In practice, the amount of money given and the number of people contributing in the case of illness is rather small. Members in the organizations perceive their association as some kind of credit institution. This perception limits the possibility of their acting as health insurance. For most people, local practices of saving and circulating money do not include health financing. Often in case of serious illness, funds from familiar methods of saving are insufficient to pay for treatment in hospital. Nonetheless, opting for membership in a *mutuelle de santé* still has not become an accepted choice in the population of Diourbel. Most people would rather demand that hospital services be free of charge, as was the case before the structural adjustment programs altered access to health care. The idea of paying for health insurance *is* widely accepted among people in the formal working sector in Senegal. For the much larger informal sector, however, it remains a challenge, since, contrary to the historical conditions that surrounded the establishment of social security in Europe, here few people have regular income, and administrative regulation is lacking. Whereas the countries of Western Europe assigned a central role to the state in social security activity, African countries have been forced to cut back or abandon the very provisions which helped richer countries build up flourishing health care systems in the past.

Conclusion

State–society relations are at stake when it comes to international organizations' requirements. In this chapter I have tried to avoid portraying what Ferguson (2006) called the vertical topography of power. Looking at actions taken by global or transnational organizations, such as the World Bank, IMF, and development agencies in the health sector, sheds light on their pervasive impact on all domains of Senegalese society. Ferguson calls into question the verticality of the relation of the state to society and argues ". . . that both the 'top' and the 'bottom' of the vertical picture today operate within a profoundly transnationalized global context . . ." (Ferguson 2006: 93). States in Africa barely exercise the power of a sovereign nation-state anymore. The introduction of health insurance in Senegal provides a good example of limited state power and the importance of the link with the transnational entities that the local voluntary associations depend on.[14] The state has been pushed back by the requirements of the SAPs demanded by the IMF and World Bank. These have imposed policies that have eroded the sovereignty of the Senegalese state in general, in terms of financing health care in particular. Voluntary associations such as MHOs in Diourbel work in the wider biomedical field because of transnational organizations such as GTZ, ANMC, and World Solidarity, which support, guide, and sponsor them. However, the purely technical and financial understanding of solidarity and support in health care financing shifts the burden of a new form of bureaucracy from the government to volunteers in the social arena. This kind of bureaucracy has been called biobureaucracy.

Kohrmann (2005) refers to institutions that "share the conceptual and practical orientation of advancing the health and wellbeing of people understood to have bodies which are either damaged, sickly or otherwise different, based on local or translocal norms of existence" by the term *biobureaucracy*, "in order to highlight the degree to which they are integrally undergirded by what has been an accelerating proliferation worldwide of the biological and biomedical sciences . . .." According to Kohrmann (2005: 34), the relationship between individual actors and biobureaucracy has been depicted by scholars over the last two decades in research on the construction of biomedical apparatuses such as psychiatric treatments, medical school curricula, and molecular research centers. In these studies, researchers have in general followed two different paths. On the one hand, there are studies of the ways in which biomedical providers, researchers, and teachers produce, shape, and extend biomedical knowledge and techniques in the global/local context. The other path is research on the experiences of the suffering and how they encounter biomedical institutions. Rarely is much attention paid to questions pertaining to the *establishment* of health protection.

The process of introducing health insurance in the informal sector in Diourbel creates a good opportunity to observe the formation of a new biobureaucracy. Bureaucrats in the realm of biomedicine frame and shape the way people are medically treated by regulating prices and ways of paying for the treatment in question. In Diourbel, lay people have to deal with issues of administration and the management of health insurance. Advertising the new idea of health protection, collecting fees, and issuing letters of guarantee seem to be obvious tasks. But activities such as bookkeeping, negotiating contracts with health care providers, or cost allocation with clients and health service providers pose a real challenge for individuals involved in the establishment of MHOs. Thus, the workshop participants must understand various terms for money; and even if the hospital's vice director has his doubts about the low level of administration, Mr. Dembele will have to continue with the planning, monitoring, and evaluation of mutual health organizations. Biobureaucracy invades the life of these people due to decisions that transnational agencies have made at the expense of state sovereignty. Thus, health insurance remains a matter of trust in people who show initiative and walk the narrow line between local achievements and international organizations' requirements.

Notes

1. "L'Atelier de formation des adminstrateurs des mutuelles de santé en planification, suivi et evaluation," held August 28–29, 2004.

2. This chapter is based on research within a joint project conducted during three stays in Senegal between August 2004 and March 2006. It was part of the research program "Local Action in Africa in the Context of Global Influences" by the Humanities Collaborative Research Centre (SFB/FK 560) at the University of Bayreuth funded by DFG (Deutsche Forschungsgemeinschaft). I am grateful to Michael Niechzial (EPOS health management) and Babacar Lô for support and discussion within the project, and to Fane Dieng for assistance and translation. I very much appreciate the comments of my colleague Alexander Schulze of the Novartis Foundation.

3. I would like to thank Susan Reynolds Whyte for pointing this out to me.

4. Sir William Beveridge was the director of the London School of Economics when he was given the assignment of preparing a report on social insurance, and he recommended provision of health care for all people, benefits during unemployment or sickness and after disability, and retirement through central taxation.

5. This has been especially true since the World Summit for Social Development, held in March 1995 in Copenhagen, when governments reached a new consensus on the need to reduce poverty and foster social integration. Establishing health insurance schemes has become part of the strategy in international development to alleviate poverty (Preker et al. 2004; Bührer 2006).

6. The FCFA (franc CFA or CFA franc) is the unit of currency in various West and Central African nations that were formerly under French colonial rule. As of 2010, the exchange rate was approximately: 1 USD = 503 FCFA, 1 euro = 655 FCFA.

7. However, according to Bärnighausen and Sauerborn (2002), in order to achieve universal coverage government action is needed to introduce a principle of compulsion.

8. In many societies livestock, land, and other means count as savings (see Shipton 1995).

9. These terms are widely used in insurance management. *Moral hazard*: insurance members make more claims because they have coverage. *Adverse selection*: mainly people with higher risk levels take membership

10. In addition, health is frequently addressed in the non-biomedical sector, which consists of a variety of different types of healers, among them diviners and *marabouts,* who use herbs, concoctions, and spiritual techniques for healing. Costs for treatment in this sector are very flexible as well. The first visit is usually for

diagnostic measures, and then healers charge for their therapy according to their clients' means. Most people in Diourbel approach the different medical sectors concurrently.

11. The Bamako initiative was launched at a meeting of African Ministers of Health in 1987. It focused on the provision of essential drugs and primary health care services.

12. Kane mentions *natt*, *tegg*, and *sani diamra* as Wolof terms and calls the organizations grassroots financial arrangements. He defines *mbootay* (an alternate spelling of *mbootaay*) specifically as financial arrangements centered around family ceremonies (Kane 2006: 99). Sow (2005) illustrates the role of these associations of support among migrants in Spain. The groups resemble Rotating Savings and Credit Associations (ROSCAs). On the anthropological dispute about the meaning of ROSCAs, see Geertz (1962) and Ardener (1964); for discussions of rotating credit schemes in West Africa see Hill (1986) and Guyer (1995).

13. I would like to thank Mamarame Seck at the University of Florida, Gainsville for his support on the meaning of Wolof terms.

14. On the relationship between NGOs in the global south and NGOs from the global north see Neubert (1997).

References

Ardener, Shirley. 1964. "The Comparative Study of Rotating Credit Associations." *Journal of the Royal Anthropological Institute* 94: 201–229.

Arhinful, Daniel K. 2003. *The Solidarity of Self-interest: Social and Cultural Feasibility of Rural Health Insurance in Ghana.* Leiden, the Netherlands: African Studies Centre.

Asfaw, Abay. 2004. *The Impact of Social Health Protection Mechanisms on Access to Health Care, Health Expenditure, and Impoverishment: A Case Study of Senegal.* Berlin: Center for Development Research (ZEF).

Atim, Chris. 1998. *The Contribution of Mutual Health Organizations to Financing, Delivery, and Access to Health Care: Synthesis of Research in Nine West and Central African Countries.* Bethesda, Md.: Abt. Associations Inc.

Bärnighausen, Till, and Rainer Sauerborn. 2002. "One Hundred and Eighteen Years of the German Health Insurance System: Are There Any Lessons for Middle- and Low-Income Countries?" *Social Science & Medicine* 54: 1559–1587.

Bührer, Franziska. 2006. "Soziale Sicherung in Entwicklungsländern als Herausforderung für Politik: Der Prozess der Förderung der, Mutuelles de Santé im Senegal." M.A. Thesis, Department for Political Sciences, University of Hamburg, Germany.

Concertation. 2004. *Inventaire des Systèmes d'assurance maladie en Afrique: Synthèse des trauvaux de recherche dans 11 pays.* Dakar, Senegal: La Concertation sur le mutuelles de santé en Afrique.

Damen, Haile Mariam. 2003. "Indigenous Social Insurance as an Alternative Financing Mechanism for Health Care in Ethiopia (the Case of Eders)." *Social Science & Medicine* 56 (8): 1719–1726.

Doetinchem, Ole, with Bernd Schramm and Jean-Oliver Schmidt. 2006. "The Benefits and Challenges of Social Health Insurance for Developing

Countries." In *Financing Health Care: A Dialogue between South Eastern Europe and Germany*, ed. Ulrich Laaser and Ralf Radermacher, 27–43. Series International Public Health, vol. 18. Lage, Germany: Jacobs Editing Company.

Drechsler, Denis, and Johannes Jütting. 2005. "Private Health Insurance for the Poor in Developing Countries?" In *Policy Insights 11: OECD Development Centre*. Electronic document: http://www.oecd.org/dataoecd/25/14/35274754.pdf.

Evrard, Dominique. 2002. "Mutuelles de Santé en Afrique: Mouvement émergent ou phénomène de mode?" Dakar, Senegal. Electronic document. http://www.masmut.be/masmut/website/uploads/pdf/20060324_309024993_anmcmouvementfr.pdf.

Ferguson, James. 2006. *Global Shadows: Africa in the Neoliberal World Order*. Durham, N.C.: Duke University Press.

Foley, Ellen E. 2008. "Neoliberal Reform and Health Dilemmas: Illness, Social Hierarchy, and Therapeutic Decision-Making in Senegal." *Medical Anthropology Quarterly* 22 (3): 257–273.

———. 2010. *Your Pocket Is What Cures You: The Politics of Health in Senegal*. New Brunswick, N.J.: Rutgers University Press.

Geertz, Clifford. 1962. "The Rotating Credit Association: A 'Middle Rung' in Development." *Development and Cultural Change* 10: 241–263.

Gueye, Amadou T., with Mamadou B. Daff, Fatou Sow, Abibou D. Camara, Aminata Sow, Jürgen Hohmann, and Michael Niechzial. 2001. "Promotion de mutuelles de santé dans la région de Diourbel. Rapport de l'étude de faisabilité technique et financière." Diourbel: Hôpital Regional de Diourbel, Senegal.

Guyer, Jane I., ed. 1995. *Money Matters: Instability, Values, and Social Payments in the Modern History of West African Communities*. London: James Currey Ltd.

Hemenway, Derek. 1997. "Senegal and Structural Adjustment: For Better or for Worse?" Department of Urban and Regional Planning, Planning for Developing Areas, Florida State University. Electronic document: http://garnet.acns.fsu.edu/~dhh4266/Senegal.htm.

Hill, Polly. 1986. *Development Economics on Trial: The Anthropological Case for a Prosecution*. Cambridge: Cambridge University Press.

Huber, Götz, with Jürgen Hohmann and Kirsten Reinhard. 2003. *Mutual Health Insurance (MHO)—Five Years Experience in West Africa: Concerns, Controversies, and Proposed Solutions*. Eschborn, Germany: GTZ.

IMF. 1998. "Senegal. Enhanced Structural Adjustment Facility. Economic and Financial Policy Framework Paper (1999–2001)." Prepared by the Government of Senegal in Consultation with the Staffs of the International Monetary Fund and World Bank. Electronic document: http://www.imf.org/external/NP/PFP/1999/senegal/INDEX.HTM.

Kane, Abdoulaye. 2001. "Les Caméléons de la Finance Populaire au Sénégal et dans la Diaspora." PhD diss., Amsterdam School for Social Science Research, University of Amsterdam.

———. 2006. "Tontines and Village Cash Boxes along the Tilonge–Dakar–Paris Emigration Route." In *Mutualist Microfinance: Informal Savings Funds from the Global Periphery to the Core?*, ed. Abram De Swaan and Marcel van der Linden, 97–120. Amsterdam: aksant.

Kawabata, Kei, with Ke Xu and Guy Carrin. 2002. "Preventing Impoverishment through Protection against Catastrophic Health Expenditure." Bulletin of the World Health Organization 80 (2): 612. Electronic document: http://www.scielosp.org/pdf/bwho/v80n8/v80n8a02.pdf.

Klocke-Daffa. 2001. *Wenn du hast, musst du geben. Soziale Sicherung im Ritus und im Alltag bei den Nama von Berseba/Namibia.* Münster: LIT.

Kohrman, Matthew. 2005. *Bodies of Difference: Experiences of Disability and Institutional Advocacy in the Making of Modern China.* Berkeley: University of California Press.

MAE. 2000. *Etude sur l'extension des assurances sociales obligatoires au risqué maladie dans le pays de la zone de solidarité prioritaire.* Paris: Ministère des Affaires Extrangères. Direction Générale de la Co-operation Internationale et du Développment DCT/HS.

McPake, Barbara. 1994. "User Charges for Health Services in Developing Countries: A Review of the Economic Literature." *Social Science & Medicine* 39: 1189–1201.

Mossialos, Elias, with Anna Dixon, Josep Figueras, and Joe Kutzin. 2002. *Funding Health Care: Options for Europe.* Buckingham, U.K.: Open University Press.

Musgrove, Philip. 1996. *Public and Private Roles in Health: Theory and Financing Patterns.* World Bank Discussion Paper No. 339. Washington, D.C.: The World Bank.

Ndiaye, Abdourahmane. 2002. "Foreign Debt, Structural Adjustment Programs, and Poverty in Senegal." Department of Economics and Management, Cheikh Anta Diop University, Senegal. Electronic document: http://www.france.attac.org/spip.php?article3095.

Neubert, Dieter. 1986. *Sozialpolitik in Kenya.* Münster, Germany: Lit.

———. 1997. "A Development Utopia Re-visited: Non-Governmental Organisations in Africa." *Sociologus* 47: 51–77.

Nolan, Brian, and Vincent Turbat. 1995. *Cost Recovery in Public Health Services in Sub-Saharan Africa.* Washington, D.C.: The World Bank.

Preker, Alexander S., with Guy Carrin, David Dror, Melitta Jakab, William Hsiao, and Dyna Arhin-Tenkorang. 2002. "Effectiveness of Community Health Financing in Meeting the Cost of Illness." *Bulletin of the World Health Organization* 80 (2): 143–150. Electronic document: http://www.scielosp.org/pdf/bwho/v80n2/a10v80n2.pdf.

———. 2004. "Rich–Poor Differences in Health Care Financing." In *Health Financing for Poor People: Resource Mobilization and Risk Sharing,* ed. Alexander S. Preker and Guy Carrin, 3–51. Washington, D.C.: The World Bank.

Schoepf, B. G., with C. Schoepf and J. Millen. 2000. "Theoretical Therapies, Remote Remedies: SAPs and the Political Ecology of Poverty and Health in Africa." In *Dying for Growth: Global Inequality and the Health of the Poor,* ed. Jim Yong Kim, Joyce Millen, Alec Irwin, and John Gershman, 91–126. Monroe, Maine: Common Courage Press.

Schramm, Bernd, with Ole Doetinchem and Marion Baak. 2004. *Social Health Insurance—Systems of Solidarity: Experiences from German Development Cooperation.* Eschborn, Germany: GTZ.

Schulze, Alexander. 2010. "Gemeindebasierte Krankenkassen im Kontext sozialer Differenzierung. Zur Charakterisierung von Mitgliedern und Nichtmitgliedern im ländlichen Mali." In *Medizin im Kontext. Krankheit und Gesundheit in einer vernetzten Welt*, ed. Hansjörg Dilger and Bernhard Hadolt, 305–328. Frankfurt am Main: Peter Lang Verlag.

Shipton, Parker. 1995. "How Gambians Save: Culture and Economic Strategy at an Ethnic Crossroads." In *Money Matters: Instability, Values, and Social Payments in the Modern History of West African Communities*, ed. Jane I. Guyer, 245–276. London: James Currey Ltd.

Sigerist, Henry E. 1943. "From Bismarck to Beveridge: Development and Trends in Social Security Legislation." *Bulletin of the History of Medicine* 13: 365–388.

Sommerfeld, Johannes, with Mamadou Sanon, Bocar A. Kouyate, and Rainer Sauerborn. 2002. "Informal Risk-Sharing Arrangements (IRSAs) in Rural Burkina Faso: Lessons for the Development of Community-Based Insurance." *International Journal of Health Planning and Management* 17: 147–163.

Sow, Papa. 2005. "Formes et comportement d'épargne des Sénégalais et Gambiens de la Catalogne (Espagne)." *Géographie et Cultures* 56: 39–56.

Steinwachs, Luise. 2006. *Die Herstellung sozialer Sicherheit in Tanzania. Prozesse sozialer Transformation und die Entstehung neuer Handlungsräume*. Münster, Germany: LIT.

Waelkens, Maria Pia, with Werner Soors and Bart Criel. 2005. *The Role of Social Health Protection in Reducing Poverty: the Case of Africa*. ESS Paper No. 22. Genf, Germany: ILO.

Weber, Axel, with Friedeger Stierle, Jürgen Hohmann, Bergis Schmidt-Ehry, and Jens Holst. 2005. *Social Protection in Health Care: European Assets and Contributions*. Eschborn, Germany: GTZ.

Wolf, Angelika. 2007. "Health Insurance—A Question of Morality?" Paper presented at the symposium Agency and Changing World Views in Africa. Apr. 26, University of Bayreuth.

Wolf, Angelika, with Michael Niechzial and Eckhard Nagel, eds. Forthcoming. *Krankenversicherung und soziale Sicherung in Afrika. Perspektiven aus Entwicklungszusammenarbeit und Wissenschaft*. Berlin: LIT

World Bank. 1987. *Financing Health Services in Developing Countries: An Agenda for Reform*. Washington, D.C.: World Bank Publications.

FOUR

Afri-global Medicine:
New Perspectives on Epidemics, Drugs, Wars,
Migrations, and Healing Rituals

John M. Janzen

Afri-global Medicine: Global Intersections

The three case studies that make up this chapter illustrate what I call "Afri-global medicine." By this I mean: on the one hand, situations in which sickness and healing in an African setting are affected, addressed, or handled by wider global forces or agencies; or, on the other hand, persons, practices, or materia medica that, having originated in an African setting, are used far from their origins yet in a manner reminiscent of, or in keeping with, their original characteristics. The first case study involves Ebola viral hemorrhagic fever outbreaks in Central Africa in the early 2000s, and the constellation of individuals and agencies that came together to deal with the epidemic. The second focuses on the effort to prospect and market pharmaceuticals derived from African medicinal plants. The third is about transplanted, transnational African refugee immigrants. Each case begins with a particular set of individuals who by their actions engage wider, global connections, exchanges, and movements.

The case studies occur within the "global now" (Appadurai 1997), in an anthropological perspective[1] where the units of study are sets of practices or supply chains of capital, labor, and community over many sites[2] (Tsing in Finkelstein and Zeiderman 2006: 23) rather than local communities or regions. Along these chains or networks of relations there arise points of difference or contradictions over the control of labor, natural resources, and the means of production. Powerful meanings, emotions, and desires arise in and around these networks and their contours.[3] People move along these networks as a result of economic opportunities or the displacement of wars. The resulting transnational kindreds become the vehicle for various mobilities: of messages about family affairs, monetary support from workers in the North to those back home in Africa, and, often, rapidly changing meanings of social roles and expectations.[4] Telephone, telex, and internet provide instantaneous global contact between the nodes of these structures of communication and trans-action. The introduction to this volume elaborates more fully on this new globalized Africanist medical anthropology.

The Conversation between Local Communities and Global Experts about Epidemics

French anthropologist Alain Epelboin and his colleagues from the Centre Nationale de Recherche Scientifique (CNRS), Doctors Without Borders (Médecins Sans Frontières), and the World Health Organization (WHO) (Epelboin and Formenty 2003), together with the survivors of Mbomo and Nkele at the Gabon/Congo border, continue to reflect on the lessons learned during those catastrophic months from 2001–2004 when, over intervals, more than a hundred people in several communities died of Ebola viral hemorrhagic fever. Epelboin wonders how the international medical team might have done things differently to prevent the next of kin of the dying—the very people they were trying to help, some of whom were presumably infected—from fleeing into the forest, or from attacking the health workers who claimed to know something about the disease. The people of Nkele, for their part, although they have memorized the mantra that they should no longer eat bush meat, and the biomedical explanation that it is a microorganism that causes the deaths, when pressed will say that the cause of the deaths was sorcery. Will Ebola strike again? How will the international experts talk to the locals and sort out some of the issues that arise when family and neighbors are dying for no apparent reason? Although the experts say that it was a virus, they are not entirely sure of the host, or exactly how it was transmitted. It is the fear of deadly epidemic outbreaks and their spread worldwide that drives inter-national health agencies (the WHO, the Centers for Disease Control [CDC], Doctors Without Borders) to travel in great haste to Central Africa, and to become involved—often in an overbearing way—with the local communities and with local and national health officials in order to do something, *fast,* to stop the epidemic. Expectations on the anthropologists who are called in to help are enormous: they are to reconstruct the pattern of transmission, to interpret the culture of the locals so that the medical experts don't transgress local etiquette and ethics, and to help however possible to bring the epidemic to a close.

HIV/AIDS and Ebola are epidemics that catch the attention of the world's experts because they are a threat to people elsewhere, in the global North. HIV/AIDS has been called a security risk to the North. Its contagion has the potential to spread silently all around. It can collapse societies and states; it invites global political chaos. Ebola outbreaks attract world attention because of the disease's rapid and extreme lethality (60–90 percent) and the fear of spreading its deadly viral infection via air travel to cities and the North.

Ebola is one type of virus in an entire class of hemorrhagic fevers that occur worldwide. Its incubation period is about five to ten days, and once infected an individual experiences severe fever, cramps, and internal bleeding, and within a few days will either die or begin recovering. Experts now suggest that most of these particular Central African epidemics were caused by individuals encountering infected primates, amongst whom the virus may be endemic. Its mechanisms of contagion allow it to spread in every direction silently. In most cases the original humans infected have been hunters, or those who eat infected bush meat, or in the case of the Kikwit epidemic, a charcoal worker who probably was exposed in the forest where he collected and processed charcoal (NOVA 1996). The next to be exposed are often family members; health workers who come in contact with the body, blood, or bodily fluids of the infected; or other hospital and clinic patients touched by these caregivers or by fellow patients. Almost all of the Central African Ebola epidemics have endangered health care workers; nurses and doctors have been infected and died. The WHO, the CDC, and national health agencies have developed measures to protect health care workers involving protective masks, gowns, and boots; rigorous disinfection of surroundings where Ebola sufferers have been; careful disposal of the clothing and material possessions of the infected; and, most challenging of all, the disposal of the bodies of the Ebola dead in ways that meet cultural expectations of appropriate burial while at the same time protecting the grieving and next of kin from further infection.

There is a wealth of good documentation on the natural history and public health of Ebola outbreaks in Central Africa. We know how many individuals were infected in each epidemic, how many died, the vector suspected, the course of spread of the epidemic, and how it was eventually contained or came to a close on its own (Waterman 1999). Table 1 shows the highlights of that documentation on Central Africa, as presented before a WHO/Pasteur Institute colloquium held to gain strategies for dealing with Ebola.

The documentation and analysis of the sociocultural dimension of Ebola epidemics in Central Africa have been far less thorough. The two engagements in Ebola outbreaks by anthropologists thus far are the work of Alain Epelboin and Pierre Formenty in the Congo/Gabon outbreaks of 2001–2004, and the work of Armin Prinz in northeast Congo and southern Sudan in 2004. In addi-

Table 4.1. Ebola Epidemics, by country and year. Infections in relation to deaths: e.g., 318/280. (Formenty, Roth, and Grein 2004; IRIN 2007)

Country	1970s	1980s	1990s	2000s
Cote d'Ivoire			?/1	
Gabon			52/?, 37/?, 6/?	65/?
Republic of Congo— Brazzaville				57/13, 143/128, 35/?
Democratic Republic of Congo	318/280, 1/?		315/245	217/103
Sudan	284/154, 34/?			17/7
Uganda				425/app. 400

tion to the important work of helping identify the pattern of infection and the ecology of infection, the unique calling and opportunity of anthropologists in these epidemics has been, in the words of Epelboin and Formenty (2003), to "humanize the taking in charge of the population" in an epidemic and to "counsel the intervention team." In other words, the unique calling and opportunity of the anthropologist has been to stage-manage the communication between the international and national experts and the local community.

This anthropological work entails answering such questions as: What exactly was the popular perception and reaction to the outbreak of this deadly disease? Who did what to whom in the early stages of the outbreak? Who became a suspected agent of the grave danger to the community in the course of the epidemic? Who controlled or sought to steer the diagnosis and negotiated understanding of the misfortune? There are hints of such behaviors in the above reports. The WHO/CNRS report suggests that the epidemics have usually come to an end because the populace of the afflicted region or communities simply flee from fear and thus no further contagion is possible. Others report that it has been most difficult to carry out public health measures of quarantine or disposal of diseased bodies because of customs that emphasize holding the sick and dying, and bathing the dead before burial and grieving. Some reports by journalists emphasize the panic and fear of illiterate peasants and the difficulty of teaching them anything, or the divided popular consensus over whether disease or sorcery is at the root of the epidemic (Agence France Presse 2004).

The French anthropologist/physician team of Epelboin and Formenty were part of a larger public health group that responded to the 2003–2004 Congo Brazzaville outbreaks. Dr. Alain Epelboin is a medical anthropologist with CNRS. Dr. Pierre Formenty, with the WHO since 1996, is responsible for research on the sociocultural background of hemorrhagic fever, and coordinator for the following viral zoonotic diseases: Ebola; Marburg, Rift Valley, and Crimean-Congo hemorrhagic fevers; Nipah virus; and Monkeypox.. He is a field epidemiologist specialized in public health (infectious diseases surveillance and outbreak response) and in medical virology, with a special focus on viral hemorrhagic fever. He is also a Veterinary Officer specialized in virology and epidemiology for domestic and wild animals.

The Epelboin and Formenty report gives us a detailed account of two interlinked outbreaks that continued for months in Mbomo and Kelle near the Gabon/Congo border. The medical team and researchers did an ethnographic reconstruction of the onset when several local school teachers were accused of having caused the Ebola and were assaulted and killed while people near the Ebola victims either fled into the forests or locked themselves in their houses. Europeans at a nearby nature reserve were charged with enriching themselves with local resources, and thus, somehow, being implicated in the Ebola outbreak.

The research/medical team's involvement came as health experts arrived to try to introduce measures that would interrupt the transmission of the virus to new cases. Apparently, in one instance rigorous quarantine measures were resisted; the affected people fled from health authorities or hid their diseased next of kin. Yet, in the other community where the anthropologist was on hand, there was a greater degree of collaboration. The difference may have been due to the anthropologist's encouragement of customary burials, including permission to put the draped corpses into coffins, and the personal possessions of the deceased on the graves, rather than to have the corpses and materials burned. These more "humane" treatments of the deceased were made possible when the public health team adopted compromise safety measures that included donning protective clothing, using extensive disinfectant sprays on funeral participants, and creating a barrier around the cemetery.

The second example of anthropological reporting on Ebola outbreaks is by Armin Prinz, Director of the Ethnomedicine Department at the Medical University of Vienna, who in 2004 was doing follow-up research among the Azande of northern Democratic Republic of the Congo. The Yambio outbreak occurred among Azande across the border in Sudan. Prinz (personal communication, 2005) sketches his remarks within the broader framework of emphasizing the importance of ethnomedicine, the importance of traditional medicine to many societies, and the chaos that has affected the traditional healing elites of the Azande society in this region.

In recent years there have been massive disturbances of indigenous health care provisioning. In northeast Congo, for example, due to the civil war and the reigning warlords' fear of the magical powers of healers, hundreds of these specialists were murdered in a grisly manner. Prinz described to me the wholesale massacre of traditional healers following the chaos of civil war, resultant disease outbreaks, and the fear of the magical power of healers. The witchcraft accusations against those who appear to know something about AIDS or other epidemics are not unrelated to this fear, nor is the resistance to public health teams' efforts to impose quarantine and other aggressive measures to contain the Ebola outbreak. Prinz is critical of Doctors Without Borders for having conducted too little ethnomedical preparatory research, resulting in families hiding their sick.

Yet the Yambio outbreak was contained in an orderly manner by the WHO under the direction of Dr. Pierre Formenty (WHO 2004). Of 17 infected, only seven died. The medical response team tried to apply the lessons learned from the recent outbreaks in Congo and Gabon. A quarantine ward was set up within the village or hospital compound where next of kin could see their loved ones. A meeting room was opened where local community people could meet with members of the health team, ask questions, and reach meaningful agreement on what was happening. Infected mattresses, treatment materials, and things that could not be disinfected were burned daily. Families were encouraged to perform the funeral rituals, but with the bodies being handled by the medical team.

Prinz, Epelboin, and Formenty compared notes in September 2004 at the colloquium on Ebola hosted by the Institut Pasteur in Paris. They, along with other colloquy participants, agreed on the importance of "ethnomedical information for the health worker, in order to explain quarantine and treatment measures to the populace, so as to be able to modify the awareness of the people's consciousness of disease on which their intervention measures are based" (Prinz, personal communication, 2005).

However, missing from these quick or emergent ethnographies of Ebola and the interventions was a grasp of the social context of the diagnostic negotiation of the emergency, particularly the framework in which such diagnosis was subject to social and political forces and how, and by whom, these were controlled (Janzen 2005). Instead, the analysis of intervention was based on a static cultural model of customary behavior that must be respected. Although the WHO-managed intervention in southern Sudan emulated a therapy management model, there was no reference in the report to the dynamic features of this way of sorting out issues (Janzen 1978). The literature on therapy man-agement in Equatorial African societies reveals that a group of kin presides over the debate about causation with the help of diviners, prophet-seers, and the biomedical establishment. In the present reports on Ebola a reader can follow the outlines of who is seeking to control or manage the diagnosis and steps of the intervention. But there is no closely focused ethnography and analysis of this process as it occurred in the patient and kin groups during the months-long unfolding of the epidemic outbreaks. One wonders whether in the next crisis interventions will again be negotiated through such a public forum.

Also missing from the ethnographic reports of these Ebola interventions is any appreciation of the etiological attributions through which a misfortune may be either seen to be "natural" (usually identified by a euphemism such as "of God") or brought on through agentative cause, i.e., by the victims them-selves or by an other, an enemy (usually identified via the euphemism "of man") (Janzen 1978: 44ff; Ngubane 1977: 22ff; Davis 2000: 94f). As widespread ethnographies have shown, single cases of affliction often shift from one type of cause to the other. Recently, depictions of such "etiological dualism" have surfaced in accounts by journalists, medical workers, and scholars of out-breaks of epidemics. In cholera and Ebola outbreaks and in areas suffering escalating deaths by HIV / AIDS, not only lay therapy managers and diviners but also living victims, survivors and their next of kin, local health work-ers, national health officials, NGO representatives, and even anthropologists may find themselves drawn into situations where accusations are leveled and assaults occur against alleged perpetrators of disease.

Current thinking amongst medical anthropologists who work in Equatorial and Central Africa is that social control is an absolutely critical factor in the etiological judgment of misfortune. Mary Douglas's (1970, 1992) work on the association of cosmologies (grid) to social authority and struc-ture (group) suggested ways of identifying degrees of chaos and of order, of control or lack of control. Where social and political decentralization prevail, or issues of danger remain ambiguous and no authorities "take charge" of the discourse of misfortune, blame-seeking runs rampant. In the Central African setting, suspicions of "sorcery" or "witchcraft" abound. (It is important to note that Douglas has long since identified similar other-blaming behavior in Western industrialized society as well.) This same process of the allocation of danger underlies the identification by health experts of at-risk categories of society; in this case, determinations are filtered through probability statistics and public health screening. Where there is greater control or more hierar-chical authority, there is a quicker willingness to allow for a "natural" illness attribution. It may also be that when the outside expert engages in discussion and negotiation with the local therapy managers as part of an "empathetic" physician-anthropologist intervention, the new knowledge thus brought to the community suffices to sway the consensus to the acceptance of a "natural" option and therefore one that allows for medical interventions—isolation, medication, and health education—rather than provokes the need for prayer, sorcery hysteria, and the urge for revenge killing.

So, the question of the social context of attempted response to misfortune, the nature of the negotiation, who is involved, and the institutionalized or de facto articulation of agency are all very important in shifting the etiological attribution from sorcery to naturally occurring affliction. Local knowledge may well include scientific understanding of public health dangers. But this knowledge, in a social context charged with high anxiety and an atmosphere of neighbor-against-neighbor, is susceptible to being overwhelmed by the perception of an antagonistic agent bent on destruction and death. By contrast, the presence of an authoritative voice or official who represents an explanation or resolution to the crisis can calm fears and persuade the local community to accept a "natural" course of treatment. The implications for health officials and communities are obviously very great, and determine whether such officials or teams will be part of the solution, or whether they are perceived to be part of the problem. The effective introduction of new public health knowledge to deal with Ebola requires an understanding of the social logic held by local kin, and a successful negotiation with local power constellations and political alignments.

African Materia Medica Meets Global Pharmaceuticals

Congolese pharmacist and author Byamungu Lufungula, of Bukavu, Eastern Congo, wondered aloud to me in late 1994 why the dozens of nongovernmental organizations (NGOs) at work in the refugee camps of Goma and along Lake Kivu had not accepted his cholera medications, given the severity of the epidemic in large refugee camps (Byamungu 1982; personal communication 1994) and the threat of outbreaks in other camps. To his dismay, they preferred medicines from Europe and the United States with which they were familiar. Byamungu, for his part, learned a lesson about the structure of global flows of medicine, pharmaceutical legitimacy and who bestows and controls it, and who may use the medicine that is thus prioritized. During those weeks and months when Bukavu was at the pivot of global attention because of the Rwandan war and its displacement into Congo, Byamungu rightly felt that he could and perhaps should have aligned his pharmaceutical production with the global distribution of medicines handled by dozens of NGOs under the umbrella of the United Nations High Commission for Refugees (UNHCR). How do anthropologists conceptualize such a range of juxtapositions as are at play in the production, use, and signification of medicines? What would be an appropriate framework that would be required for Africans' community of healers, herbalists, pharmacists like Byamungu, and entrepreneurs to globally validate the tradition of Central African materia medica? Beginning "from the ground up and out" this case study illustrates the global linkages between African healers, drug analysts, businessmen, and the multinational drug companies and their users. Linkages extend from rainforest to global marketplace, illustrating circuits of exchange to the full scope of drug globalization.[5]

The much-vaunted knowledge of Central African medicines, knowledge waiting to be developed by a range of national and international researchers and entrepreneurs, is held in the minds of *banganga* such as those featured in *The Quest for Therapy* (Janzen 1978). Mama Mankomba combined the sap of her well-used finger cactus tree with soap and seven other plants to treat congestive swelling. Kitembo called himself an *nganga nkisi* and prided himself on his vast knowledge of the plants of the wild. Nzoamambu, also an *nganga nkisi,* who was featured in an entire chapter of *Quest,* operated fulltime as an *nganga,* both at his home and on his occasional sorties to cities of the region, principally Matadi. His village was a richly planted herbarium of medicinal plants that he used regularly. Already in the early twentieth century, the colonial government was on to the *banganga* and their knowledge; colonial science sought to research and valorize this knowledge through publications such as De Wildeman's monograph (1935).

Urban *banganga* did not wait for research and licenses to validate their work. Many, like Tambwe Antoine of Lubumbashi and Kinshasa, forged ahead with a vast knowledge of medical materials available on the market, as well as eager urban customers ready to submit to a range of treatments such as injections of herbal medications and various surgeries. Tambwe resupplied his stocks from the pan-African merchants at the Central Market in Kinshasa, both those from Lower Congo, who sold mainly plant materials, and those in the Hausa section, whose merchants sold West African arid-lands medicaments. In the late twentieth and early twenty-first centuries, much of African medicine could be found in the markets of metropolitan centers.

There are many trained African pharmacists who research medicinal plants in order to help their fellows and to make good on the lucrative market for medicine. One such pharmacist from the Lower Congo is Batangu Mpesa, former parliamentarian, founder of the Centre de Recherche Pharmacologique de Luozi, and publisher of his own research journal, *Bilongo*. In recent decades,

Mpesa avidly sought to further his business by bringing raw materials to the Program for Pharmaceutical Chemistry at the University of Kansas. Anti-diarrheal medicines were at the top of his list for development, and indeed, the brand name Manidiar is on the market and available in his pharmacy in Kinshasa.

Byamungu, in Bukavu, eastern Congo in the Great Lakes region, oper-ated a more impressive establishment throughout the 1990s and 2000s, with 25 employees and a production list of 25 medicines sold in three pharmacies in Bukavu, Uvira along Lake Tanganyika to the south, and Goma at the north-ern edge of Lake Kivu. Following his pharmacological training in France, Byamungu conducted research in the 1980s under the aegis of a national institute on medicinal plants and therapeutic rites of the Kivu (1982). When the Rwandan war broke out and Rwandan refugees flooded across the bor-der into Congo (then Zaire) Byamungu offered his medicines—especially for infantile diarrhea and cholera—to medical personnel in charge of the camps all around him. But his generous offer was rejected by skeptical NGOs who did not have time for unproven local products. Their supply networks came from the North; Africa was the victim, the target, not the source of relief assis-tance. Still, Byamungu continued his work supplying the local market with medicines that sold alongside the pharmaceuticals imported from the North. The need was great, and pharmacies and hospitals often lacked medicines, a picture that is unfortunately widespread across Africa.

Regional and national research institutions are common in Africa. In the Great Lakes region, Bukavu in Eastern Congo and Butare in Rwanda are well known. These institutes work together with local healers and develop their own products from extensive gardens such as the one on the shores of Lake Kivu. One of the premiere research institutes is the Traditional Medicine Research Unit, an institute of Muhimbili Hospital in Dar es Salaam.

A healthy dynamism reigns in the world of medicines in Central Africa. Although healers are eager to be recognized and taught the ways of modern medicine in order to be granted legitimacy by their governments, they are sus-picious of research institutes and entrepreneurs who seek their knowledge for their own schemes and enrichment. Everywhere I spoke with healers about this, I heard the same refrain.

Which brings me to Shaman Pharmaceuticals. Shaman Pharmaceuticals, Inc. of San Francisco was a NASDAQ-listed company (under the moniker SHPH) from 1989 to 2004, during which time it enjoyed up to about 50 mil-lion USD from investors. Its bold experiment in reconciling bioprospecting and successful commercial drug development from rainforest herbaria with bioconservation was as intriguing and seductive as it proved economically unfeasible (Clapp and Crook 2002). The company's brief career in the world of corporate high finance, global networking, research, testing, and patenting of new products appeared to fulfill the promise of miracle cures long thought to exist in the minds and gardens of tropical Africa's healers. Yet the rockiness of the road to actual understanding of a given treatment—the tests and the clinical trials required for such medicines to be approved by government regulators, the capital needed to finance the researchers and the trials—suggests that it will be difficult for another enterprise to succeed where Shaman failed. Meanwhile, it appears that national agencies like Zimbabwe National Traditional Healers Association (ZINATHA) (Simmons 2006) and the Pharmacopeia Centre in Rwanda (under the auspices of the Institute of Scientific and Technological Research), along with many independent pharmacist-entrepreneurs like Byamungu and Batangu, are developing and marketing products without the extensive clinical trials necessary to pass muster at the U.S. Food and Drug Administration.

The field of this case study is a marvelous one for further research on all aspects. The lens of globalization theory provides the needed framework to understand the issues: the genius and science of African medical knowledge and practice; conversations and working relationships between healers and research institutes, pharmacists, and their financiers; legitimation structures and symbols of African medicine and biomedicine; local, regional, and global medicine flows and markets, and how they intersect and compete.

Post-war, Post-flight Trauma Healing at Home and Abroad

Farah Abdi, President of the Somali Foundation of Kansas City, who was wounded in the war in Mogadishu and is now wheelchair-bound, argues that Somalis and other forced immigrants from Africa in the United States and other Northern countries should adjust to life in America (or their other host country), learn the language, learn to drive, learn the skills needed to become productive in their new settings, and above all educate their children and help them find their way. Yet, as he readily admits, immigrants to cities of the North continue to be haunted by their memories of flight from their shattered homes and lives. Many have tried to track and reconnect kin scattered in dozens of cities and countries worldwide. Their lived worlds span from the now demolished or abandoned house they knew in Mogadishu to the apartment in which they now live temporarily. Telephone calls, emails, periodic cross-country drives, letters—these constitute the fabric of their lives. Where and what is home today? For Farah, Somalia is the individuals and the network of people he helps; to nourish his own imagination, he has mounted a collage of photos of Somalis and Somalia on the wall of the Foundation office in the basement of the Saint Alois Catholic Church in Kansas City. From 2004–2006 the Kansas African Studies Center conducted a project on and with new African immigrants in Kansas (KASC 2005–2006) to explore how anthropologists, other scholars, and supportive groups can play a constructive role in analyzing and interpreting the experience of forced migration, the trauma and adventure it entails.

Post-war, post-flight trauma and healing have concerned an increasing number of Africanist anthropologists. Sadly, the African continent has seen and continues to see entire regions engulfed in conflict. Most of these conflicts and their aftermaths are globalized. They are based on or embraced by international alliances. They are fueled by the international arms and mineral trades. Their victims are ministered to by international relief agencies. The global media may or may not publicize the conflict—as they did the Rwandan genocide and the current Darfur situation—to make it a cause célèbre. The inevitable civilian and military victims become far-flung refugees. Anthropological writings, scholarly research, and applied engagements focus on displacement, refugee camps, trauma, migration, and resettlement (Agier 2002; Foner 2003; Holtzman 2000; Malkki 1995a, 1995b; Janzen, Ngudiankama, and Filippi-Franz 2005). It is not simple to focus this vast and variegated field into a case study in globalized African medical anthropology. I offer several strands of my own research and writing, dealing first with the Rwandan genocide and war, then refocusing on recent work among new African immigrants in the United States.

The first of these strands I would identify as the ethnographic imperative (Janzen and Janzen 2000) of anthropology in the documentation of distress within major conflicts and displacements of entire communities. "Trauma" is a limiting code word in some circles, and we must try not to restrict our inquiry, as anthropologists, to something that is narrowly construed to be a diagnostic label in Western biomedicine or psychology. Christopher Colvin (2006: 166–184) has shown how a narrow trauma narrative model controlled by psychological therapists in the South African setting was inadequate to provide groups of citizens a sufficient framework for relieving their suffering that resulted from Apartheid. Our own work, reflecting the wider scope of anthropology, demonstrates how ethnography based on an invitation to sufferers of conflict and violence to "tell their story" can be met by a considerable eagerness that leads to much valuable human communication. In the Rwandan post-war, post-genocide setting our narrators often seemed driven by a kind of compulsion to "tell their story" so that the world would know. We felt under an ethical obligation to record and publish these accounts (Janzen 1999,

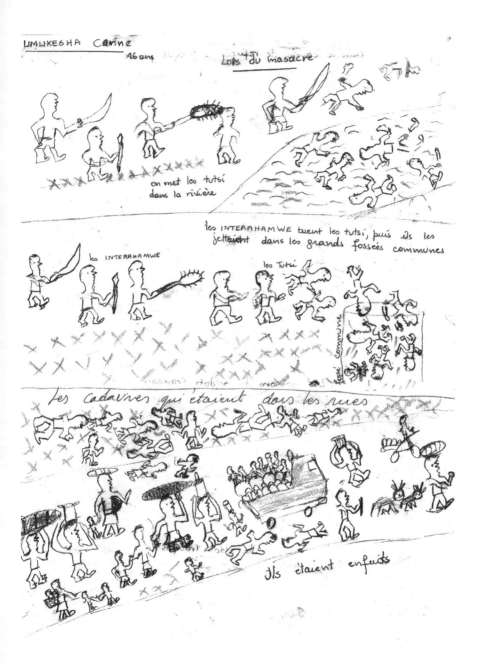

Fig. 4.1. Genocide and Flight, by Carine Umukesha, Kayenzi Commune, Rwanda. Pencil and colored pen on paper. December 1994. Reinhild Janzen commissioned this and other children's drawings from Rwandan children in Rwanda and Congo. Top panel: During the massacre they threw the Tutsi into the river. Middle panel: The Interhamwe killed the Tutsi, then they threw them into big communal pits. Lower panel: The cadavers were in the streets [as the masses] took flight [before the Rwandan Patriotic Front soldiers].

2003; Janzen and Janzen 2000; Janzen, Ngudiankama, Filippi-Franz 2003). This ethical imperative goes hand in hand with an "ethnographic imperative" that obliges anthropologists working in settings of postwar violence to engage a broad range of community members to tell their story, thereby reinvesting their dehumanizing experiences with a semblance of humanity.

This type of ethnography may be construed broadly enough to include drawings such as those by the Tutsi girl Carine, who was taken in by her Hutu neighbors after her parents were killed. Carine's drawings vividly capture the horror of the genocide in Rwanda and the memories of many victims who survived (figure 1).

A second perspective I have gleaned from my work in the Great Lakes region is that in most settings there was differential trauma—violence, suffering, displacement, the perception of a ruptured life. I am referring not just to the fact that we visited several communes, including those that had experienced disruption, violence, internal tearing asunder, and dislocation (that is, refugee flight), as well as those that had been spared such totalistic horror. Mainly I refer to the palpable divergence within communities in kinds of trauma, evident to me in the tone of voice of the narrators (Janzen 1999). It was as if a self-actualizing differentiation came about from the context of the violence. Most marked were the differences in bearing of those—such as the woman who risked her life to shelter her attacked neighbor—who had a kind of radiant defiance and ebullience, versus those who had succumbed to the propaganda of hate and had participated in the violence to save their lives. These latter individuals demonstrated a kind of confused agitation evident in a voice that seemed to cover the sense of regret, guilt, self-justification, doubt, and condemnation of history, and, no doubt also fear and loss of self-confidence.

Among other voices in the camps of the eastern Congo were those who had perpetrated violence for ideological reasons; those who had simply fled; those who were victimized and in deep grief and shock. There are many nuances around these and some other types of "moral-emotional" stances (Janzen 1999).

A third perspective emerges from this work, having to do with the compelling evidence that if such trauma as is described above is not resolved and/ or healed (and trauma healing often comes through conflict resolution), the conflict will in all likelihood be perpetuated into further cycles of violence: as survivors seek revenge, as perpetrators continue the original campaign or seek to cover their tracks by silencing those who know their deeds, or as victim-perpetrators act out their duplicitous compulsions in search of relief. This differentiation of trauma can be perceived across all segments of a postwar popu-lation, whether they are at home, have returned from flight, are still in limbo, or have emigrated to a new country and are trying to make their lives over.

The globalized nature of African war and its aftermath, and other forms of distress that lead to migration, is evident in the numbers of African-born individuals who reside in the U.S. According to the American Public Health Association, citing the U.S. census, more than 600,000 African-born immi-grants from all over the continent are now in the U.S.: from Sudan, where thousands have fled civil war and the repressive regime; Somalia, following civil war and the collapse of the state; Nigeria, because of ethnic violence and government repression; Rwanda and Burundi, following ethnic cleansing and genocide; Congo/Zaire, in the shadow of government repression, economic hardship, and civil war. Increasingly familiar in these groups are the stories of hardship and persecution; flight and arrival in the United States; the quest for a means of livelihood and the struggle to become established in a new home (Holtzman 2000). For many there is the gnawing question of return, although that happens only rarely (Janzen 2003). Farah Abdi, President of the Somali Foundation of Kansas City, described his community in a meeting in May, 2006.

> The immigrants who have come from East Africa are mostly refugees. My own country, Somalia, has been in a state of civil war since 1991. The economy and the government infrastructure have collapsed. The refugees who come here today are victims of armed conflict, rape and torture. They have spent years in refugee camps living under substandard conditions before they were given the opportunity to come to the United States. As a result, many of the refugees experi-ence post-traumatic stress disorder. (KASC New African Immigrants Project 2005–2006)

Traumas and the resulting memory constructions in immigrants should concern scholars, practitioners, and policy makers alike, for they affect the manner in which these new residents and citizens relate to their nations of origin and to their newly adopted home. Unresolved traumas and lingering memories of conflict not only threaten to exacerbate the cycles of violence within the immigrants' societies of origin, but also have the potential to bleed into American society (Janzen, Ngudiankama, and Filippi-Franz 2005). Constructive resolution or healing of such traumas lessens the potential of continuing chronic conflict. More research is needed, especially for the United States (Chavez 2003; Hirsch 2003). Refugee and immigrant communities that have been in the U.S. for decades offer guidance for new research. Several studies with southeast Asians who arrived in the U.S. in the 1970s as victims or survivors of war, attack, loss of next of kin, flight, and the refugee experience showed that these immigrants manifested symptoms and signs of "fright," "soul loss," and fear of persecution at the hands of old enemies and rivals. In the Kansas City Hmong community, which had converted to Christianity in Laos, the traumas of war, flight, and loss were addressed with intense prayer and fellowship gatherings (Capps 1994). Hmong-specific syndromes such as "fright" and "soul loss" were handled with traditional treatments and the maintenance of strong clan ties, combined with "making it" in American society. Elsewhere, in larger Hmong communities, lingering trauma and the challenges of a new land were addressed with shamanism, spirit rituals, and avoidance of old rivalries. For Vietnamese Americans, signs and symptoms of the war were "nightmares," "recurring same bad dreams," "headaches," and "anxiety attacks" associated with physical reminders of the original trau-matic experiences. Growing up in America did not fully resolve these trau-matic flashbacks. In fact they sometimes worsened in adulthood. Recurrent traumatic associations were greatly relieved through the disciplined practice of martial arts and the creation of community around this practice (Choby 2000). The Somali and Great Lakes/Congolese vignettes that are featured in joint work (Janzen, Ngudiankama, and Filippi-Franz 2005) represent a range of religious responses to trauma experience and memory that can serve as a basis for further research and action.

In our project on comparative religious healing and restoring commu-nity, Janzen, Ngudiankama, and Filippi-Franz (2005) identified several lines of inquiry that could be pursued in evaluating the extent and nature of the work at hand. As already mentioned, there is the basic ethnographic task of identifying how traumatic experiences of war, loss, displacement, and dis-orientation are dealt with in a new land. The people in our focus—in Great Lakes, Congolese, and Somali societies—described such signs and symptoms of trauma as recurrent nightmares, fears, sense of isolation, sexual impo-tence, feelings of guilt, and despondence. Some were brought to clinics by counselors or family members. The majority were never seen by professional therapists; rather, family and community members act as therapists. The role of congregations—mosques and healing churches—is especially important, given that families often are too traumatized or internally conflicted to heal themselves. In Gozdziak and Shandy's (2002) study of situations of forced migration, religion plays a significant role in helping adherents deal with the transition of migration—if the religious fabric is not destroyed by the conflict that drives them from home. Ngudiankama's work (2001) with Congolese refugees in London and Washington, D.C. recognizes the embracing and discerning community as an important resource for healing.

A second line of inquiry explores what happens when the syndromes of trauma cannot be handled within the tradition-appropriate means in family, community, or congregation. What are the consequences of sufferers' avoidance, denial, repression, or lingering trauma that is too painful to confront? Or if the tradition-appropriate methods of dealing with issues are shattered, no longer useable because of mistrust, conflict, or other institutional displacement? This appears to be the case with many Somali refugees. By selecting the road of least resistance, by default, such individuals may come to believe that their best option is to move on in life in the new society. "Simply becoming American" is tempting for some. The complex emotions surrounding unresolved trauma may, however, with reinforcement from others in the community, fuel the recourse to vengeance against antagonists, either directly or indirectly through financial and political support of ongoing conflict in the former home. Recognition of this dynamic process on the part of community members and health officials can be an important contribution to the welfare of new immigrants to the U.S. Yet it is important that refugees—especially traumatized ones—be able to take charge of decisions, to deal with their life issues and challenges on their own. Empowerment is a key to the ability to overcome trauma. There are no pat recipes for this, for just as experiences of violence differ, so the resources and resolutions differ for each case (Verwey 2001).

As Farah Abdi characterizes the Somalis of Kansas City, the refugees typically lived in traditional farming communities before the war. Illiteracy was common in those communities. Now, after they have arrived in the United States with few or no possessions and no income, they have to compete in a society where they cannot speak the language and do not have the skills to get good-paying jobs. They need interpreters to understand official documents and school documents, and to meet with health care providers. They need transportation to go to work, childcare, school, and doctors' offices. They need to learn the English language and how to drive a car. And they need advocates for their health care and workers' rights (Abdi in KASC 2005–2006).

In 1999, a group of refugees decided to help. They created Somali Foundation, a social services agency dedicated to helping the East African refugee community in Kansas City. Somali Foundation is a totally grassroots organization, established and sustained by the refugee community. It situates itself at the center of this desire to "move on" yet at the same time to assert Somali identity and community. Its mission is to assist East African refugees to achieve economic self-reliance, adjust socially to the United States, and keep honoring their cultures by providing social services, vocational training, information, and support.

In our inquiry we explored involvement in a religious congregation as a way of coming to terms with war trauma, painful memories, and their attendant symptoms. Both Islam (in the case of the Somalis) and Christianity (in the case of the Great Lakes/Congolese individuals), imbued with strong themes from Central African traditional religion, provide the forms of this orientation. New religious communities and identity may offer some an avenue in the quest for trauma healing.

Farah Abdi puts health care at the top of his list of ways that the Foundation serves the community.

> Health care access: We provide translation/interpretation and transportation to refugees when they need to see a doctor. Our translators are trained in the JVS Bridging the Gap program for medical and social translation. Our staff and volunteers are available after hours in case of an emergency situation or special need. Health education: We offer educational events as part of our community luncheon series. Recent events have focused on diabetes, cardiovascular disease, HIV/AIDS, tobacco use prevention and female circumcision, which is still a large problem in Africa. (Abdi in KASC 2005–2006)

English language classes, driving classes, women's programs, youth recreation, cultural celebrations, foods, cultural competence assistance, and translation and advocacy complete Abdi's list of ways that the Foundation helps immigrant Somalis. Fundamentally, the Foundation asserts Somali self-reliance. Farah Abdi closed his remarks at the May 2006 meeting by stating, "We are refugees helping other refugees."

What the Case Studies Have in Common: New Perspectives on Globalization

These cases and reflections on earlier research in globalization stress the importance of contextual reasoning around social, economic, and political circumstances, and of historical reasoning around events, relationships, and structural transformations. There is evidence in all three cases of the establishment of globalizing frameworks, the creation and flow of symbolic and cultural capital, and the movement of people within these frameworks. Ebola epidemics, the production and trade of drugs, and wars and humanitarian disasters become the sites where frameworks emerge for global interaction. Media create images of corpses, medical teams, and yellow bands that define quarantine zones. Medicinal plants, research journals, bottles and pills, and trademark labels become the stock in trade for the global drug exchange. Transnational migrants are in some ways the most evident symbols of globalization, as they arrive on the shores and in the cities of the North, become taxi drivers, restaurant owners, mosque and church builders, and, quickly, middle-class professionals who are in a position to send remunerations to their families in Africa.

Issues of power and control emerge in each of the cases. Who is responsible for the epidemics? Who controls and benefits from the sale of drugs? Who determines where refugees and migrants go, what privileges they enjoy? With all of these issues, particularly the last one, processes of exclusion and inclusion, and of resistance, need to be studied. Also of concern are the conditions that give rise to constituencies formed in reaction to their exclusion from rights and privileges, with corresponding identities, grudges, and scores to settle—publics that Appadurai (2006) calls "predatory identities." How are these formations avoided?

Conversations across boundaries are particularly interesting, as we have witnessed in the case studies: between international health experts on the one hand, and local communities and health agencies on the other in the Ebola outbreaks; among African healers, pharmacists, researchers, business entrepreneurs, and national institutes in relation to multinational drug researchers and manufacturers; between refugees and émigrés and all the agencies they interact with (relief workers, NGOs, national immigration officials, and foreign cities) as they take up residence in other lands.

These conversations and encounters also demonstrate the creative ways that globalization operates at both the far reaches of the unfamiliar and in the re-creation of the local. Individuals like Byamungu in Bukavu and Farah Abdi in Kansas City occupy strategic points on international networks, yet they also are situated within regional and national networks. They build institutional frameworks and understandings. They become power brokers in their own communities and beyond, in the wider society. What is most "new" in this perspective is the reflexive self-consciousness among such African actors of their place in the global redefinition of society, economy, culture, and of course, medicine and healing.

Notes

1. Globalization, transnational studies, the cross-border analysis of society and culture, and the circulation of cultural meanings, objects, and identities in diffuse time-space have long occupied anthropologists, at least since Emmanuel Wallerstein's "world system" in *Africa and the Modern World* (1986), Eric Wolf's

"center and periphery" in *Europe and the People without History* (1982), and George Marcus' "Ethnography in/of the World System: The Emergence of Multi-Sited Ethnography" (1995). More recently, Arjun Appadurai, in *Modernity at Large: Cultural Dimensions of Globalization* (1997) and *Fear of Small Numbers* (2006), seeks to understand "the global now." See also Beaujard (2006) for new formulations on globalization in health and development issues, and, in Africanist medical anthropology, Tracy Luedke and Harry West's *Borders and Healers* (2006).

2. James Ferguson recommends taking "relations as primary, rather than objects," and "re-conceptualiz[ing] objects as sets of practice"(Ferguson in Finkelstein and Zeiderman 2006: 23), whereas Anna Tsing, an economic anthropologist, advocates examining "[supply] chains of capital, labor, and community" (Tsing in Finkelstein and Zeiderman 2006: 23).

3. The Nike swoosh is one of the great examples of a globalized symbol that has been created to generate a significance for a commodity that is totally separated from the sweat shops that produce it, the shipping chains that deliver it, and the sales that give it value (Tsing in Finkelstein and Zeiderman 2006: 24). Using a similar perspective, van der Geest and associates have studied the construction of metaphors by which medicines are given their signification along the course of their development and use: before a sale, as used and understood in treatment, and in the post-treatment follow-up assessment of the efficacy of the intervention (van der Geest and Whyte 1989; van der Geest, Whyte, and Hardon 1996; Whyte, van der Geest, and Hardon 2002). Studies of this global media anticipate and follow the circulation of goods, symbols, and metaphors as they create powerful associations, meanings, and desires in people who usually cannot begin to afford them.

4. Appadurai (2006: 131ff) has emphasized the new quality of this modernization whose outcome is neither teleological nor predictable: it may offer both alienation bred of anger and predatory marginalized identity, and an opportunity for creative "grassroots globalization" that may provide solutions to local challenges as global connections and resources are brought together.

5. This is the same world in which the South African government stood up to the pharmaceutical giants and intimidated them into allowing generic ARVs into the African market to deal with the horrendous HIV/AIDS epidemic. That story is reviewed by, among others, Didier Fassin (2007: 66–70).

References

Agence France Presse. 2004. "Un an après, le village de Mbomo vit toujours dans la crainte d'Ebola. CONGO (BRAZZA)—16 décembre." Electronic document: http://www.lintelligent.com/gabarits/articleAFP_online .asp?art_cle=AFP43304unanaalobed0.

Agier, Michael. 2002. "Between War and City: Towards an Urban Anthropology of Refugee Camps." Ethnography 3 (3): 317–341.

Appadurai, Arjun. 1997. Modernity at Large: Cultural Dimensions of Globalization. Minneapolis: University of Minnesota Press.

———. 2006. Fear of Small Numbers: An Essay on the Geography of Anger. Durham, N.C.: Duke University Press.

Beaujard, Philippe. 2006. "Globalization and Re-qualification of Societies and Territories." Research Theme, Centre d'Etudes Africaines, University of Paris. Electronic document: http://lodel.ehess.fr/ceaf/document .php?id=280.

Byamungu Lufungula wa Chibanga-banga. 1982. Plantes médicinales, les rites thérapeutiques, et autres connaissances en médecine des guerisseurs au Kivu. Kinshasa, Democratic Republic of the Congo: Centre de Médecine des Guerisseurs.

Capps, Lisa. 1994. "Change and Continuity in the Medical Culture of the Hmong in Kansas City." Medical Anthropology Quarterly 8 (2): 161–177.

Chavez, Leo R. 2003. "Immigration and Medical Anthropology." In American Arrivals: Anthropology Engages the New Immigration, ed. Nancy Foner, 197–228. Santa Fe, N.M.: School of American Research Press.

Choby, Alexandra. 2000. "Trauma Memory and Healing in Vietnamese-Americans." M.A. Thesis, Department of Anthropology, University of Kansas.

Clapp, Roger Alex, and Carolyn Crook. 2002. "Drowning in the Magic Well: Shaman Pharmaceuticals and the Elusive Value of Traditional Knowledge." Journal of Environment & Development 11 (1): 79–102.

Colvin, Christopher. 2006. "Shifting Geographies of Suffering and Recovery: Traumatic Storytelling after Apartheid." In Borders & Healers, ed. Tracy J. Luedke and Harry G. West, 166–184. Bloomington: Indiana University Press.

Davis, Christopher. 2000. Death in Abeyance: Illness and Therapy among the Tabwa of Central Africa. Edinburgh: University of Edinburgh Press, for the International African Institute.

De Wildeman, E. 1935. A Propos de Medicaments Indigènes Congolais. Bruxelles: Institut Royal Colonial Belge, Section des Sciences Naturelles et Medicales. Memoires, Tome III, Fascicule 3.

Douglas, Mary. 1970. Natural Symbols: Explorations in Cosmology. New York: Random House.

———. 1992. Risk and Blame: Essays in Cultural Theory. London: Routledge.

Epelboin, Alain, and Pierre Formenty. 2003. "Anthropologie appliquée en situation d'épidemie: Ebola au Congo en 2003." Electronic document: http://www.pathexo.fr/pages/Ebola/Epelboin.htm.

Fassin, Didier. 2007. When Bodies Remember: Experiences and Politics of AIDS in South Africa. Berkeley: University of California Press.

Finkelstein, Maura, and Austin Zeiderman. 2006. "The Practice and Politics of Global Fieldwork: Keynotes from James Ferguson and Anna Tsing." Anthropology News (Sept.): 23–24.

Foner, Nancy, ed. 2003. American Arrivals: Anthropology Engages the New Immigration. Santa Fe, N.M.: School of American Research Press.

Formenty, Pierre. 2004. "Leçons apprises lors des dernières épidémies d'Ebola en Afrique." Electronic document: http://www.pathexo.fr/pages/Ebola/Formenty.htm.

Formenty, Pierre, Cathy Roth, and Thomas Grein. 2004. "Institut Pasteur. Les épidémies de fièvre hemoragique à virus ebola en Afrique Centrale (2001–2003). Quelles stratégies adopter pour controller les futures flambées?" Paris: Atelier sur les fièvres hemorragiques virales, Institut Pasteur. Sept. 7–8. Electronic document: http://www.pathexo.fr/pages/Ebola/program.html.

Gozdziak, Elzbieta M., and Dianna J. Shandy, eds. 2002. "Editorial Introduction: Religion and Spirituality in Forced Migration." Special Issue: "Religion and Spirituality in Forced Migration," Journal of Refugee Studies 15 (2): 129–135.

Hirsch, Jennifer S. 2003. "Anthropologists, Migrants, and Health Research." In American Arrivals: Anthropology Engages the New Immigration, ed. Nancy Foner, 229–258. Santa Fe, N.M.: School of American Research Press.

Holtzman, John. 2000. Nuer Journeys, Nuer Lives: Sudanese Refugees in Minnesota. Needham Heights, Mass.: Allyn & Bacon.

IRIN (United Nations Office for the Coordination of Humanitarian Affairs). 2007a. "Suspected haemorrhagic fever claims 100 in Kasai." August 30. Electronic document: http://www.irinnews.org/Report.aspx?ReportId=74029.

———. 2007b. "DRC [Ebola] Outbreak Contained." November 4. Electronic document: http://www.irinnews.org/report.aspx?ReportId=74300.

Janzen, John M. 1978. The Quest for Therapy in Lower Zaire. Berkeley: University of California Press.

———. 1999. "Text and Context in the Anthropology of War Trauma: The African Great Lakes Region 1993–95." Suomen Antropologi 24 (4): 37–57.

———. 2003. "Illusions of Home in the Story of a Rwandan Refugee's Return." In Coming Home: Toward an Ethnography of Return, ed. Ellen Oxfeld and Lynellyn Long, 19–33. Philadelphia: University of Pennsylvania Press.

———. 2005. "Etiological Dualism in Ebola Public Health Crises in Central Africa." Paper presented at the African Studies Association Meetings, Ethnographic Turns and Cognitive Dissonance: Exploring Science, Magic, Healing, and Race, a panel directed by Helen Tilley. Washington D.C., Nov. 18.

Janzen, John M., and Reinhild Kauenhoven Janzen. 2000. Do I Still Have a Life? Voices from the Aftermath of War in Rwanda and Burundi, 1994–1995. University of Kansas Monographs in Anthropology 20. Lawrence, Kans.: University of Kansas.

Janzen, John M., Adrien Ngudiankama, and Melissa Filippi-Franz. 2005. "Religious Healing among War-Traumatized African Immigrants." In Religion and Healing in America, ed. Linda Barnes and Susan Sered, 159–172. New York: Oxford University Press.

KASC (Kansas African Studies Center). 2005–2006. "Identity, Voice, and Community among New African Immigrants to Kansas." Kansas Humanities Council Project Interviews and Proceedings. Unpublished.

Luedke, Tracy J., and Harry G. West. 2006. Borders and Healers: Brokering Therapeutic Resources in Southeast Africa. Bloomington: Indiana University Press.

Malkki, Liisa. 1995a. Purity and Exile: Violence, Memory, and National Cosmology among Hutu Refugees in Tanzania. Chicago: University of Chicago Press.

———. 1995b. "Refugees and Exile: From 'Refugee Studies' to the National Order of Things." Annual Review of Anthropology 24: 495–523.

Marcus, George. 1995. "Ethnography in/of the World System: The Emergence of Multi-Sited Ethnography." Annual Review of Anthropology 24: 95–117.

Ngubane, Harriet. 1977. Body and Mind in Zulu Medicine. New York: Academic Press.

Ngudiankama, Adrien 2001. "Concepts of Health and Therapeutic Options among Congolese Refugees in London: Implications for Education." PhD diss., University of London.

NOVA. 1996. "Ebola: The Plague Fighters." 60 min. VHS Film.

Simmons, David. 2006. "Of Markets and Medicine: The Changing Significance of Zimbabwean Muti in the Age of Intensified Globalization." In Borders & Healers, ed. Tracy J. Luedke and Harry G. West, 65–80. Bloomington: Indiana University Press.

van der Geest, Sjaak, and Susan Reynolds Whyte. 1989. "The Charm of Medicines: Metaphors and Metonyms." Medical Anthropology Quarterly 3 (4): 345–367.

van der Geest, Sjaak, Susan Reynolds Whyte, and Anita Hardon. 1996. "The Anthropology of Pharmaceuticals: A Biographical Approach." Annual Review of Anthropology 25: 153–178.

Verwey, Martine, ed. 2001. "Trauma und Ressourcen / Trauma and Empowerment." (Special Issue) Curare 16.

Wallerstein, Immanuel. 1986. Africa and the Modern World. Trenton, N.J.: Africa World Press.

Waterman, Tara. 1999. "Tara's Ebola Site." Honors thesis, Department of Human Biology, Stanford University. Electronic document: http://www.stanford.edu/group/virus/filo/refs.html.

Whyte, Susan Reynolds, Sjaak van der Geest, and Anita Hardon. 2002. Social Lives of Medicines. Cambridge: Cambridge University Press.

Wolf, Eric R. 1982. Europe and the People Without History. Berkeley: University of California Press.

World Health Organization. 2004. "Ebola in Yambio." Electronic document: http://www.who.int/features/2004/ebola/en/.

FIVE

AIDS Policies for Markets and Warriors: Dispossession, Capital, and Pharmaceuticals in Nigeria

Kristin Peterson

Dispossession and Its Organizational Strategies

Most of the literature on globalization that theorizes flexible capital, flows (media, migration, technology), global cities, cosmopolitanism, and local–global relationships proceeds from an analysis of finance and manufacturing capital.[1] Such paradigms account for accumulation, speed, and the migratory patterns of both people and technology via capital circulating among cybernetic and physical spaces. As one imagines the enormity of capital movement, what is said of the spaces and places that are emptied out, from which these voluminous forms of capital are originally extracted? As it is widely recognized that the African continent continues to provide raw material in the form of oil, minerals, and cash crops to the rest of the world in crumbling and non-reproducible ways, can there be an analysis of an emptied-out space as the left-behind effect of such movement? Can there be an accounting of this space that is connected to but defies overlap with other spaces in the transnational realm; an account that, though cannot always imagine how raw material and capital are transformed and consumed beyond its boundaries, is not parochial in the estimation of its own loss?

When it comes to theorizing Africa's relationship to globalization, there is remarkably little said other than that Africa is simply marginalized in the global political economy.[2] However, Africa is being rigorously "reinscribed" in the world via trade, development, and economic policies that suggest an importance greater than simple marginalization. How African states comply with the World Trade Organization (WTO), for example, will largely determine the role and activities of trade and global governance in ways that are yet to be imagined, as well as in ways that are alarmingly on the horizon, such as the slow and rigorous wiping away of the generic drug industry via legal measures found in numerous free trade agreements.

This chapter assesses a form of "lively capital" that begins with the following assumptions: wealth accumulation as described by analyses of speculative and manufacturing capital, global cities, etc., cannot solely account for the contours or performance of global capitalism and Africa's relationship to it. Rather, Africa is an imperative and integral part of current processes of globalization that include the continent's cultural and economic representations, the building of new capital markets, and the redirected efforts of foreign aid that are increasingly being tied to global securitization. Instead of thinking about globalization as a unitary capitalism, I am more interested in theories of capital that may better capture and complicate Africa in the world, as more than one capitalism is at play and at stake here.[3] In these paradigms, therefore, more attention needs to be paid to *wealth extraction* and *dispossession,*[4] whereby emptied-out material space is generated by both extractive industries and overlapping configurations of policy making and capital mobility. This dispossessed space provides the seams upon which emergent and competing kinds of capital, as well as social and institutional exchange, find their roots and grow. In this particular instance, they manifest as varying forms of pharmaceutical capital, whose circulation and existence are tied to oil, debt, and military economies.[5]

By describing the institution of pharmacy (defined as the discipline of drug dispensation and composition), and to a lesser extent drug manufacturing, in Nigeria as exemplary of emptied-out space, I am not referring to *terra nullius,* which would imply sheer absence in a colonial imaginary—an absence that has in fact been conceived in the past, the modern ghost of which is invoked by the pharmaceutical industry as "lack of infrastructure," used as a prime reason to refuse adequate drug price reductions. Nor am I suggesting that the colonial state was a robust entity that extended its drug distribution efforts beyond the citizen to the subject, a task now begging the attention of the postcolonial state. Rather, I am referring to two means of dispossession: the first is the 1986 International Monetary Fund's (IMF) structural adjustment program (SAP) that was strongly tied to a rise of militarism in Nigeria and a protracted pro-democracy movement. The SAP initiated the massive emptying out of existing health institutions and pharmacy and disabled drug manufacturing (via currency devaluation, wage decreases, state privatization and dismantling, etc.).[6] Other therapeutic institutions emerged to replace the dying ones, and with them new professional and patient agencies, strategies, and subjectivities came into being, literally enveloping older forms. The second is a more refined form of dispossession that attempts to dismantle the generic drug industry's market viability through two routes: trade-related intellectual property law and specific AIDS treatment policies, both of which emphasize and privilege proprietary transnational drug companies and the circulation of their products.

By exploring the near death of an industry and the subsequent rise of neoliberal health policies, I show how wealth extraction and other forms of dispossession are preconditions for generating contradictory *imperatives of capital* as they relate to old battles over the social contract, but also how they are largely being reterritorialized in these new scenarios (Ferguson 2005). Marx described two competing forms of capital, one that perpetuates further production (1977) and the other that perpetuates further circulation (1959). More recently, David Harvey's important insights on capital mobility, described as "accumulation by dispossession" (2003: 137–182), rethink the importance of primitive accumulation since 1973—a process that (in contrast to Luxemburg's [1968] formulations, yet following Arendt [1968]) remains an important strategy for capitalist expansion in the twenty-first century.[7] Using Marx and Harvey[8] to frame the larger politics and stakes, I would argue that what we are seeing in these dispossession/reinvestment strategies is the combination of territorial and capital logics with policy logics that specifically merge in the context of AIDS. Here, I refer to the financial interaction among and capital movement facilitated by policy organizations as well as financial institutions overseeing the implementation of policy. Policy organizations, the state, corporations, and AIDS activists brought together by AIDS make *implicit agreements* with each other that generate very particular kinds of capital flows. In this context, implicitness represents the very crux of policy logics reacting to neoliberal strategies and reform. That is, health care systems as means of comprehensive care are increasingly overlooked in favor of policies that address "the gaps" in care, such as prevention and treatment for HIV. Nonexistent robust health systems infrastructure is a prerequisite for implementing policy that addresses these infrastructure gaps. This has led to new ideas about health, bodies, and surveillance collated by a myriad of consenting actors and institutions that generate abstractions and analysis of "the gaps." As a result, the "gaps" in health care systems are transformed into a system itself, for which humanitarian and government organizations deploy millions of dollars dedicated to new infrastructure while comprehensive health systems are left to wither in neglect; it is a scenario where the logics of health and economic crises both presuppose and require each other. The phrase "implicit agreements" thus points to how economic and health abstractions become naturalized as normative social and institutional exchange. The policy-driven capital form is thus simply a question of how capital naturalizes its own mobility and operation.

Until the recent implementation of the U.S. President's Emergency Program for HIV/AIDS Relief (PEPFAR) for select states including Nigeria, most AIDS development agencies have favored HIV prevention policies over widespread treatment. This means that in Nigeria, for example, HIV education and prevention programs function as an AIDS humanitarian apparatus that provides protectionist measures for the oil extraction industry. That is, long-term and sustainable AIDS treatment polices would require, first and foremost, converting oil wealth[9] into funding for treatment for the nearly five million who are HIV-positive and many more who are infected with numerous other infectious diseases. Fundamentally, any attempt toward widespread treatment necessitates reconfiguring the relationship between African states and their corporate partners, between external debt and foreign aid, between African states and their creditors. Because Africa's creditors are also Africa's AIDS donors (World Bank, Paris Club members, the United States), it is perhaps no coincidence that a very particular biopolitical regime manages HIV bodies as well as relationships between the state, humanitarian, and international financial institutions.

In these interdependent contexts, the state's role is to facilitate, orchestrate, and permit "accumulation by dispossession to occur without sparking a general collapse" (Harvey 2003: 115)—constituting the general gist of an IMF SAP. While Roitman (2005), Mbembe (2001), Bayart (1997), Ake (1996), and Brotherton (2008) have all demonstrated how the state in Africa[10] does act in its own interests, turning dispossession into new kinds of accumulation, I would furthermore suggest that the state's technological capacities are shifting into other technological priorities that inscribe new patterns of capital flow and formation. In such cases, the state and capital are not always at odds with one another: it is not always the case that the state erodes while capital flourishes. Certainly for Nigeria, the primary source of accumulation is not based on wage labor, but rather government contracts and oil rent politics through which accumulation is fundamentally channeled via the state, so that the state and capital actually rearticulate each other.[11] If anything, there can exist stringent and lax laws in the same space that enable and disenfranchise certain capital manifestations, where the state's own interests are both fulfilled and erased.[12] This is a contradiction that largely emerges in the aftermath of a state privatization and is particularly visible within Nigeria's current efforts to be more squarely inserted into global markets.

This rest of this chapter describes the shrinkage of pharmacy and decline of drug manufacturing since IMF structural adjustment, and the resultant lack of available quality drugs. It also describes the excess of counterfeits, illegal drug markets, self-medication, and drug-labeling problems as material-ity and practice produced in a "post"-IMF space. It then examines how two treatment policies (one Nigerian, one from the U.S.) map onto these spatial environments. Special attention is paid to the merging of security and health discourses in the implementation of these treatment policies. Here "house-hold security" loses ground in the context of AIDS to "national security," giving rise to new policy logics that bypass the aftermath of health care infra-structure dispossessions. Ultimately, I argue that the 1986 IMF SAP in Nigeria constitutes a particular historical moment that emptied out Nigerian and other African pharmacies while inaugurating new protectionist measures for the global circulation of pharmaceuticals, wherein new markets and security cultures thrive.

Franz Fanon wrote "it was not the organization of production but the persistence and organization of oppression which formed the primary social basis for revolutionary activity" (Fanon 1966: 88, cited in Robison 1997: 134 and discussed by Gordon 2004).[13] In following Fanon, and in viewing *dispossession* as a form of *oppression*, I argue that dispossession is the primary organizational strategy that generates the protectionist measures that alter health and medi-cal practices, including drug production and consumption. The very drive of this dispossession is in the implicit agreements made among institutions to enable capital to thickly accumulate in ways that contradict the interests of public health. It may be counterintuitive to imagine that state and other forms of dispossession negate capital accumulation and wealth.[14] Indeed, dispos-session ultimately curtails incentives for foreign direct investment when state services like electricity no longer function properly and social conflict carries on amidst scarce resources. But in what follows I will show how dispossession actually serves as a productive contradiction in a Marxist sense. Here, the AIDS policy is a pivoting anchor that enables the subsidizing of new drug markets, and, particularly for Nigeria, keeps the flow of oil wealth sustained in ways that continually reproduce national and international elites. In the process, the state both consumes and negates its own interests, and the population must negotiate a therapeutic economy and knowledge that edges on a dangerous medical pluralism.

Emptying Out Pharmacy, Dismantling Drug Manufacturing

In the mid-1980s, the Nigerian pharmaceutical manufacturing industry comprised over 50 manufacturing firms that produced generics for malaria and other pertinent endemic parasites and diseases. By 1996, ten years after structural adjustment implementation, nearly two thirds of the industry had bottomed out. Two IMF austerity measures (among others) were instrumental in this decline. The first was a high tax placed on imported raw materials. The tax was viewed as a step in increasing local production of raw materials, justified by the IMF as the need to wipe out "non-essential" state imports. The second was the devaluation of the currency (the naira), which cut earning power across the country in half within the first month of structural adjustment implementation (it further declined after that). This had two effects. One, it eliminated purchasing power for local manufacturers, who could no longer invest or reinvest in raw material production. As of now, 100 percent of all raw materials for drug manufacture are imported to Nigeria at extraordinary costs, defying the IMF's original claims about providing impetus for self-sustainability. Two, the purchasing power of the consumer was also devastated, such that those who sought out generic Nigerian drugs either had to pay much more, or were pushed to seek other alternatives such as traditional medicine and the generally untrustworthy entrepreneurs who claim to have a cure for AIDS. Traditional medicine has always comprised part of the therapeutic economy; it is estimated that currently 70 percent of the population seeks out traditional healers as primary health care providers due to their familiarity and more flexible rates (Maiwada 2004). This figure correlates with most estimates that 70 percent of the population lives on less than 1 USD per day.

Both private capital flight[15] and the national debt repayment are derived almost exclusively from oil wealth, and both represent primary forms of wealth extraction. State privatization, trade liberalization, the removal of petroleum subsidies, and the devaluation of the naira led to decreased earnings, and food prices nearly quadrupled. Nigeria faced increased black market expansion, heightened poverty, increased crime, food riots, and worker strikes. Primary health care services collapsed—which impeded the IMF's stated goal of building self-reliance—while the Fund envisioned total cost recovery from patients who could not afford even basic food commodities (Salako 1997). In Nigeria, capital investments and recurrent payments such as salaries, essential drugs, and facilities maintenance were suspended (Samba 2004). With the introduction of user fees and the sale of drugs liberalized, the public consumption of drugs drastically declined. By 1990, the domestic production of pharmaceuticals ceased almost entirely not only in Nigeria but throughout Africa; most pharmaceutical and medical supply industries were pushed into bankruptcy; and medical workers fled to the private sector both within and outside of Africa (Samba 2004).

The SAP also impacted drug distribution systems, which were already facing great difficulties and challenges.[16] Nigeria's original drug dispensation program was based on a colonial administrative system where drugs were transported to central stores and dispensed by government pharmacists. Following the civil war (1967–1970) and the oil boom of the 1970s, there was massive hospital and health care expansion. Additionally, overseas manufacturers found the 70 million–person market to be lucrative and started to pack and distribute imported drugs in Nigeria. Companies such as Pfizer, Abbott, Glaxo, Wellcome, and Roche came to Nigeria and manufactured drugs (Ovbiagele 2000). The colonial system of drug dispensation could not meet the needs of an expanding health care system and the government was slow to react. Steeped in postwar reconstruction efforts, it could not immediately reconstitute or expand the regulatory structures to forestall the growing chaos of drug distribution (Ovbiagele 2000). With an oil bust producing a severe economic crisis, the government took a desperate measure that liberalized drug import policies via an "import license" whereby non-pharmacists could freely import drugs and sell them at huge profits. As a result, massive numbers of fake drugs entered the country and, together, military and civilian counterparts took over drug markets. It was not until 1990 that the National Drug Policy was executed, giving rise to the National Agency for Drug Administration and Control (NAFDAC), Nigeria's drug regulatory agency, which remains to this day highly underfunded.

By 2005, Nigeria had accumulated a total debt of 36 billion USD; finally, the country threatened to repudiate what it deemed an illegitimate accumulation of debt by corrupt military leaders who did not pay as scheduled, while late payment fines and arrears amounted to billions even though the principle had been paid off at least three times. By 2001, with the end of military rule, payments made annually to foreign creditors were in the sum of 2 billion USD while only 300 million USD was allocated toward the entire national health care budget, a budget designated for 120 million people. The health budget of 2001 was 1.9 percent of the total national budget [7 USD per capita] (WHOSIS 2001).[17]

In the same year, *nearly half* of all drugs in circulation were found to be counterfeit or substandard (Taylor et al. 2001). Such drugs are mostly found in the tens of thousands of drug markets across the country. The 2001 statistic on fake and substandard drugs may be declining, as the former director of Nigeria's drug regulatory agency (NAFDAC), Dora Akunyili, started a campaign to confiscate and burn fake drugs in great public displays before the media. As a result, she and many NAFDAC workers have been attacked in markets; there have been several car bombs and assassination attempts on their lives, as well as the burning down of the NAFDAC headquarters in 2003. Market sellers in open drug markets have rarely been prosecuted in the past despite good laws on the books, and in using their own union for protection they are fighting the prospect of unemployment. Whether or not Akunyili's efforts were effective, the public attention brought to fake and counterfeit drugs marks a shift in consciousness on the presence of fake drugs in the country.

In contrast to the numerous illegal drug markets, pharmacies are very few and over 90 percent of them are in the urban areas, 30 percent of which are concentrated in the city of Lagos. Out of the 36 states, only six have more than 100 pharmacies, and five states have fewer than 15, which are meant to serve up to millions of people (PCN 2000) out of a population of 130 million.[18] There are nearly four times the number of registered pharmacists as there are pharmacy premises, perhaps pointing to the problems of gaining startup capital and steady electric supplies. For years few hospitals in Nigeria have been actually registered to dispense drugs. Rather, doctors dispense drugs and are not keen on turning over dispensing responsibilities to pharmacists, a situation which some regulatory officials who spoke to me have resigned themselves to as a fact of life.

As the profession has declined, pharmaceutical practice itself has changed. Even in the urban areas where pharmacies are accessible, the process of drug dispensing is highly mystified for many patients. The names and dosages of drugs prescribed to patients are rarely labeled (Taylor 1998), and this lack is not only common practice but in fact the policy of many hospitals and pharmacies. For example, I was in Owerri, in the eastern part of the country, with Mary, a nurse and AIDS activist. We went to see her family in a nearby village, and when we arrived we found that her mother-in-law was ill. The next day we took her to the hospital in town, where she waited most of the day to see a doctor. After she finished up we walked with her to the hospital pharmacy, where she picked up her prescribed medication. There was a sign posted next to the pharmacy window in both English and Igbo that encouraged any questions about the drugs they were receiving. Mary's mother-in-law received her drugs in a plastic bag marked in pen with the number of pills she should take per day. The name and dosage of the drug was not listed. Mary went back to the pharmacy and asked them to label it "correctly." The conversation escalated in the street, with Mary yelling at two hospital administrators on their non-labeling policy and a couple dozen patients gathered around to hear it out. They calmly told Mary that too many patients self-medicate and that is the reason why they cannot label prescriptions, to which Mary countered, "and what happens when your patients have adverse side effects or allergic reactions to prescribed drugs? How will any medical worker ever know what was prescribed when the patient has no idea? And what if the patient dies? Then what?" To these questions, there was no response.

Indeed, the fear of self-medication (the most common method of treatment) of controlled products is the most common justification pharmacists give for non-labeling. But conversations I had with many pharmacists indicate that something else is at work, which is perhaps the desire to keep knowledge of drugs circulating only among pharmacists. Many articulated what seemed like a mantra that self-medication must be prevented by this means. Very few wanted to explore the notion of assisting a very large self-medicating population (Bright and Taylor 1999).[19] The profession of pharmacy, long held in esteem, has been increasingly denigrated due to the inhospitable climate of drug distribution and difficulties in competing against "illegitimate" businesses. Perhaps non-labeling acts as a reconfiguration of expertise where making certain knowledge secret gives a sense of authority back to a profession that no longer commands legitimacy or status. Revealingly, one of the newsletters of the Pharmacists' Counsel of Nigeria stated at the 1999 annual meetings that a newly institutionalized prefix, "Pharm," would precede Mr. and Mrs. prefixes. This prefix is now used as common practice among pharmacists. Together, the mystification of drug knowledge and new titles establish a sense of control over professional loss.

Of course, the control of knowledge does not preclude any patient from seeking the information she wants. Patients often obtain their knowledge of drugs from market sellers, most of whom are not trained as pharmacists. I have walked through the Lagos drug markets, where both controlled and uncontrolled substances can be found, and where there are usually no ideal conditions for storing and keeping drugs. I have watched buyers give sellers a list of symptoms for which the seller proceeds to find the appropriate medication in his supply.[20] Moreover, hospitals and clinics also get their supplies from these markets; pickup trucks with hospital logos regularly pull up to restock their supplies.[21] So, not only do patients prefer to buy in markets, but so do physicians. In Lagos a report estimated that 58 percent of all physicians purchase from drug markets as their vendors of choice because of availability and ease (PGM-MAN 2001), despite the fact that some of these markets contain substandard or counterfeit drugs.

Many people I interviewed seeking drugs preferred to buy them in the markets. This form of self-medication also saves money, because going to a doctor for treatment and care can generate additional costs. Drug availability even extends to roadside "hawkers" who sell medications of all sorts in traffic jams and along busy and commercial roads, literally appearing and disappearing with the traffic itself. Sellers are also found on public transport. While taking buses to other parts of the country, I encountered traveling drug salesmen on board who take turns wooing the crowd by offering candy and not-very-funny jokes about gender relations and then launch into the efficacy of their wares. The crowd on such bus rides evolves from boredom and annoyance into enthusiasm and consumer passion. Pain pills, antibiotics, acne busters, and aloe vera were offered for sale, and I even bought some imported Indian *Neem* toothpaste. Manthia Diawara has argued that:

> West African markets provide a serious challenge to the scheme of globalization and structural adjustment fostered by the World Bank and other multinational corporations that are vying to recolonize Africa. . . . [W]hat makes these traditional schemes of globalization special is the structural continuity they maintain with contemporary markets in opposition to the forms and structures of modernism that the nation-states have put in place in West Africa since the 1960s. (Diawara 1998: 114–115)

Indeed, economics are largely controlled and determined inside the markets (stationary and mobile) and not the banks. Diawara rightly claims that this poses a challenge to financial institutions that see the nation-state as the only legitimate vehicle through which to conduct business (1998: 116). Diawara describes a typical scenario: state officials depend upon markets to cope with the struggling economy because currency can be exchanged there at higher rates than banks offer, low civil service wages can be enhanced by bribes, and the markets may even provide forms of emergency cash to a strapped government (Diawara 1998: 116). This is a system of recycling indebtedness that actually helps to stabilize a financial crisis (Diawara 1998: 117) and is tied to a conglomeration of state practices where notions of the public and private are highly blurred.

The extent of counterfeit, fake, and substandard drugs located in the markets and on the streets actually represents a remarkable contradiction. On the one hand, the dispossession of the Nigerian pharmaceutical industry's capacity to, at best, carry out good manufacturing practices, freed up space for new, mostly imported, drug products to take root—drugs that can bypass regulatory organs of the state. During the 1990s, these drugs competed especially with global company products that had distribution outlets in the country. In the process of an IMF-generated dispossession that would lay the ground for new proprietary pharmaceutical capital, counterfeit drugs, which made up about 80 percent of the national drug market, became the thorn in the proprietary distribution agenda. In this sense, the drug markets provided the very challenge to state privatization and neoliberal reform that Diawara claims above.[22] For Diawara: "as postmodern reality defines historicity and ethics through consumption, those who do not consume are left to die outside of history and without human dignity. The traditional markets are the only places where Africans of all ethnic origins and classes, from the country and the city meet and assert their humanity and historicity through consumption (1998: 120–121)." On the other hand, there are a great number of counterfeits and fakes that can create severe side effects and injury, which puts the "right to consume" in jeopardy and thus the role of both the state and the market in question. The "right to consume" needs to be situated in the context of the "right to produce" and the "right to regulate," which together make for a messy configuration; and as these rights of the individual and the nation-state surface, forms of medical pluralism continue to thrive.

At the very same time that fake and counterfeit drugs were wildly out-competing the global proprietary drugs in Nigeria (and counterfeits of all sorts were doing the same in other parts of the world), demands for increased intellectual property protection began to be made by private industry and Western governments via the WTO. As stated above, NAFDAC has made moves to break down drug markets in the interest of both protecting propri-etary drug businesses (an agenda that was explicitly emphasized to me) and public health. This certainly does protect the intellectual property rights of the global proprietary industry. But it is starting to give an unexpected boost to the local generic industry, whose products were also widely copied during the 1990s. In the context of this rebirth, a different form of dispossession is creeping in that poses threats to the local manufacturing industry. This clear-ing is making room for U.S.-subsidized proprietary antiretroviral drugs via the politics of trade-related intellectual property law as well as AIDS treatment policies. But this more refined emptying out may actually destabilize the very new capital forms that are just beginning to be cultivated in this dispossessed drug landscape.

AIDS Treatment Policies and New Capital Imperatives

In Nigeria there are two major antiretroviral treatment policies. One is the Nigerian government's, which uses only generic drugs produced in India by Ranbaxy and Cipla for the 20,000 enrolled patients (out of four million HIV-positive people, 400,000 are estimated to be in immediate need of ARVs). The second uses both generic and proprietary drugs that are being supplied by PEPFAR—the largest international health initiative ever to target a single disease. In Nigeria, PEPFAR subsidizes and distributes U.S. proprietary drugs to over 100,000 patients.[23] Over 20 million USD was allocated to PEPFAR in Nigeria for fiscal years 2004–2006. There is no long-term plan of sustainability for either program. The initial PEPFAR plan was to allocate drugs and treatment for five years, later extended by the Bush administration up through 2013. In the meantime, the Nigerian government plan is slowly yielding ground to PEPFAR, as it is less expensive to patients than the government's program.

Both programs involve different treatment regimens, are differently subsidized, and are highly politicized. As a Nigerian government supplier, Ranbaxy cornered the generic market in the early 2000s, and their drug prices actually exceeded the cost of similar generics. And there have been tensions: while at the 2004 Nigerian National AIDS conference, I witnessed a confrontation between Ranbaxy and Nigerian AIDS activists over the fact that the company was selling ARVs at their booth without a prescription. There are numerous other incidences that indicate that Ranbaxy does not want the more extreme problems of drug distribution in Nigeria to be widespread public knowledge, particularly the issues that surround counterfeits. The company must contend with a popular Nigerian opinion held over since the SAP that the majority of counterfeits are made and exported from India and China (generics and fakes can often be confused as the same, but fakes are often referred to as "India" drugs). Moreover, the Nigerian government has been accused of poor distribution and operations, the worst of which was a two-month-long drug shortage in 2002 due to bureaucratic complications—another reason that PEPFAR is gaining ground.[24]

PEPFAR constitutes the largest rollout of public health funding in history. It follows a particular policy logic initiated by Bill Clinton, who declared HIV/AIDS a national security threat in the mid-1990s. Since then, the rationales of health and security policies have increasingly merged in several different international arenas. For example, the U.S. Africa Command (AFRICOM) integrates staff structures from the U.S. Department of the State, the U.S. Agency for International Development, and humanitarian organizations into existing military structures to conduct tasks ranging from managing AIDS to sharing intelligence. Indeed, the Office of the U.S. Global AIDS Coordinator, which heads PEPFAR, has been moved out of U.S. offices managing traditional development work and now answers to the State Department under the Secretary of State. Furthermore, the U.S. Department of Defense has a large role to play in the PEPFAR countries, including Nigeria, which occupies a high spot on the list of U.S. security concerns. In Nigeria, not only does the Department of Defense have well-endowed AIDS projects,[25] but so too does the Henry M. Jackson Foundation, a philanthropic organization dedicated to subsidizing what it calls "military medicine," which largely constructs infectious disease as part and parcel of security discourse.

Stefan Elbe (2005) shows how these events reflect the ways a range of actors (international organizations, governments, and NGOs) are cast in the name of the survival of communities, economics, militaries, and governments. Key here is how such mobilization is engaged by the language of security and emergency, which as Alan Ingram (2007: 516) describes "takes HIV/ AIDS out of the sphere of 'normal politics' and creates obligations to respond in ways that are adequate to the new salience of the problem." As a result, policy becomes less directed toward civil society and more directed toward security and intelligence (Elbe 2005; Ingram 2007). Vinh-Kim Nguyen sums up much of the substance of these new rationales and deployments through his term "experimentality," which he describes as exercising

> . . . a new form of legitimate domination through highly mobile, disaggregated and mutable governmentalities. The latter are biological and political technologies for constituting populations and transforming subjectivities in a focused manner around a particular predicament of government. These predicaments are framed in humanitarian terms and call for urgent measures designed to save lives and prevent suffering, which is understood as an immediate and embodied (or even biological) phenomenon. (Nguyen 2007: 1)

Aside from the general merging of health, development, and security organizations and rationales, Nigeria occupies a very particular place in these new activities because it is a country that is viewed by the U.S. as strategic to both peacekeeping operations in Africa and, more importantly perhaps, to security efforts related to oil supplies throughout the Bight of Benin. Oil is crucial because it constitutes a significant chunk of the country's income; several authors (Apter 2005; Okonta and Douglass 2003; Watts 2001; Zalik 2004; Ingram 2007) have demonstrated how security and oil are abstracted, and how private forms of health development erase the politics and violence of extraction. That is, in order for the rationales and linkages of partnership development (Zalik 2004) and security to actually take hold and play out, HIV prevention and treatment policies must be rationalized as normative in precisely the same way as oil extraction and security paradigms. Translating these paradigms into policy requires a particular form of management: indeed, PEPFAR under the Bush and now Obama administrations mirrors the ways in which the Iraq and Afghanistan wars are managed—largely contracted and outsourced to private partners. The indirect result is that just as West African security expansion is facilitated by U.S. anti-terrorism efforts and the search for steady oil supplies, it may also be expanding off the back of subsidized pharmaceutical products that rely upon AIDS treatment policies for their mobility and consumption.

One of the early predecessors to the Bush administration's PEPFAR initiative was a lesser-known program that may mark the beginning of multilateral AIDS policy networks: the UN Accelerated Access Initiative (AAI), a joint 2000

UNAIDS/WHO/proprietary pharmaceutical industry initiative[26] that utilized public relations firms to bilaterally negotiate the reduction of high and out-of-reach drug prices in Africa. In exchange, stringent intellectual property laws were conceptualized, proposed, and often implemented for African states in a manner that favors and protects multinational pharmaceutical companies' business practices there. After a coalition of drug companies withdrew a well-known suit against South Africa in 2001, claiming that its 1997 Medicines Act violated WTO regulations on compulsory licensing and parallel importation—an act that South Africa never even acted upon—companies taking part in the AAI began to heavily recruit many African countries to negotiate bilateral confidential agreements, with the apparent aim of wiping out the generic drug industry. Two years into the program, ACT UP Paris (ACT UP Paris 2002) reported that UNAIDS and the WHO, which orchestrated the negotiations, never provided any technical assistance to participatory countries in protecting intellectual property law or creating guidelines on relations between countries and companies where the WHO and UNAIDS had forfeited their power (indeed, the companies ultimately took advantage of this freedom to bypass UN oversight) (ACT UP Paris 2002). Health Gap Coalition declared "UNAIDS drug access policies are currently being structured, by and large, in response to big pharma's displeasure" (2000).

Even as these negotiations were hailed as some of the best and only options to provide access to treatment—even though only 0.1 percent more people were put on treatment (ACT UP Paris 2002)—other issues were crucially erased. At the end of this program, drug prices were not heavily slashed, but the AAI served as one of the now many existing gateways for the proprietary pharmaceutical industry to outcompete generics, by making policy that eradicates the generic industry. Such policies and actions shape the compilation of future drug markets, not simply in Africa, but throughout the world.

In addition to bilateral intellectual property negotiations, the Trade Related Intellectual Property (TRIPs) Agreement of the WTO, to which Nigeria is a signatory, gives proprietary pharmaceutical companies exclusive 20-year manufacturing, pricing, and distribution rights on their drug patents. The U.S. government's Agency for International Development (USAID) funds the Commercial Law Development Program (CLDP), an initiative of the U.S. Department of Commerce, to "assist" Nigeria in complying with TRIPs. The CLDP sponsored several meetings jointly with the Nigerian Intellectual Property Law Association between 2000–2004. At these meetings, there were many panels and instructions on how to comply with the TRIPs/WTO geared around how Nigeria can "be on the right side of globalization." Consistently, the discourse, without any explanation, enforced the idea that the stronger a country's intellectual property (IP) law, the more economically viable and powerful it becomes in the global economy. Compared to the vast numbers of IP lawyers in the U.S. and European patent offices who have access to world-wide databases that can easily determine if an invention is new or discern an IP violation, the Nigerian patent office awards a patent simply if the two-page application form is filled out correctly. Such disparities in technology and expertise can hardly be expected to compete internationally or instantly to instantiate power in the global economy.

The U.S. submitted its own drafts of a new Nigerian intellectual property law to the Nigerian government in 2002. I acquired these drafts, which clearly showed that the U.S. desires a law that favors U.S. businesses while wiping out all legal provisions that could allow import of less expensive generic drugs. At the "final" drafting meeting, AIDS activists (with technical support from international actors like Médecins Sans Frontières [Doctors without Borders] and Ralph Nader's Consumer Project on Technology) muscled their way into the meeting to demand the inclusion of "health care safeguards," which were then incorporated into the draft. This was perceived as a great victory. However, less than a year later, the CLDP returned to Nigeria, apparently (according to rumor at least) under the instructions of the U.S. Trademark and Patent Office, which viewed the new Nigeria IP draft as not meeting U.S. desires. A new secret meeting took place without activists' or govern-ment health officials' knowledge. But the meeting became known when its "successful conclusion" was announced on national television. I acquired this latest IP draft—which may or may not be the official document, because in the past, several drafts have been known to be in circulation among Nigerian and U.S. officials who have thus generated confusion over the "real" docu-ment. However, lawyers at Médecins Sans Frontières in Europe analyzed it and found that "data exclusivity" measures were included that, in short, effectively reduce the generic drug industry's capacity to quickly manufacture gener-ics coming off-patent. Such provisions already carried out in other free trade agreements allow proprietary drug companies to keep data confidential. Such an act actually undermines the original intent of the patent, a concept meant to exchange inventive data for short-term exclusive marketing. Moreover, it may be a strategy that slowly begins to wither away the public domain. That is, without the data in hand, a generic company is restricted from developing the technological design to engineer a generic product, a delay that can essen-tially extend the life of a patent.

USAID simultaneously provides a great deal of funding to a number of local AIDS NGOs to carry out prevention and education programs. To some AIDS activists, there is the appearance of a USAID policy contradiction, given that it supports AIDS activism yet also works to severely curtail drug access.

But there may not in fact be a contradiction, as prevention and education campaigns are located in the realm of individual empowerment and responsibility, drawing attention away from the legal structures that generate obstacles to pharmaceutical flows. AIDS activists and NGOs have objected to the relationship between the Nigerian and U.S. governments. But this relationship demonstrates a conflict that the state itself has with multilateral organizations. That is, at global trading negotiations the Nigerian state opposes U.S. and European stances on treatment access, but at the same time it attempts to meet the pressure to comply quietly behind the doors of federal ministries. This contradiction is an outcome of an increasingly common strategy utilized by the U.S. whereby it capitalizes on the lack of communication between ministries, and between ministries and Nigeria's Geneva representatives. Bilateral and regional (trade or otherwise) agreements thus become the alternative avenue and means for compliance when global negotiations continually fail to meet U.S. goals. Yet, what does it mean exactly for Nigeria to buy generic drugs for its own national antiretroviral program while at the same time it cooperates with the U.S. government to legally wipe out generic drug access? Such an action will effectively make its own antiretroviral program illegal. Nigeria still has not complied with TRIPs, and it is not clear when or if that will happen. The outcome of compliance or noncompliance will greatly determine the future of drug access in the country.

Conclusion

The "implicit agreements" made among multilateral institutions fundamentally drive a political economy that relies on dispossession as it primary organizational strategy. Unlike the massive state and economic adjustments made under the IMF that literally teeter economies on the edge of collapse, a sustained dispossession is very particular and targeted; it takes place amidst already chaotic economic and social environments and therefore must operate in more delicate ways that do not threaten the existing thresholds of disintegration. The most particular example is found in struggles over intellectual property designs, struggles that do not necessarily destroy entire economies, but rather target specific industries that are viewed as especially competitive. Likewise, the massive introduction of free ARV drugs that will not be sustained over time will have a similar impact on this industry.

While dispossession on a large scale produces sustained clearings for new transnational capital to take root, I have tried to demonstrate here that, as Janet Roitman would put it, there is something far more productive in the margins. But at the same time, dispossessed capital and its new formations and mobilities have to rely on other orchestrations of individual and institutional struggle and consent—orchestrations that should suggest just how we might rethink political economy. Rationales for public health and imperatives of capital, humanitarianism efforts and security cultures combine and conflict, but ultimately show that the AIDS crisis itself is the greatest thorn in any country's national neoliberal agenda—or perhaps its greatest opportunity.

Notes

1. Some of the literature on the global and globalization that informs my thinking here: on the global city: Sassen (2001); cosmopolitanism: Cheah and Robbins (1998) and Derrida (2001); globalization, transnationalism, global networks: Grewal and Kaplan (1994), Appadurai (1991, 2001), Jameson and Miyoshi (1998); neoliberalism: Comaroff and Comaroff (2000); finance markets: Lee and LiPuma (2002).

2. Notable recent exceptions include Ferguson (2006), Mbembe (2001), Cooper (2002), and Moore (2005). James Ferguson (2006) in particular has referred to Africa as the "inconvenient case" that runs against contemporary works on globalization that describe unencumbered transnational flows; particularly provocative is his analysis of the way that capital does not flow but "hops" through privatized spaces, especially oil extraction (Ferguson 2006).

3. I acknowledge Kaushik Sunder Rajan for helping me think through this argument.

4. I acknowledge Donald Moore, who spoke to me about how "emptying out" as a form of dispossession is generated by political technologies that contribute to creative destruction accompanied by consequential material realities.

5. Few of the globalization paradigms in circulation today entirely apprehend the complicated ways that African states are positioned in these scenarios. That is, global cities, finance markets, and widespread manufacturing bases do not exist on this continent in the congruent ways found elsewhere in the world; and local–global relationships do not adequately capture the nature of states where kinship, private, and public forms of power comingle (Ake 1996).

6. Contrary to widespread popular dissent, the IMF negotiated a SAP with then-head of state General Ibrahim Babangida shortly after he took over by coup d'état. This event marked the beginning stages of a protracted pro-democracy movement that coexisted with a heightened culture of militarism characterized by the quest for wealth and violence. With rising poverty and lack of security, a culture of militarism lingers now into the current civilian era and significantly informs retrospective debates and discourses about IMF fallouts such as governance and the politics of health care, pharmacy, and drug manufacturing.

7. Elyachar (2005), Roitman (2005), and Moore (2005) examine the micropolitics of dispossession and the various forms of reinvestment and political stakes in Egypt, the Chad Basin, and Zimbabwe, respectively.

8. George Caffentzis (1995) makes an almost identical argument about structural adjustment and dispossession in Africa in which he traces their dramatic impact on social transformation.

9. According to official statistics, oil wealth makes up over 46% of Nigeria's GDP and accounts for 85% of the country's foreign exchange (World Bank 2004).

The rumor on the street in Lagos is that up to 40% of Nigeria's crude oil goes missing each year.

10. Brotherton (2008), however, refers to the Cuban state.

11. For more recent excellent analyses on oil in Nigeria see Watts (2001, 2004), Apter (2005), Naanen (2004), and Okonta (2004).

12. One quite formidable contradiction of state absence / state power erupted in 1996 when the pharmaceutical giant Pfizer conducted a clinical trial during a massive meningitis outbreak in Kano using the drug Trovan. After 11 children died, FDA inspectors examined documents from Nigeria and found nearly four dozen discrepancies (*Washington Post* 2000). Nigeria's drug regulatory agency was never informed of the trial and therefore did not monitor it (personal communication). The families of the children sued Pfizer, leading to years of disagreement over which country had the authority to hold the trial; ultimately it was held in a New York City federal court after years of dispute. A 75 million USD settlement with the State of Kano was reached July 30, 2009.

13. I first found an analysis of this quote in Avery Gordon's introduction to Cedric Robinson's *The Anthropology of Marxism* (2001), which is reprinted in Gordon's *Keeping Good Time* (2004).

14. Although, James Ferguson (2005) points to how these scenarios become possible when capital hops rather than flows into privatized sectors, like oil extraction.

15. Robertson (n. d.) estimates that "capital flight from Nigeria alone vary [*sic*] from $50 billion, to 135–150 billion, to 3,000 billion British pounds" (5).

16. For work on drug distribution systems in Nigeria, see Anyika (1999), Ezeanya (2000), Fashesin (1998), and Ovbiagele (2000).

17. The 2006 Nigeria debt cancellation deal involved forgiving all but 12 billion USD owed to Paris Club members. This deal included adhering to the controversial IMF Support Policy Instrument, which is extended to countries not needing IMF loans but who nonetheless seek IMF endorsement, signaling an easier release of funds from multilateral donors and banks. This mechanism extends older forms of legitimacy making in the context of debt (not necessarily credit) worthiness. In return, countries must adhere to the usual privatization schemes geared toward foreign direct investment. Nigeria agreed to completely privatize the national energy sector and reorganize its banking sector, among others, in exchange for the deal.

18. In fact, one pharmacist who has worked in the national inspectorate estimated to me that 95% of all registered pharmacies would not actually pass inspection, but manage to get their licenses in exchange for money to "look the other way" as he put it.

19. A survey by Bright and Taylor (1999) showed that irrespective of socio-economic stratum, rates of self-medication are very high, recording 75% as the lowest figure. It concluded that if pharmacists refuse to assist the self-medicating population, then morbidity, mortality, iaotrogenicity, and other adverse effects will increase. Their statistics on reasons for self-medication are worth reporting here: cheapness: 32.9%; effectiveness: 71.35%; sure relief or cure: 85.23%; time saving: 66.19%. Respondents with clear knowledge of local pharmacists: 88.79%; respondents who would ask for pharmacist intervention: 52.49%; respondents who would see doctors first if ill: 9%; respondents who feel they do not need a pharmacist: 36.11%. See also Ekanem (1997) on the rational use of malaria drugs.

20. See Atueyi (1999) on drug education in Nigeria.

21. For a variety of compelling research on hospital pharmacies, see Chukumerije (1982); Eniojukan, Alebiosu, and Oni (1997); Eniojukan and Adeniyi (1997); Ohaju-Obodo, Isah, and Mabadeje (1998); Taylor (1998).

22. Importantly, Julia Elyachar (2005) shows how in the aftermath of structural adjustment the poor—their networks and social practices—have been incorporated into the rhetoric and logics of free market expansion by the World Bank and others that use an explicit neoliberal vision (and not other alternatives) to implement such policies and practices.

23. There are several other international bilateral treatment programs that are also part of this mix.

24. It should be noted that at least one indigenous Nigerian drug manufacturing firm was poised to begin producing anti-HIV medication. The subsidization of both U.S. and Indian products has essentially eliminated the prospects of Nigerian manufacturing at this time.

25. The other top two PEPFAR countries that get D.O.D. funding are Tanzania and Kenya, perhaps as part of anti-terrorist efforts since the 1998 U.S. embassy bombings in those countries.

26. It was made up of the Joint United Nations Programme on HIV/AIDS, the World Health Organization, and five companies: Boehringer Ingelheim, Bristol-Myers Squibb, Glaxo Wellcome, Merck, and Hoffmann-La Roche.

References

ACT UP Paris. 2002. "'Accelerating Access' Serves Pharmaceutical Companies While Corrupting Health Organizations." Electronic document: http://www.globaltreatmentaccess.org/content/press_releases/02/051502_APP_PS_WHO_ACC_ACC.html.

Ake, Claude. 1996. *Democracy and Development in Africa.* Washington, D.C.: Brookings Institute.

Anyika, E. N. 1999. "Eclipse (Model) of Pharmacy Practice and the Ethical Distribution System." *West African Journal of Pharmacy* 13 (2): 1–4.

Appadurai, Arjun. 1991. "Disjuncture and Difference in the Global Economy." *Public Culture* 2 (2): 1–24.

———. 2001. *Globalization.* Durham, N.C: Duke University Press.

Apter, Andrew. 2005. *The Pan-African Nation: Oil and the Spectacle of Culture in Nigeria.* Chicago: University of Chicago Press.

Arendt, Hannah. 1968. *Imperialism: Part II of the Origins of Totalitarianism.* Orlando, Fla.: Harcourt Trade Publishers.

Atueyi, I. 1999. "Drug Information, Education, and Communication." *West African Journal of Pharmacy* 13 (2): 10–13.

Bayart, Jean-Francois. 1997. *The Criminalization of the State in Africa.* Bloomington: Indiana University Press.

Bright, A. O, and O. Taylor. 1999. "A Socio-economic & Demographic Assessment of the Extent of Self-Medication in Nigeria." *West African Journal of Pharmacy* 13 (2): 74–77.

Brotherton, Sean. 2008. "'We Have to Think Like Capitalists But Continue Being Socialists': Medicalized Subjectivities, Emergent Capital, and Socialist Entrepreneurs in Post-Soviet Cuba." *American Ethnologist 35* (2): 259–274.

Caffentzis, Constantine George. 1995. "Fundamental Implications of the Debt Crisis for Social Reproduction in Africa." In *Paying the Price: Women and the Politics of International Economic Strategy,* ed. Maria Rosa Dalla Costa and Giovanna Dalla Costa, 15–41. London: Zed Books.

Cheah, Pheng, and Bruce Robbins, eds. 1998. *Cosmopolitics: Thinking and Feeling Beyond the Nation.* Minneapolis: University of Minnesota.

Chukumerije, A. A. 1982. "Shortage of Drugs in Nigerian Hospitals." *Nigerian Journal of Pharmacy* 13 (6): 13–21.

Comaroff, Jean, and John Comaroff. 2000. *Millennial Capitalism and the Culture of Neoliberalism.* Durham, N.C.: Duke University Press.

Cooper, Frederick. 2002. *Africa since 1940: The Past of the Present.* Cambridge: Cambridge University Press.

Derrida, Jacques. 2001. *On Cosmopolitanism and Forgiveness.* New York: Routledge.

Diawara, Manthia. 1998. "Toward a Regional Imaginary in Africa." In *The Cultures of Globalization,* ed. Fredric Jameson and Masoa Miyoshi. Durham, N.C.: Duke University Press.

Ekanem, O. J. 1997. "On Rational Use of Antimalarial Drugs." Paper presented at Malaria Society of Nigeria Symposium. June 19.

Elbe, Stefan. 2005. "AIDS, Security, Biopolitics." *International Relations* 19 (4): 403–419.

Elyachar, Julia. 2005. *Markets of Dispossession: NGOs, Economic Development, and the State in Egypt.* Durham, N.C.: Duke University Press.

Eniojukan, J. F., and A. Adeniyi. 1997. "Community Pharmacists and Primary Health Care Programmes: the Nigerian Experience." *Nigerian Journal of Pharmacy* 28 (2): 21–24.

Eniojukan, J. F., O. Alebiosu, and A. S. Oni. 1997. "Hospital Pharmacy in Nigeria: Practice and Progress." *Nigerian Quarterly of Hospital Medicine* 7 (1): 69–73.

Ezeanya, C. C. 2000. "Drug Distribution Channels in Nigeria." *Pharma News* 22 (3): 11.

Fanon, Franz. 1966. *The Wretched of the Earth.* New York: Grove Press.

Fashesin, O. 1998. "Unethical Drug Distribution as a Double Edged Sword." *Nigerian Journal of Pharmacy* 29 (3): 140–143.

Ferguson, James. 2005. "Seeing Like an Oil Company: Space, Security, and Global Capital in Neoliberal Africa." *American Anthropologist* 107 (3): 377–382.

———. 2006. *Global Shadows: Africa in the Neoliberal World Order.* Durham, N.C.: Duke University Press.

Gordon, Avery. 2004. *Keeping Good Time: Reflections on Knowledge, Power, and People.* Boulder, Colo.: Paradigm Publishers.

Grewal, Inderpal, and Caren Kaplan. 1994. *Scattered Hegemonies: Postmodernity and Transnational Feminist Practices.* Minneapolis: University of Minnesota Press.

Harvey, David. 2003. *The New Imperialism.* Oxford: Oxford University Press.

Health Gap Coalition. 2000. "Questioning the UNAIDS/Pharmaceutical Industry Initiative: Seven Months and Counting . . ." Electronic document: http://

www.globaltreatmentaccess.org/content/press_releases/00/121300_
HGAP_PS_UNAIDS.pdf.

Ingram, Alan. 2007. "HIV/AIDS, Security, and the Geopolitics of U.S.–Nigerian
Relations." *Review of International Political Economy* 14 (3): 510–534.

Jameson, Fredric, and Masao Miyoshi. 1998. *Cultures of Globalization.* Durham,
N.C.: Duke University Press.

Lee, Benjamin, and Edward LiPuma. 2002. "Cultures of Circulation: The
Imaginations of Modernity." *Public Culture* 14 (1): 191–213.

Luxemburg, Rosa. 1968. *The Accumulation of Capital.* Trans. A. Schwartzschield.
New York: Monthly Review Books.

Maiwada, Jude. 2004. "70% of Nigerians Patronize Traditional Medicine
Practitioners." *Nigerian Newsday,* August 11.

Marx, Karl. 1959 [1867]. *Capital: A Critical Analysis of Capitalist Production.* Ed.
Frederick Engels, translated from the 3rd German edition by Samuel
Moore and Edward Aveling. Moscow: Foreign Languages Publishing
House.

———. 1977 [1894]. *Capital: A Critique of Political Economy,* vol. 3. Ed. Frederick
Engels, trans. Ben Fowkes. New York: Vintage Books.

Mbembe, Achille. 2001. *On the Postcolony.* Berkeley: University of California Press.

Moore, Donald. 2005. *Suffering for Territory: Race, Place, and Power in Zimbabwe.*
Durham, N.C.: Duke University Press.

Naanen, Ben. 2004. "The Political Economy of Oil and Violence in the Niger
Delta." *ACAS BULLETIN: The Warri Crisis, the Niger Delta, and the Nigerian
State* 68.

Nguyen, Vinh-Kim. 2004. "Antiretroviral Globalism, Biopolitics, and Therapeutic
Citizenship." In *Global Assemblages Technology, Politics, and Ethics as
Anthropological Problems,* ed. Aihwa Ong and Stephen Collier, 124–144.
Oxford: Blackwell.

———. 2007. "Experimentality: Massive AIDS Intervention in Africa as Military
Therapeutic Complex." Paper presented at the Experimental Systems
Conference, University of California, Irvine, April 14, 2007.

Ohaju-Obodo, J. O., A. O. Isah, and A. F. B. Mabadeje. 1998. "Prescribing Pattern
of Clinicians in Private Health Institutions in Edo and Delta States of
Nigeria." *Nigeria Quarterly Journal of Hospital Medicine* 8 (2): 91–94.

Okonta, Ike. 2004. "Death-Agony of a Malformed Political Order." *ACAS
BULLETIN: The Warri Crisis, the Niger Delta, and the Nigerian State* 68.

Okonta, Ike, and Oronto Douglass. 2003. *Where Vultures Feast.* London: Verso.

Ovbiagele, Godwin. 2000. "Decorous Drug Distribution Channels: Challenges of
the Democratic Dispensation." *The EKO Pharmacist* (Nov.): 19–38.

PGM-MAN. 2001. "Dangers Posed to Life and the Economy by Drugs and
Medicines from Illegal Sources." A Presentation at the Public Hearing
of the Health and Social Services Committee, Federal House of
Representatives, National Assembly, March.

Pharmacists Council of Nigeria (PCN). *PCN List of Registered Pharmacies, Lagos:
Nigeria.* Archives of the Pharmacists Council of Nigeria, Abuja, Nigeria.

Robertson, A. P. No date. "Corruption, 'Shadow Revenues' and Capital Flight."
Unpublished manuscript.

Robinson, Cedric. 1997. *Black Movements in America.* New York: Routledge.

———. 2001. *Anthropology of Marxism.* Surrey, U.K.: Ashgate Publishing Ltd.

Roitman, Janet. 2005. *Fiscal Disobedience: An Anthropology of Economic Regulation in Central Africa.* Princeton: Princeton University Press.

Salako, Lateef. 1997. "Health for All Nigerians—So Far, So What?" *Nigerian Quarterly Journal of Hospital Medicine* 7 (3): 199–206.

Sassen, Saskia. 2001. *The Global City: New York, London, Tokyo.* Princeton: Princeton University Press.

Samba, Ebrahim Malick. 2004. "African Health Care Systems: What Went Wrong?" *News-Medical.net.* December 8, 2004. Electronic document: http://www .news-medical.net/?id=6770.

Taylor, O. 1998. "Dispensing Practices in Private and Government Health Facilities in Lagos State." *Nigerian Journal of Pharmacy* 29 (1): 63–67.

Taylor, R. B., O. Shakoor, R. H. Behrens, M. Everard, A. S. Low, J. Wangboonskul, R. G. Reid, and J. A. Kolawole. 2001. "Pharmacopoeial Quality of Drugs Supplied by Nigerian Pharmacies." *The Lancet* 14 (July):V358.

Washington Post. 2000. Editorial: "The Body Hunters: Testing Amid an Epidemic." December 17: A01.

Watts, Michael. 2001. "Petro-Violence: Community, Extraction, and Political Ecology of a Mythic Commodity." In *Violent Environments,* ed. Nancy Lee Peluso and Michael Watts, 189–212. Ithaca, N.Y.: Cornell University.

———. 2004. "Resource Curse?: Governmentality, Oil, and Power in the Niger Delta, Nigeria." *Geopolitics* 9 (1): 50–80.

World Bank. 2004. *World Bank Annual Report.* Washington, D.C.: World Bank.

World Health Organization Statistical Information System (WHOSIS). 2001. "Statistics by Country-Nigeria." Electronic document: http://www3.who .int/whosis/country/indicators.cfm.

Zalik, Anna. 2004. "The Niger Delta: 'Petro Violence' and 'Partnership Deve

PART 2

Alternative Forms of Globality

Assisted Reproductive Technologies in Mali and Togo: Circulating Knowledge, Mobile Technology, Transnational Efforts

Viola Hörbst

Aissetou (43), an academically trained Malian, was working for an NGO and was economically independent. She married Moustaffa (45) in 1999. Although both had already had children with other partners, Aissetou and Moustaffa were seeking to have children together. Thus, they began trying to conceive shortly after the wedding. Aissetou visited a gynecologist, who discovered that one of her tubes was blocked. Soon after this, she had an operation in France. Later, in 2004, two myomas were removed in Dakar, Senegal. Aissetou had known about in-vitro fertilization (IVF) for many years as a general possibility for treating female infertility. But it was only in 2005 that a conversation with a Malian friend who was then living in Canada gave her the idea that this might be an option for her. He recommended a Canadian clinic, which she contacted in 2005.

Until this conversation, Aissetou had had doubts about whether IVF could really work and wanted to try what for her seemed more obvious forms of treatment. Nowadays she considers this to have been a serious waste of time that eventually exacerbated her problems. She wanted to go to Canada, but was unable to get a visa from the Canadian embassy in Bamako. She therefore changed her plans and went to Germany instead, where she had relatives. Her husband joined her there for a week, during which an intracytoplasmic sperm injection (ICSI) was carried out. Unfortunately, the procedure failed to result in pregnancy.

Although assisted reproductive technology (ART) such as intrauterine insemination (IUI), IVF, and ICSI is cost-intensive and offers relatively low success rates (no higher than a 30 percent chance per attempt of bringing a healthy baby home), it is a tempting prospect for members of sub-Saharan societies like Aissetou and Moustaffa, since ART procedures offer an infertile couple the chance to raise their own genetic or biological offspring. ART procedures represent biomedicine's best solutions for conditions like severe oligospermia, azoospermia, and blocked fallopian tubes, which have high prevalence in West Africa (Mayaud 2001: 75ff, 87). While 8–12 percent of couples worldwide are believed to be struggling with fertility problems, in Mali an estimated 23.6 percent of women are suffering from secondary infertility and 10.4 percent from primary infertility (Rutstein and Shah 2004: 25, 15). Like Aissetou and Moustaffa, there are other relatively affluent couples in Mali trying to get the money together to undergo ART procedures, mainly in Europe, neighboring African states, Canada, or the U.S. But the costs are a considerable burden even for affluent Malians. Depending on national markets, the type of procedure and the amount of pharmaceuticals needed, the sum necessary for one ART cycle varies roughly between 1,800 and 10,000 USD. In addition to the cost of the procedures themselves, there are further financial obstacles, as demonstrated in the case of Fanta and Mohammed.

Fanta (35), educated in administration but unemployed, had been married since 1998 to Mohammed (43), who worked as a journalist and instructor. Fanta had visited a variety of public and private clinics in Bamako since 1999. After years of ineffective treatments she went to Dakar, where one of her cousins lived. He referred her to a private clinic where they found nothing wrong with her. Mohammed then was asked to provide a spermogram, which was performed in Bamako. The results, which showed severe oligospermia, were then faxed to Dakar. The doctor recommended that Mohammed undergo treatment in Dakar, which he did six months later, but still Fanta did not conceive. Then, Fanta explained, "The doctor in Dakar said we should return for IVF. Well, the costs, we evaluated the costs, which were a bit too high for our pocket. [. . .] It was around 3 million FCFA [app. 4,800 euro or 6,200 USD], plus two air tickets and accommodation—we would have to stay in a hotel, and so on." In the meantime Fanta had visited another gynecologist in Bamako: "She told me that IVF was necessary, either in Senegal or in France, but preferably in France. I said, ah the costs [. . .]. If we have to go to France, that is even more expensive than Senegal." Mohammed wanted Fanta to wait a bit to save up the money needed, but in the meantime they heard about a private clinic in Bamako offering ART as well, so they went there. "I told myself, why go to Senegal when it can be done here too?" After six months of hormone treatment for Mohammed, an IUI was scheduled. The gynecologist had brought the pharmaceuticals used for Fanta's hormonal preparation for IUI from France. Unfortunately, the IUI was unsuccessful. Another IUI was recommended, but Mohammed lost his job and the couple could not afford a second try.[1]

Getting these amounts of money together means having access to financial resources, which cannot be reduced to a question of class. While education plays a significant role in getting a job with a regular salary (whether providing funds to be disbursed in advance or used to get bank loans), utilizing social capital is another crucial factor. Above all, this is linked to family ties, where structural positions between people are highly important. If, for example, a younger brother or sister has a good job in Mali or overseas, they can be asked to help to pay for the treatment. Nevertheless, the majority of infertile couples in Mali cannot afford ART abroad or in Mali. In most cases the costs have to be borne privately, as there is no area-wide health insurance or a specific national program for funding ART.

In the international sphere, the right to reproduction was acknowledged as a basic human right at the International Conference on Population and Development (ICPD) in Cairo in 1994. Since then, infertility problems and access to adequate treatment have been formally recognized on international health agendas (Inhorn and Bharadwaj 2007: 1; Daar and Merali 2002: 19). While infertility rates are high in Mali, they occur in a context of underdevelopment, where a decrease in overall high birth rates (an estimated 6.6 children per woman) is a high priority for international policy makers and donor organizations (Mariko and Berthé 2007: 52). Infertility's devastating social consequences and the need to enhance the available treatments are easily overlooked. The issue of infertility treatment has not become an important topic on Malian political agendas, although Mali (as well as Togo) agreed with the ICPD statement.

Due to structural adjustments since the late 1980s, the Malian health system has changed from cost-free medical care to a "participative" health system where patients have to pay (Giani 2006: 83). Between 1970 and 1988 the national budget for the health sector decreased from 9 to 4 percent of the total national budget. The general impacts of these structural adjustments were expansion of the private health sector, at least in Bamako, and loss of confidence in the quality of treatment and technical equipment at public facilities, where all patients must pay for low-budget medicine if they are to have any at all. Additionally, social connections and bribes to health personnel are often mentioned as necessary for getting treatment at public institutions (see Jaffré and Olivier de Sardan 2003; cf. Masquelier, chapter 8 in this volume). By contrast, the private sector's reputation with the general population has improved with regard to equipment, work ethics, and quality of services. These changes have become pronounced in the field of reproductive care, as public hospitals often lack technical equipment and so send their patients to private clinics for ultrasound scans, hormone tests, etc. High-tech solutions like ART are simply not available in the public sphere. One professor of the gynecological department at the university clinic Point G has been saying for several years that they will set up an ART program, but they have not yet done so.

In contrast to the marked doubts and reservations with regard to infertility and ART that pervade the policies of national, international, and transnational institutions, gynecologists in the private sector are very interested in reproductive options.[2] There are now more than two dozen infertility clinics in sub-Saharan Africa (Pilcher 2006: 976). Some of them are situated in French-speaking West African countries like Cameroon, Senegal, and Togo, and IVF babies have already been born in this region. There are a few private gynecology clinics providing IUI in Mali, but only one of them also offers IVF, and ICSI was not yet available in 2008. Drawing from the views of gynecologists and patients in Mali and Togo, in this article I will focus on how transnational social fields are involved and activated in the ART process in the private health sector and in patients' use of ART. I will also sketch the desires, needs, and intimacies of the people concerned and the resulting social drive for this kind of procedure from these different perspectives.

Research Methods and Theoretical Approaches

My reflections and insights are based on fieldwork I carried out in Bamako and partially in Dakar (Senegal) and Lomé (Togo) between 2004 and 2008. My research focused on the life experiences of infertile couples, and on different treatment perspectives and activities in the traditional, religious, and biomedical fields. The data were collected through participant observation at private clinics; (in)formal talks (partially recorded) with biomedical and paramedical professionals, Islamic religious leaders from different subgroups in Mali, and several focus groups (women and men, both workers and students); and through interviews with state health institutions and the National Ethics Council. I worked with 17 Malian and five Togolese patients (in some cases, both partners, in others only the wife or only the husband) with retrospective, prospective, and concomitant experience of ART, and with seven Malian patients (again, some couples and some individual spouses) who would probably never be able to afford to undergo these procedures. Where level of education, occupation, property, and affluence were concerned, the majority of the interviewees can roughly be grouped as members of the middle or lower upper class.

Although infertility and ART treatment are delicate social issues in Mali and Togo, in comparison with other places (cf. Inhorn and Bharadwaj 2007: 4f), my exchange partners' desire for secrecy and confidentiality in most cases did not exclude follow-up interviews or regular visits to their homes. This may have been due to my position as an outsider in the complex Malian social system, which makes it quite difficult for those suffering from infertility to find people with whom they can talk openly about their difficult situation.

From a theoretical point of view, my research combines different perspectives on the handling of infertility and ART on local and translocal levels to show the mutual influences between these two levels. This coincides with a "multiple level approach," as proposed by van der Geest et al. (1990), which examines the different meanings of medical phenomena at different levels of social organization. My research was based on the idea of medicoscapes, inspired by Appadurai, and stresses that medical issues cannot be regarded within locally isolated frames of reference. Medicoscapes embrace worldwide landscapes of heterogeneous actors (people, states, institutions, and organizations; ideas and ideologies; practices and things) which may show up in specific locations but simultaneously connect spatially distant locations (Hörbst and Wolf 2003: 4; Hörbst and Krause 2004: 55). With its focus on the positioning and interrelatedness of different kinds of actors, the concept of medicoscapes embraces globalization processes and simultaneously overcomes territorial and national restrictions on culture and society, while still maintaining an understanding of the significance of specific locations (Hörbst and Krause 2004: 559). In the dissemination of ART, different actors, such as biomedical experts, service users, and medical institutions in different nations of the world are linked together, thereby forming loosely knit, diffuse, and fluid transnational networks. The processes of introducing and using ART in these transnational networks are shaped by economics; national and international politics; and various regimes of knowledge, sociocultural practices, moral orders, and different priorities of interests.

This approach clearly corresponds to a transnational perspective for overcoming the idea of the "container society" without abandoning the binding forces of the nation state. Transnational social fields which "connect actors, through direct and indirect relations across borders" (Levitt and Glick Schiller 2004: 6) are a tool that can be used to conceptualize "the potential array of social relations linking those who move and those who stay behind" (Levitt and Glick Schiller 2004: 6). Thus, in this chapter on the practice of ART in francophone West Africa I look at social relations in the private health sector on a personal level, and at their influence and agency within globalization processes in the field of medicine. I focus on the "migration" of assisted reproductive technologies and the role that medical professionals' transnational connections and clients' transnational networks play in the process of introducing ART in Mali and Togo. This transnational view helps to develop insights into the process of spreading ART in West Africa, even though current priorities in international and national health policies have so far neglected infertility and its biotechnological solutions.

Marital Childlessness, Gendered Accusations, and Competing Solutions

Even when marriage partners have children from other relationships, as in the case of Aissetou and Moustaffa (above), marriage in Mali or Togo typically entails a desire for and expectation of children from marriage partners. Involuntarily childless Djeneba (35), who trained as a journalist, explained:

> I would say for me, for us, [having children] gives sense to our lives, because a child allows you to give more sense to everything you are doing in your life. Without one, for us, it is senseless to work hard like that, to save all that money, even though we can satisfy our needs, if there is not an heir, all that . . . well. If there is no one to educate either . . . Particularly in Africa, your lineage must always be perpetuated. Hence, it is very important for us, and for our families, too; it contributes to the family's delight. This all comes together. [. . .] Thus, if you have a child, they tell you, yes, you have at least accomplished your social duty.

As in other African countries,[3] having children is not a question of choice or decision but a social need internalized in such a way that it takes the form of a "cultural imperative" (Inhorn and Bharadwaj 2007: 1) enacted by the marriage partners, extended families, and the surrounding society (Hadolt and Hörbst 2010). Children are seen as a kind of exchange gift from the newly married woman to her husband's family. Although children tend to have strong emotional bonds with their mothers, they are seen as belonging to the patrilineage. If a marriage does not result in procreation, the woman is generally held responsible—in particular by the husband's family, as Modibo (53), working as an accountant in an international NGO, described: "If we see that it isn't working out, well I understand it, but my kin, they don't understand. They don't see it from my point of view and they will always oppose my wife and think that it is her fault. But it is me; you see the [medical] results. There is a disorder on my level which my family does not know about." Whether or not women are the reason for childlessness, comments to them generally start a couple of months after the wedding:

> Particularly your sisters-in-law, the younger sisters of your husband, will tease you [. . .]. They say, "Ah, now you have to give a good return for the money, the bride price, we invested in you. It was very expen-

sive and when will you start to give us the fruits of our investments?"
[. . .] These are the pressures, and particularly the mothers-in-law,
your husband's mother and your husband's aunts. But particularly my
husband's mother pressured me to give her a homonym [namesake]
by her son.[4]

Such harassment occurs in daily life, but especially at baptisms and marriages, and may involve snide remarks about the woman's "unworthiness" or
comments like "my son is sleeping with a man" which refer to the childless
women as "not being a full female person." Living conditions (in the family's
compound or in an individual house), the absence of co-wives, the existence
of children from other relationships, or the existence of other family members
who suffer from the same problem can at least reduce the amount of mockery
aimed at female in-laws within the husband's family.[5]

Male-factor infertility, as in Modibo's case, is rarely at first sight assumed
to be the cause of marital childlessness in mainstream narratives. Rather, it
is pushed aside and considered something "unthinkable," particularly within
the husband's patrilineage (Hörbst 2008). As in many other regions of the
world, male infertility is often equated to impotence, thereby affecting a man's
personal and sexual identity (cf. van Balen and Inhorn 2002: 5; Inhorn and
Bharadwaj 2007: 6; Inhorn 2006b: 219, 229; Schuster and Hörbst 2006: 7). As
Boubakar, an academic who has suffered from azoospermia for 20 years, put
it, "Without children, you are not a man."

As regularly pointed out to me, male infertility is regarded as an absolute
disgrace and a source of shame for a man and his family. Consequently, in Mali
some men refuse to undergo sperm tests and often hide a negative diagnosis
from their kin (Hörbst 2010). Out of nine couples with male-factor infertility
in my study, only three of the men informed specific family members whom
they trusted not to disclose their insufficiency. Modibo, for example, admitted:
"I keep it to myself, but if someone [in the family] had the courage to ask me,
I would tell him."

Because of the imagined equation between infertility and impotence,
admitting to the former leads to "emasculation" by the social environment
(van Balen and Inhorn 2002: 5; Dyer et al. 2004: 966; Inhorn and Bharadwaj
2007: 8). Childless women in Mali are also denied the status and prestige of
being "real" women and are confronted with social "de-feminization," as
women have to bear children to attain full female personhood. But there is
perhaps one crucial difference, which seems to make male infertility especially
shameful. While female sexual capability is bodily visible during pregnancy,
male sexual capability is linked to erection, which is not shown in public, as
well as to the power to impregnate women. Both factors only become indi-

rectly visible in public through a woman's swelling belly. If a man's wife fails to become pregnant, his sexual potency and ability to achieve erection, which is not seen publicly, will be doubted, and rumors may start.[6]

Even in cases where male factors are the reason for a couple's childlessness, in many families and in the neighborhood the woman keeps being harassed. At the same time, women are the ones who are repeatedly encouraged and pushed by family members to undergo different procedures. Therefore, on different counts, extended families (patrilineal and matrilineal) not only form a passive background or a configuring context but also constitute a specific pushing factor for couples in general and women in particular to repeat different procedures again and again.

As in many sub-Saharan African societies, Malian women, men, and couples affected by infertility are confronted with a choice of social strategies for remedying childlessness, such as fostering children, extramarital sex, and polygyny.[7] About 90 percent of nearly 11 million inhabitants in Mali are nominally Muslim, and the Qur'an (sura 4:3) allows the majority of men to marry up to four wives if they have the financial resources to provide for them. Thus, polygyny seems to be an ideal solution for marital childlessness—at least from the husband's and his family's point of view. In contrast, many women in infertile marriages fear co-wives and regard them as increased pressure.[8] Regarding polygyny, Djeneba says:

> With the Muslim religion, the husbands are sometimes obliged to marry another woman under pressure from their parents or because of their own wish to continue their lineage [. . .]. This is even the vision of society, which encourages this. Very rarely, husbands accept their wives as they are and do not remarry. Perhaps this may be 2 in 100. It is very, very rare that husbands don't give in to pressure from the family, no. If this is the case, you will find that it is probably the husband who has a problem, too. But even if the husband is the problem, he will be tempted to marry a second wife before deciding to accept that he really has a problem himself.

For an infertile husband who knows his diagnosis, pressure from his family to take a second wife poses a danger. If his second wife does not get pregnant soon, rumors may start concerning his capability. At the same time, his first wife may officially disclose that he is the cause of her childlessness. Thus, the husband is somewhat at his wife's mercy, as she has the power to either protect him or expose him to the greatest disgrace (Hörbst 2008).

Keeping a secret is a highly idealized and valued topic in Malian narratives, especially when it comes to gender relations and family affairs (Grosz-Ngaté 1989: 174f). In popular discourse, women are assumed to disclose secrets readily and are feared for this reason. Contrary to this image, with one exception, all the women in my study whose husbands were the reason for the couple's childlessness kept their secret, some of them even from their mother, sisters, and close friends. Fanta explained her reasons:

> On the one hand, this would stop [my in-laws] from teasing me, but on the other hand they won't ever keep quiet. On the contrary they would talk about my husband. I prefer to take the responsibility instead of him. [. . .] It is too hard for him. I know this could even impact on his work. I know that women can suffer on this level but men can't at all. [. . .] It is between us, the doctors—they know, I know it, and he himself knows it. I think this is enough.

By keeping the secret and shielding their husbands from mockery, Fanta and the other women also strengthened their marital bond while in many cases shouldering ongoing stigmatization.

However, if male-factor infertility is the reason for a couple's childlessness, resorting to extramarital cohabitation could be at least a theoretical possibility for the wife. In Mali there is an option which was described to me by many Malians as being a "traditional" one. As Djeneba stated: "In some families, [. . .] if they know or assume that the elder brother can't father children, then the younger brother sleeps with his elder brother's wife." Any child resulting from such a union officially counts as the infertile husband's offspring, since he is married to the mother and thus the child is legitimately related to the patrilineage (cf. Clarke 2008: 163). Without genetic testing, no one could tell who actually fathered the child. According to infertile women, healers in Bamako who assume that the husband is the cause of childlessness also recommend clandestine extramarital sex to women.[9] But these options seem easiest to handle within a field of diffuse assumptions, secrecy, and uncertainty, particularly as long as the husband has not yet performed a spermogram, because then the woman's risks of disclosure is not as high as it would be if the husband knew his diagnosis.

Most of the women participating in my research excluded the option of extramarital sex for themselves, giving love or religion as reasons, even though many men may have sexual intercourse outside marriage. Additionally, fear of malicious gossip from their social environment and fear of being discovered kept them from choosing to have extramarital sex in order to "find a child." Furthermore, they were afraid that a husband—in the event of marital arguments—might reveal to others that he was not the biological father of the child, which could result in withdrawal of material support and negative social consequences for the child as well as the wife. One woman also feared her co-wife or her husband might demand genetic testing if she became pregnant.

Only Seynabe (34), an IT specialist, expressed a slightly different opinion: "If tomorrow I could tell him that I was pregnant, I am convinced that he would probably be angry with me, but I am sure that in the long run he would accept the child as our child. Because one thing is clear. I would never do it only for me but for both of us. Anyway, that's my point of view. It is as simple as that."

Another strategy mentioned in the literature for dealing with marital infertility (Sako 1989: 66f; Brand 2001: 241) is parenting foster children, which is a common social practice in West Africa, including Mali. Most couples I worked with had been given children by relatives. Taking a younger brother's child is similar to the "traditional way" in which a younger brother clandestinely impregnates the wife of his older but infertile brother. However, it does not involve the cohabitation necessary in the "traditional" solution and thus overcomes possible religious and emotional barriers, at least from the husband's perspective. But all the women felt ambivalent about foster children and feared that the identity of the children's biological mother would not be kept secret. At the same time, foster children, although loved and cared for, do nothing to alleviate the position or stigmatization of a wife within her husband's family, as Odile (29) pointed out. Odile had been childless for five years before she conceived a baby after three ICSI procedures carried out in Senegal. "It's different, because you know [foster children] will go away one day. Particularly it is different, because everyone within the family knows they are not your own children—thus it is no solution." From the point of view of affected women in Bamako, foster children neither offer a solution to unwanted childlessness, nor do they stop them from desperately looking for their own offspring. As part of this quest, social and therapeutic methods may be used simultaneously and traditional remedies may be approached at the same time as biomedical treatments, often overlapping. Whenever infertile women and men have financial resources, they visit different "traditional" practitioners such as phytotherapists, marabouts, or hunters in Bamako and in remote areas. These therapies include taking phytotherapeutic and mineral products, washing the body with these substances, saying prayers, wearing small objects, making sacrifices to ancestors and charged objects, and taking pilgrimages to tombs or powerful places.

Most women and men suffering from infertility will also consult different public biomedical institutions and/or private clinics. Here, biomedical diagnosis (such as hormone analyses, ultrasound scans, and hysterosalpingography), hormone treatment, or surgical procedures (such as laparoscopy, tubal insufflation, and intrauterine hormone cocktails) are performed. Often diagnoses and treatments are repeated by different gynecologists, even though they have already been performed several times.[10]

For many, these attempts to conceive are a desolate journey, sometimes going on for years without success, often with thousands of dollars spent on various therapies, including, for some, ART.

Experts' Interest and Efforts to Establish ART in West Africa

The road to ART in Nigeria, where research and equipment were initially funded by public resources and institutions, is described by Giwa-Osagie (2002: 23; see also Pilcher 2006: 276) as the common model for establishing ART in sub-Saharan Africa. In contrast, in Mali and Togo ART procedures depend on the efforts of gynecologists in the private health sector, as state institutions are not involved and do not provide structural support to private agents or treatments. Knowing that elite members travel to Europe or neighboring African states to undergo IVF or ICSI, gynecologists see a profitable market in ART. They assume that the reduced costs of local ART due to lower medical fees and no travel, visa, or other expenses would be attractive to many couples, even those belonging to the upper classes. Drawing on intertwined humanitarian, biomedical, and economic considerations, gynecologists are hoping to enlarge the spectrum of clients with access to ART, thereby also enhancing their business opportunities.

As the introduction of ART goes hand in hand with the need to purchase cost-intensive high-tech equipment, forming a consortium of gynecologists in order to share the costs would facilitate its progress. However, gynecologists unanimously explained to me that many colleagues in Mali and Togo did not even refer patients to them and preferred to send them to other countries instead. Therefore, building a consortium is not feasible in Mali or in Togo, due to the fear of envy, rivalry, and resulting problems. Additionally, they confirmed the tendency for experts in the public sector to regard those in the private sector as rivals or opponents (cf. Giwa-Osagie 2002: 26). This also hinders national public–private partnerships, which are recommended for facilitating ART in low-resource countries (Daar and Merali 2002: 20).

Without the options of private–private or public–private partnerships, how is the introduction of ART in Togo and Mali taking place?

The owner and director of a private Togolese infertility clinic, Dr. T, studied medicine in France, where he then specialized in gynecology. After having completed some years of internship at French clinics and a French sperm bank, he returned to Lomé with his wife, a pediatrician, in 1983, to work in his father's private general medicine practice. Combining the fields of gynecology and pediatrics, they then founded the current private clinic together. As Dr. T had always been interested in the field of infertility and had worked for a long time at a French sperm bank where IUIs were performed, he continued to carry them out in Lomé. "But I had no IVF," he told me.

In 1986, while attending an international gynecology conference in Martinique, Dr. T ran into a French infertility specialist to whom he mentioned his idea of introducing IVF at his Togolese clinic. His French colleague was interested, but due to political unrest in Togo, Dr. T and his friend put the idea on hold and did not revive it until 1994. They then developed a "private transnational partnership," in which the French specialist assisted as a counselor. In the first years, the French specialist and his team, financed by Dr. T, came to Lomé regularly for a few weeks at a time to supervise puncture and transfer. Additionally, Dr. T and his biologist stayed at the French gynecologist's private clinic for a couple of weeks for training. In 1997 the first IVF baby was born at the clinic. In 1998, Dr. T decided to add ICSI to his services. For this technique he contacted the head gynecologist of another French ART centre, who also came to Togo to provide training. Since 1999 Dr. T has successfully performed ICSI and cryopreservation of sperm and embryos, as well as running a donor program for sperm and oocytes. Patients come from Togo, Benin, Ghana, Burkina Faso, Mali, and Ivory Coast, and some are Togolese living in Europe. Dr. T negotiated a special price with French laboratories for the pharmaceuticals used for hormonal stimulation, so he offers some at cheaper rates than in France. The equipment needed for the laboratory was purchased tax-free, though transport costs added up.

In contrast to Dr. T's success establishing ART services at his clinic in Togo, the director of a private Malian clinic, Dr. M, was still struggling with the process of introducing ART when I worked with him. He studied medicine in Kiev, where he also specialized in gynecology. When he came back to Mali in the late 1980s, he worked at a university clinic before founding a private practice specializing in gynecology in Bamako in 1993, which he enlarged step by step. Since then, he has not worked in the public sector in Mali. At the end of 2003, Dr. M began working with his biologist, who had studied in Bulgaria. Second-hand equipment was purchased from a retired French gynecologist, a room was reconstructed and dedicated to ART procedures, and the laboratory budget and staff were increased. In 2005, Dr. M and his biologist used his personal connections in the Netherlands to enroll in a Dutch development evaluation program for technology: a retired Dutch biologist examined the clinic's technological equipment, which was then improved based upon his recommendations. The Dutch specialist promised to get sponsoring from a Dutch university for ten IVF attempts, but this has not yet happened. While they have been successfully and routinely performing IUI since 2004, in 2008 they were still trying to achieve success in IVF.

Besides access to private financial resources, in both Mali and Togo personal transnational networks are an important prerequisite for establishing contact with retailers, and particularly for gaining access to skills and practical know-how about ART. Many gynecologists in francophone West Africa have at least bilateral contacts, as the majority of them trained abroad. In Mali, for example, biomedical experts' mobility is closely linked to former colonial relations and affinities stemming from Mali's early postcolonial socialist era. In addition to France, nations like the former German Democratic Republic, USSR, Poland, and Bulgaria were involved in gynecological training for Malians, as gynecology and obstetrics only began to be taught in Bamako's medical school in the 2000s. While France still plays a major role in higher education for Malians, the countries of the former Eastern Bloc have lost their importance. In their place, countries like Ivory Coast and Senegal are gaining in significance, as are (due to religious affiliations) North African nations like Algeria and Morocco. Malians also study in Canada and the United States.

Dr. M from the Malian private clinic and his biologist did several internships in Canada and Germany,[11] as well as in France, the primary place for professional networking. Through his Togolese colleague Dr. T, Dr. M completed his first internship at the infertility center of the French gynecologist who supports the Togolese clinic. Now Dr. M is also a member of international and French gynecologists' associations, regularly receives information and instructions on new issues online, and participates in exchange platforms with international colleagues. Additionally, he attends gynecological conferences in France each year, and travels to France roughly every three months. When Dr. M returns from these trips, he brings back pharmaceuticals for hormonal stimulation and sells them to patients at net cost price in order to facilitate access and reduce the costs of ART treatment.[12]

Looking at experts' activities in the domain of ART, it becomes clear that the flow of material, financial capital, ideas, contacts, and knowledge—special characteristics of transnational processes, according to Glick Schiller and Levitt (2006: 5)—is initiated and maintained by individual efforts to overcome local social constraints as well as financial and political barriers. The medical experts participate in transnational professional fields, which can be regarded as forming part of different transnational social fields and simultaneously embodying being transnational (cf. Levitt and Glick Schiller 2004: 6f) through their professional engagement.

Moreover, Dr. M and Dr. T tend to consider themselves members of a global biomedical scientific community that actively shapes and is shaped by the latest advances in medical knowledge and practice. As part of this worldwide inter- and trans-national knowledge scheme, they want to achieve biomedical advances despite belonging to developing nations. As Dr. T spells out: "There was the first case of IVF that occurred before I finished my studies in France. Louise Brown was born in Great Britain and Amandine four years later in France, in 1982—roughly the time I left France. [. . .] And yes, at that moment I wondered whether we could get this advanced technology one day in our country."

Both gynecologists participate in the distribution of information on ART not only during patient consultations, but also in public through the national media. In interviews and discussions on these topics, they try to initiate a public debate on infertility and its social handling while simultaneously promoting their own business interests. In the Malian case, for example, a five-minute documentary on female and male infertility treatment at Dr. M's clinic has been produced and is shown repeatedly on Malian national TV. This has attracted many patients to the clinic, even from Chad and Burkina Faso. Due to their briefness and entrepreneurial interest, these media events emphasize the success of ART by downplaying or ignoring constraints, risks, and barriers like advanced age, hyperstimulation, or high costs. Thus they support the miracle image of ART and create high expectations in patients. If these treatments fail, both Dr. T and Dr. M told me that patients accuse them personally of having taken them in.

Patients' Access to Globally Circulating ART Ideas and Practices

The majority of the couples participating in my research had access to information about ART via family members living outside Mali, and roughly half of them also received pharmaceuticals sent by these migrants. They were therefore participating in transnational social fields, even though half of them had never been to Europe themselves (Levitt and Glick Schiller 2004: 6). The other half had studied or lived some time overseas and/or worked at international NGOs during the time of my research. They directly embodied "being" transnational. Besides these sources, globally circulating information on ART makes its way to Malians through other channels: gynecologists, documentary programs on French TV, or rumors about well-known Malian artists and politicians who are thought to have undergone these procedures. Only some of the participating women, men, and couples also consulted French internet sites on medical issues. Thus, personal networks, mouth-to-mouth propaganda, and informal popular discourses are highly important in the distribution of basic information on "test-tube" babies.

When ART procedures are performed abroad, travel costs, etc. pose a considerable obstacle, so people take advantage of (temporary) employment, professional secondments (temporary post transfers), scholarships, studentships, or business visits. Family members or friends living abroad may not only provide substantial financial resources but are crucial in selecting the country or city for an ART procedure. As in Fanta's case, sketched in the introduction, most of the women, men, and couples participating in my research would have preferred to undergo ART procedures in Mali, because of lower costs and higher emotional comfort in respect to social life and communication. Only two respondents mentioned lack of experience and lower technical standards in Malian clinics as a crucial factor for seeking clinics abroad. Some patients who underwent IUI or IVF in Mali activated members of their overseas networks to send them the required medicines, which were not available in Mali or only at a higher price. Alternately, some patients had begun hormonal treatment in France and then completed it in Mali. Thus, varying forms of transnationally practiced procedures seem to emerge in the context of ART, just as they do in other medical contexts.

Both gynecologists and patients draw on globally circulating ideas and practices to which they have access in different ways. On both levels, the circulation of ideas, practices, technologies, medicines, and people is triggered by the hope of overcoming infertility. This circulation in turn raises those hopes. Concerning infertility and its treatments, these transnational activities challenge ideas about gender and family relations and even right and wrong (Levitt 2007: 3). Transnationally exchanged ART ideas and practices, as appealing as they are, in combination with economic interests challenge the social norms and moral convictions of the gynecologists and their patients.

Patients' Views on ART Practices

With regard to the patients' perspective on assisted reproductive technologies like IUI, IVF, and ICSI, it seems that men in general are more hesitant to use them than women. Some men expressed the idea that Islam would disapprove of ART in general,[13] while others feared third-party manipulation of the sperm in the laboratory and subsequent biological/genetic uncertainty regarding the child's origin. Nevertheless, the majority seemed to accept homologous forms of ART using gametes from the marital partners.

Procedures using donor sperm were rejected by nearly all the men in my study. In their explanations, some of them referred to the "immoral practices of the West," where they felt that ART was practiced without any ethical limits. According to them, Islam in general rejected ART using donor gametes in order to prevent future problems of incestuous relations between resulting offspring, and placed the insertion of extra-marital gametes on a level with adultery.[14] In addition to religious ethics, some men spoke of personal emotional ties and referred to genetics. For example, Tidiane (43), an IT specialist suffering from severe azoospermia, shared:

> I need to have a child because I want to have one with her. Today. You know? If the problem lay in her and not within me, I would not be tempted to have a child with someone else. This is not my goal. It is because she is important in my life. If we did [ART via] donor sperm or with an oocyte of another woman, this would go beyond my vision. I don't like that. Moreover, I tell myself, it is simple—we live in a society where it is easy to take a child from a brother or a cousin. You can do this; this is easy.

For Tidiane, having children with another man's sperm via ART would be similar to having foster children. Foster children would not only be the easier way, but they would stem from his consanguine kin rather than an unknown donor, and would thus enable him to indirectly continue the patrilineage, one of men's specific reproductive aims (Hadolt and Hörbst 2010). Under Muslim rules, a child has to be legitimately related to the patrilineage (cf. Clarke 2008: 163), which is achieved through marriage. But if the husband knows he is the one diagnosed as sub- or in-fertile, for him to achieve a child "legitimately related" to the patrilineage requires his biological substance. Thus, with biomedical diagnosis the legitimacy of a child's relationship to the family is translated into biological terms.

In contrast, the women seemed to be more pragmatically oriented. Only one of the devout Muslim women in my study had any reservations against homologous ART, while the majority of them would accept insemination with donor sperm or IVF via donor ova, at least as a last resort. Tidiane's wife Seynabe explained: "I believe, contrary to him—perhaps it is because I am a woman that I think so—I don't see any problem at all in using an in-vitro system with his sperm or someone else's. To make a baby in an assisted way, whether it was his or not, I personally feel that if this is a baby and I have it from the first day until the ninth month and I deliver this baby, this would be our baby." Houwa (40), working as a paramedic staff member at a public clinic, suffered from ovarian aging and was preparing to undergo IVF with ova from her younger sister. She said: "If I carry the child to term, I say now that it will be mine. Perhaps 10 percent to 15 percent I would think is from my younger sister. [. . .] The idea is to know the joy of motherhood, the joy of carrying a child."

Here, the childless women argued that to carry a fetus for nine months and give birth to it allowed them to nourish and communicate with the baby, even if it came from another woman's ovum. Through pregnancy and birthing these babies became their "own" babies in a corporal sense. While through ART with donor ova these women would become biological rather than genetic mothers, it would enable them in particular to be pregnant—in the public eye, the only means of definitely overcoming social stigmatization and exclusion. Children stemming from ova donation and the husband's sperm would come from the husband's patrilineage and thus fulfill the husband's aim of continuing the male line. In contrast, only children originating from donor sperm would not genetically achieve this aim (Hadolt and Hörbst 2010).

Influences on Consultation and Therapy

Gynecologists in Mali and Togo are participating in transnational bio-medical knowledge schemes, but at the same time they argue that ART has to be appropriated, due to social and cultural configurations in West African nations. Since there are not yet any specific state laws regulating ART in Mali or Togo, the handling of these procedures is left to the gynecologists. As regards questions of medical ethics in ART, gynecologists are bound by their own moral and medical convictions as well as business interests. When speaking to me they emphasized that their practices were based on European standards and ethical arguments. On some points they seemed to follow the ethical guidelines and laws of the countries in which they received their training (cf. Giwa-Osagie 2002: 25). In Mali and Togo, no more than three embryos are transferred at one time, and surrogacy is not practiced in either country.[15] In Togo, ICSI is available, and thus most IVF are changed into ICSI. Heterologous forms of ART with egg and sperm from unknown donors are carried out in Togo as well, whereas in Mali only IVF via egg donation from known donors had been performed as of 2008.

Concerning consultation, the gynecologists also followed the paradigm of informed consent, which is highly favored in Euro-American biomedical circles. The Malian and Togolese gynecologists handed out consent forms for ART procedures for the patients to sign. Moreover, they pointed out the generally low success rates and the possibility that procedures might have to be repeated, and clearly explained the need for financial resources. Generally these gynecologists expected their patients not to be well informed and routinely explained the physiological features of human fertilization, the disorders involved in their specific case, and the different treatment options by using diagrams. They supported the image of an open dialogue where the patient was thoroughly informed. However, there were limits. They did not spell out the risks of hyperstimulation or side effects from pharmaceuticals in detail.

Other limits were social in nature. For example, communication varied depending on whether the women or men came on their own or with their partners. In the latter case, often only the husband spoke during the consultation and was the one exclusively addressed by Dr. M when he gave explanations or asked which treatment option should be followed. Under social gender norms and civil law, the husband, as head of household, is officially in charge of making decisions for the wife. If sperm analysis showed male-factor infertility, then Dr. M made an appointment only with the man to explain the diagnosis and allow him to decide if, how, and when to inform his wife. In follow-up consultations where both partners came, he usually pointed out that both partners were needed in order to conceive and emphasized any smaller problems with the woman. Being part of Malian society, Dr. M knew and conformed to these social norms in consultations. In doing so, he also enhanced his social reputation and prestige. Being recommended to others as a "respectful doctor" contributed to his business success.

When women were present in consultations without their husbands, they communicated more actively, although they rarely contradicted the doctor. They raised questions, though seldom about treatment details such as its course, risks, side effects, or if it was performed with or without anesthetic.

This issue might not only be linked to questions of medical authority and sociocultural norms in communication—especially from women toward men—but to language and comprehension problems as well. In many consultations at which I was present, Dr. M and his patients spoke either French (Mali's official language) or Bamanankan (a lingua franca in Mali), or switched between these languages. This switching seemed to depend only partially on the patient's educational background, as even with those with a higher educational background who would speak French more routinely he often spoke Bamanankan. However, even when speaking in Bamanankan, Dr. M used French technical biomedical terms to explain physiological and pathological human reproduction processes and technological procedures. By doing so he demonstrated his medical competence and authority to the patients, but hampered patients' understanding and also prevented them from asking further questions. In various interviews it turned out that the patients had not understood the issues correctly, as in Modibo's case. While I was at the consultation with Modibo, IUI and ICSI were explained to him. In our talk afterwards he admitted that he roughly knew how IUI was conducted but he did not understand ICSI, which he then asked me to explain to him, along with how it differed from IVF. Although he had been told during the consultation that IUI success rates are not 100 percent, he said, "We will do an IUI [. . .]. It is expensive, but it is quicker and the result is concrete."

But these aspects are also connected to the pragmatic, result-oriented attitude of men and women in Bamako. They predominantly wanted to conceive a baby in accordance with their gender-specific reproductive aims, but the procedures' technical details seemed to be of secondary interest to most patients and were perceived as being the doctor's affair. The social reputation of the gynecologist and the patients' individual confidence in him seemed to be more important for many patients than understanding in detail what he was actually doing.

As briefly outlined above, in his consultations Dr. M not only negotiated moral and sociocultural norms with transnationally acquired ideas about good practice, but also business interests and professional aims, such as his need for success with IVF. Having experimented with IVF for five years, and having confirmed his competence in this field, Dr. M openly stated in 2008 that he desperately needed the birth of an IVF baby to counter rumors of failure that were being spread by envious colleagues and patients with whom IVF had failed.

Dr. M doubted that a success would be possible with classic IVF, because of two factors.

> First, if the husband hears that the fallopian tubes are blocked, instead of giving the money for the woman's fertilization he will marry a second wife. Second, those women who are in a position to co-finance and/or to convince their husbands to pay for IVF in the case of blocked fallopian tubes are generally too old for positive results to be likely. But, if the man himself is the cause, then he is prepared to do anything. [. . .] They will pay, they will get the money together.

As no satisfying social strategies were available for infertile men, ICSI would allow Dr. M to achieve an IVF baby much more easily. Therefore, he was planning to purchase the equipment to provide ICSI.

Until this aim was achieved, Dr. M was taking another route to increase his chances of success. In contrast to his first statements in 2005, when he told me that he did not perform heterologous forms of IVF, he began to suggest that older women try IVF using a donor ovum from a sister, cousin, or niece. Using donor ova was possible because there were as yet no laws and no official religious guidelines banning the practice in Mali. To avoid conflict with colleagues and religious voices, Dr. M did not mention this possibility in public. It was a secret between him, his biologist, and the women he suggested it to. Asked about his moral constraints as a Muslim, Dr. M rejected religious interpretations that could limit the acceptability of heterologous practices of ART. Instead, he argued that, according to Muslim rules, the origin of a child was judged by its father and therefore, in his opinion, using donor ova was not such a big problem as using donor sperm. Moreover, he argued that he wanted to help infertile women over the age of 40 to escape their devastating social situation.[16]

The anticipation and (partial) reflection of socially different procreative agendas for males and females in Mali is negotiated along with transnationally acquired biomedical practices, various local frames of reference, and scientific and entrepreneurial interests. In his legitimizations Dr. M invoked, conflated, and blurred different voices and languages referring to morality, religion, patients' social needs, science, and international treatment standards. The ways Dr. M juggled these different aspects and switched between them showed what it meant to be transnational but at the same time to practice locally, and where these forces intersected.

Global Entanglements, Transnational Activities, Local Appropriation

Taking a look at the local Malian arena regarding infertility and ART brings out complex entanglements of different actors and forces. When these fields are followed beyond local influences, a dynamic picture emerges showing how infertility and ART are merged in medicoscapes spanning the world. In the absence of state regulations and public support in Mali and Togo, families, affected couples, and gynecologists handle biomedical knowledge and the technological possibilities of ART by negotiating different frames of reference. The regulatory gaps allow gynecologists to promote ART measures in line with their own moral convictions and business considerations. Nevertheless, gynecologists always have to take into account that their social and professional reputation might be endangered by negative rumors spread by patients or colleagues. Gynecologists base their style of consultation and treatment on social norms and family values, juggling these factors with transnationally acquired ideas of good biomedical practice and know-how, religious convictions, and economic and entrepreneurial questions. My case studies show how the use of ART is adapted and appropriated to local specificities in terms of economic, religious, moral, sociocultural, and gender-specific considerations and professional interests. But how are biomedical knowledge, practice, and ART options affecting sociocultural configurations and family values?

First, biomedicine contests the prevalent tendency to blame women for infertility. In couples suffering from male-factor infertility, knowing their husbands to be the cause of the problem seems to be a source of release and resilience for women, enabling them to handle the ongoing stigmatization within their families. Although neither secrecy management within families nor mainstream narratives that blame women seem to be directly affected by biomedical diagnosis and therapy, there is a possibility that biomedicine will influence this field in the long run, depending on the way state politics, religious opinion leaders, gynecologists, and perhaps Malians suffering from infertility inspire and actively influence public discourse.

Second, nearly all women keep the diagnosis of male-factor infertility secret within and beyond their extended families. By doing so, they seek to strengthen marital bonds against family interests and they gain a certain power over their husbands. To some degree this effort is indirectly strengthened by the gynecologist, who emphasizes the couple's cohesion as the basis for finding a solution.

Besides these influences, ART offers hope of genetic/biological offspring for marriage partners. Due to high costs and competing social solutions such as polygyny, ART in female-factor infertility seems feasible only when the marriage bonds are highly valued and/or women have financial resources at their own disposal. Concerning power relations between extended family, husbands, and wives in case of diagnosed male-factor infertility, ART and biomedical diagnosis seem to increase the couple's cohesion, thereby curtailing to a certain degree the large influence of patrilineage on marital procreative agendas. These subtle processes are encouraged by the transformative potential of biomedical diagnosis and ART.

The process of introducing ART in Mali and Togo is not taking place through activities between states, international institutions, and organizations. It is, instead, being mediated by actors through their participation in transnational social and professional fields. Transnational professional fields are characterized by affiliations through profession and expertise. These contacts are acquired and advanced by education or employment abroad, and through international conferences where West African ART pioneers connect with international ones. In contrast, transnational social fields center on (kinship) ties with emigrants living abroad. Nevertheless, they also embrace professional connections acquired through appointments at international NGOs or other organizations. Both transnational fields are informal and dynamic spaces for acquiring information, knowledge, and know-how, and for purchasing medical materials such as pharmaceuticals and technical apparatus.

My case studies also show how transnational social and professional fields are central to the establishment of ART in Mali and Togo. Access to transnational social fields and especially transnational professional fields within biomedicine is not only essential for acquiring skills and purchasing technologies, but also for building personal business relations in health-related fields. Furthermore, the example of introducing ART in Mali and Togo highlights how transnational processes are operating within medicoscapes due to the neglect of infertility as an important issue on national and international health agendas.

Seen within a global frame of reference, individual transnational health care activities in Mali and Togo characterize the arena of ART infertility treatment. While gynecologists belong mainly to the more affluent social milieus and are part of Mali and Togo's (educational) elite, in trying to establish ART in their country they find themselves at the bottom of global professional hierarchies that mirror overall global hierarchies. This perception then reinforces individual forms of transnationalism for African middle and upper-class members suffering from infertility and gynecologists working within this field. The lack of collaboration from the national public sector obstructs the introduction of ART and reduction of the costs of the reagents and medicines needed for it by bulk purchase, an area where the stronger negotiating powers of the public sector would be helpful. In this sense, the disengagement of national and international policies directly and indirectly impinges on the equity and accessibility of ART for less affluent people (cf. Giwa-Osagie 2002: 23).

Through individual transnational relations ART procedures are made available in francophone West Africa. For those who have access to financial resources and who belong to transnational social fields, it is increasingly becoming part of their therapeutic visions and itineraries. But at the same time, social and economic inequalities and inequities are reinforced and reconfigured for those who learn that ART might offer a solution to their infertility problem, but who will never be able to afford these procedures. Some Malians suffering from infertility call their condition a "disease of the poor," as they know that better therapies and procedures are available but also that there is no way to claim them either from the Malian state or the international community. Entangled with the socio-cultural necessity of producing children, this experience creates intense personal frustrations, which in turn increase loss of confidence with regard to the state, its power in administration, and its capability to care for its citizens' health. Additionally, this triggers despair and anger with regard to their own position within a wider world, in which transnational and global connectedness becomes ever more important for being able to take advantage of the new opportunities promoted by biomedical professionals.

Acknowledgments

I am grateful to the German Research Association for funding this research between 2006 and 2008. I further wish to thank everyone who worked with me during this time, particularly the Malian and Togolese gynecologists, and especially all the women and men plagued by childlessness. To protect their privacy all persons in this article have been anonymized. My gratitude also goes to the editors and two anonymous reviewers as well as to Susan Reynolds Whyte, Rene Gerrets, Kristine Krause, Kerstin Pinther, and Swenja Poll for comments and inspiration concerning earlier drafts of this article.

Notes

1. In general, IUI is carried out in cases of male subfertility, failure in sperm–mucus interaction, and immunologically caused sterility of the couple. In Mali such an intervention costs between 1,500 and 2,700 USD (medical fees and pharmaceuticals included); in Togo 1,150–2,150 USD; and in Germany 800–2,000 USD (when not covered by health insurance but paid for privately by the patients). IVF is carried out in cases of blocked tubes, adverse conditions after amputation of tubes, endometriosis, male subfertility, and immunologically caused sterility. The total costs for IVF (medical fees and pharmaceuticals included) in Mali range between 3,300 and 4,000 USD; in Togo come to around 3,750 USD; and in Germany around 5,700 USD. ICSI is carried out in case of male sub- or infertility, and total costs (medical fees and pharmaceuticals included) are around 4,350 USD in Togo and around 9,000 USD in Germany. Donor sperm is mainly used in cases of azoospermia, when no premature sperm can be harvested in the testicles; costs remain roughly the same in this case. Donor ova are mainly used in women with reduced ovarian capacity or women already in menopause. Costs are added for preparing the donor and the receiver of the ova but no average amounts are available (for indications see http://www.repromedizin.de/fileadmin/ethik/rl-befruchtung-2005_11_15.pdf [accessed June 17, 2010]; the costs for Germany were given in personal communication by the president of the Bundesverband Repromedizinischer Zentren in Deutschland e.V.).

2. Following Steven Vertovec, the term *international* in this article is used to refer either to interactions between national governments or to bi- and multilateral policies. The term *transnational* is applied to "linkages and ongoing exchanges among non-state actors based across national borders—business, non-government-organisations, and individuals sharing the same interests" (Vertovec 2009: 3).

3. See the edited volume by Inhorn and van Balen (2002), particularly the contributions of Leonard (2002), Feldman-Savelsberg (2002), and Gerrits (2002) on infertility in sub-Saharan African countries.

4. Formally structured relations between different generations and genders predominantly define social family texture. Although different frames of reference (Loimeier et al. 2005) like Islam or Western secular ideals of democracy are referred to in many situations, these intra-family interrelationships are widely accepted, respected, and enacted in daily life.

5. For more information on social stigmatization as experienced and perceived by afflicted women, see Hörbst (2006: 39).

6. Cf. Inhorn 2006b concerning the handling of male-factor infertility in Egypt.

7. Divorce does not seem to be of great importance for men in cases of female-factor infertility.

8. For further discussion on Islam, infertility, and ART see Inhorn (2005, 2006a, 2006b), as well as Clarke (2008), and Hörbst (2009).

9. Women discreetly using these options have every reason not to disclose it to anyone; thus there are limits to fieldwork concerning this point.

10. For shortcomings in gynecological infertility management in sub-Saharan Africa, see Sundby and Larsen (2006).

11. In return for giving me permission to conduct fieldwork at his clinic in 2004–2005, this gynecologist asked me to facilitate contacts with a German IVF clinic. Together with his biologist, he took up an internship in Munich in 2005.

12. This became problematic due to heightened security on flights in Europe following the thwarted terror attempts on July 7, 2005 in England, as only personally needed drugs and up to 100 ml of liquids have been allowed on airplanes since then.

13. Notions which are not correct for Islam either in Mali or in other regions. For discussion on this issue see Inhorn (2005, 2006a, 2006b).

14. For differences between Sunni and Shiite regulations as well as between religious regulations and practical achievements see Inhorn (2005, 2006a, 2006b) and Hörbst (2008, 2009).

15. The crucial importance of pregnancy for women seems to rule out surrogacy.

16. Since the end of 2009 Dr. M and his biologist have been offering ICSI as well as IVF using anonymous donor ova, while anonymous sperm donation is only performed when the men themselves request it. In 2010 the first Malian IVF- and ICSI-babies were born.

References

Brand, Saskia. 2001. *Mediating Means and Fate: A Socio-political Analysis of Fertility and Demographic Change in Bamako, Mali*. Leiden, the Netherlands: Brill.

Clarke, Morgan. 2008. "New Kinship, Islam, and the Liberal Tradition: Sexual Morality and New Reproductive Technology in Lebanon." *Journal of the Royal Anthropological Institute* 14: 153–169.

Daar, Abdallah, and Zara Merali. 2002. "Infertility and Social Suffering: The Case of ART in Developing Countries." In *Current Practices and Controversies in Assisted Reproduction*; report of a meeting on "Medical, Ethical, and Social Aspects of Assisted Reproduction" held at the WHO headquarters in Geneva, Switzerland, Sept. 17–21, 2001; ed. Effy Vayena, Patrick J. Rowe, and P. David Griffin, 15–21. Geneva: WHO.

Dyer, S. J., N. Abrahams, N. E. Mokoena, and Z. van der Spuy. 2004. "'You Are a Man Because You Have Children': Experiences, Reproductive Health Knowledge, and Treatment-seeking Behaviour among Men Suffering from Couple Infertility in South Africa." *Human Reproduction* 19 (4): 960–967.

Feldman-Savelsberg, Pamela. 2002. "Infertility an Unrecognized Public Health and Population Problem? The View from the Cameroon Grassfields." In *Infertility Around the Globe: New Thinking on Childlessness, Gender, and Reproductive Technologies,* ed. Marcia C. Inhorn and Frank van Balen, 215–232. Berkeley: University of California Press.

Gerrits, Trudie. 2002. "Infertility and Matrilineality: The Exceptional Case of the Macua in Mozambique." In *Infertility Around the Globe: New Thinking on Childlessness, Gender, and Reproductive Technologies,* ed. Marcia C. Inhorn and Frank van Balen, 233–246. Berkeley: University of California Press.

Giani, Sergio. 2006. "La santé communautire au Mali, entre mondialisation et décentralisation." *Documents et Travaux sur le Savoir Local* 3: 83–91.

Giwa-Osagie, Osato F. 2002. "ART in Developing Countries with Particular Reference to Sub-Saharan Africa." In *Current Practices and Controversies in Assisted Reproduction;* report of a meeting on "Medical, Ethical, and Social Aspects of Assisted Reproduction" held at WHO headquarters in Geneva, Switzerland, Sept. 17–21, 2001; ed. Effy Vayena, Patrick J. Rowe, and P. David Griffin, 15–21. Geneva: WHO.

Glick Schiller, Nina, and Peggy Levitt. 2006. "Haven't We Heard This Somewhere Before? A Substantive View of Transnational Migration Studies by Way of a Reply to Waldinger and Fitzgerald." Working Paper 06–01, Center for Migration and Development, Princeton University. Electronic document: http://cmd.princeton.edu/papers/wp0601.pdf.

Grosz-Ngaté, Maria. 1989. "Hidden Meanings: Explorations into a Bamanan Construction of Gender." *Ethnology* 28 (1): 167–183.

Hadolt, Bernhard, and Viola Hörbst. 2010. "Problemlagen, Anwendungskontexte, Nutzungspraktiken. Assistierte Reproduktionstechnologien in Mali und Österreich." In *Medizin im Kontext. Krankheit und Gesundheit in einer vernetzten Welt,* ed. Hansjörg Dilger and Bernhard Hadolt, 89–110. Frankfurt am Main: Peter Lang Verlag.

Hörbst, Viola. 2006. "Infertility and In-vitro-Fertilization in Bamako, Mali: Women's Experience, Avenues for Solution, and Social Contexts Impacting on Gynaecological Consultations." Special Issue: "Reproductive Disruptions: Perspectives on African Contexts," *Curare* 29 (1): 35–46.

———. 2008. "Male Infertility in Mali: Kinship and Impacts on Biomedical Practice in Bamako." In *Muslim Medical Ethics: From Theory to Practice,* ed. Jonathan Brockopp and Thomas Eich, 118–137. Columbia: South Carolina Press.

———. 2009. "Islamische Grundsätze und die Handhabung assistierter Reproduktionstechnologien in Bamako, Mali." In *Reproduktionsmedizin bei Muslimen: säkulare und religiöse Ethiken im Widerstreit?* ed. Thomas Eich, 48–64. Electronic document: http://www.heceas.org/media/Islam_Medizinethik_08.pdf.

———. 2010. "Male Perspectives on Infertility and Assisted Reproductive Technologies (ART) in Sub-Saharan Contexts." In *Social Aspects of Accessible Infertility Care in Developing Countries,* 22–27 (special publication by the journal *Facts, Views, and Vision in ObGyn*). Wetteren, the Netherlands: Universa Press.

Hörbst, Viola, and Kristine Krause. 2004. "'On the Move'—Die Globalisier-ungsdebatte in der Medizinethnologie." *Curare* 27 (1–2): 41–60.

Hörbst, Viola, and Angelika Wolf. 2003. "Globalisierung der Heilkunde: Eine Einführung." In *Medizin und Globalisierung. Universelle Ansprüche—lokale Antworten,* ed. Angelika Wolf and Viola Hörbst, 3–30. Münster: Lit Verlag.

Inhorn, Marcia C. 2005. "Religion and Reproductive Technologies: IVF and Gamete Donation in the Muslim World." *Anthropology News* (Feb.): 14–18.

———. 2006a. "Introduction to Medical Anthropology in the Muslim World." Special Issue: "Medical Anthropology in the Muslim World: Ethnographic Reflections on Reproductive and Child Health," *Medical Anthropology Quarterly* 20: 1–11.

———. 2006b. "'The Worms Are Weak': Male Infertility and Patriarchal Paradoxes in Egypt." In *Islamic Masculinities,* ed. Lahoucine Ouzgane, 217–237. London: Zed Books.

Inhorn, Marcia C., and Aditya Bharadwaj. 2007. "Reproductively Disabled Lives: Infertility, Stigma, and Suffering in Egypt and India." In *Disability in Local and Global Worlds,* ed. Benedicte Ingstad and Susan Reynolds Whyte, 78–106. Berkeley: University of California Press.

Inhorn, Marcia C., and Frank van Balen. 2002. *Infertility around the Globe: New Thinking on Childlessness, Gender, and Reproductive Technologies.* Berkeley: University of California Press.

Jaffré, Yannick, and Jean-Pierre Olivier de Sardan. 2003. *Une médecine inhospitalière. Les difficiles relations entre soignants et soignés dans cinq capitales d'Afrique de l'Ouest.* Paris: Karthala.

Leonard, Lori. 2002. "Problematizing Fertility: 'Scientific' Accounts and Chadian Women's Narratives." In *Infertility Around the Globe: New Thinking on Childlessness, Gender, and Reproductive Technologies,* ed. Marcia C. Inhorn and Frank van Balen, 193–214. Berkeley: University of California Press.

Levitt, Peggy. 2007. "Culture, Migration, and Development: Rethinking the Connections." Electronic document: http://peggylevitt.org/pdfs/Levitt-cultureanddevelopment.pdf.

Levitt, Peggy, and Nina Glick Schiller. 2004. "Conceptualizing Simultaneity: A Transnational Social Field Perspective on Society." *International Migration Review* 38: 1002–1039.

Loimeier, Roman, Dieter Neubert, and Cordula Weißköppel. 2005. "Einleitung: Globalisierung im lokalen Kontext—Perspektiven und Konzepte von Handeln in Afrika." In *Globalisierung im lokalen Kontext. Konzepte und Perspektiven von Handeln in Afrika,* ed. Roman Loimer, Dieter Neubert, and Cordula Weißköppel, 1–30. Münster: Lit.

Mariko, Soumaila, and Issa Bara Berthé. 2007. "Fécondité." In *Mali. Enquête Démographique et de Santé (EDSM-IV),* ed. Salif Samaké, Seydou Moussa Traoré, Souleymane Ba, Étienne Dembélé, Mamadou Diop, Soumaïla Mariko, and Paul Roger Libité for Cellule de Planification et de Statistique, Ministère de la Santé, Direction Nationale de la Statistique et de l'Informatique, Ministère de l'Économie, de l'Industrie et du Commerce, 49–61. Bamako, Mali: Macro International Inc. Electronic document: http://www.measuredhs.com/pubs/pdf/FR199/FR199.pdf.

Mayaud, Philippe. 2001. "The Role of Reproductive Tract Infections." In *Women and Infertility in Sub-Saharan Africa: A Multi-disciplinary Perspective*, ed. J. Ties Boerma and Zaida Mgalla, 71–108. Amsterdam: Royal Tropical Institute.

Pilcher, Helen. 2006. "Fertility on a Shoestring." *Nature* 442 (3): 975–977.

Rutstein, Shea O., and Iqbal H. Shah. 2004. *Infecundity, Infertility, and Childlessness in Developing Countries; DHS Comparative Reports No. 9*. Calverton, Md.: ORC Macro and the World Health Organization.

Sako, Aminata. 1989. "Conséquences Socio-Culturelles et Economiques de la Stérilité Féminine au Mali." Medical Thesis, L'Ecole de Médecine et de Pharmacie du Mali, Bamako.

Schuster, Sylvie, and Viola Hörbst. 2006. "Introduction." Special Issue: "Reproductive Disruptions: Perspectives on African Contexts," *Curare* 29 (1): 5–17.

Sundby, Johanne, and Ulla Larsen. 2006. "Health Care Services for Infertility in Sub-Saharan Africa: The Case of Moshi in Northern Tanzania." Special Issue: "Reproductive Disruptions: Perspectives on African Contexts," *Curare* 29 (1): 47–59.

van Balen, Frank, and Marcia C. Inhorn. 2002. "Introduction. Interpreting Infertility: A View from the Social Sciences." In *Infertility Around the Globe: New Thinking on Childlessness, Gender, and Reproductive Technologies*, ed. Marcia C. Inhorn and Frank van Balen, 3–32. Berkeley: University of California Press.

van der Geest, Sjaak, Johan D. Speckmann, and Pieter H. Streefland. 1990. "Primary Health Care in a Multi-Level Perspective: Towards a Research Agenda." *Social Science & Medicine* 30 (9): 1025–1034.

Vertovec, Steven. 2009. *Transnationalism*. London: Routledge.

SEVEN

Flows of Medicine, Healers, Health Professionals, and Patients between Home and Host Countries

Abdoulaye Kane

This chapter examines the flows of medicine and health care services both biomedical and traditional between the villages of the Senegal River Valley and the Haalpulaar[1] immigrant communities in France. Haalpulaar migrants in France are intervening in their home communities to help ensure that people at home have access to health care. Both individual and collective forms of agency grow in the process of medicine transfers between the two places. On the one hand, individuals abroad send biomedical medicine to their rural homes, and family members send traditional medicine to France. On the other hand, Haalpulaar migrants' associations like Thilogne Association Developpement (TAD) and Fouta Santé are improving access to health care in the Senegal River Valley through remittances of biomedicine and medical equipment as well as the organization of annual health caravans with the participation of French health professionals and local partners.

In the first section, I will look at the circulation of medicine between France and the Senegal River Valley villages. Medicine is part of the flows that characterize African transnational practices. The circulation of biomedicine and traditional medicine between the two spaces indicates that migrants want to take advantage of both systems. I will also examine the ambivalent attitude of Haalpulaar migrants toward utilizing biomedicine by exploring the various conspiracy theories around suspicious death. I next examine the role of village associations in meeting the challenges of providing access to health care to their communities of origin. I will look at the case of Thilogne Association Developpement, in particular, by reviewing their interventions from the early 1980s up to 2006. The last section of the chapter will highlight the achievement of Fouta Santé in mobilizing resources and expertise for the local hospitals and health facilities in the Senegal River Valley towns and villages.

The Circulation of Medicine, Experts, and Patients

Appadurai's (2001) influential argument characterizes life in the contemporary world as one of flows shaped by objects in motion. "These objects include ideas and ideologies, people and goods, images and messages, technologies and techniques" (Appadurai 2001: 5). The circulation of money, electronics objects, images, goods, and material culture has attracted the most attention because of the economic bias in the study of migration. Some researchers have analyzed the circulation of such things as food and clothes, or music and videos, conveyed from sending areas to global cities as indicators of migrants' willingness to maintain their cultural identity (MacGaffey and Bazenguissa-Ganga 2000). Other researchers are interested in the changing meaning of such commodities when they cross ethnic and national boundaries. Material goods from host countries brought back home enhance migrants' social status in their community of origin, while objects taken from home countries become part of the re-creation of a home away from home in host countries (Copeland-Carson 2004; Kane 2005; Geschiere and Meyer 1999).

This growing literature on the circulation of objects between Europe and Africa has so far overlooked the medicine traveling between diasporic communities and their places of origin. Sending biomedicine home has become as common as sending money home. I came to realize the importance of medicine remittances through my personal experiences traveling between France and Senegal. During my frequent trips between these two countries, I was often used as a carrier for all kinds of objects, including medicine being remitted by migrants to people at home. In 2004, when leaving Paris for Senegal, my mother-in-law gave me leftovers of her prescription and over-the-counter medicines for her 85-year-old mother in Thilogne. Although she has no professional background related to health, she explained to me, as if she were an expert, how her mother should use the medicine. Puzzled, I ask her whether it was safe for her mother to take these medicines. She replied that it was not the first time she had sent medicine to her. She continued: "she is used to most of these medicines. She asks me on the phone to send her more every year."

The medicines she gave me included painkillers, anti-inflammatory ointments, cold and cough syrups, anti-diarrheal medicines, etc. Besides occasionally sending these medicines with others such as myself, she goes back home every two years with a bag half-full of medicine that she distributes to her family and in her neighborhood. She explains that whenever she goes back, people come to see her to ask her if she has pills for headaches, diarrhea, colds, and malaria. Family, friends, and neighbors expect that she, like all other migrants visiting their Senegalese homes, will bring medicines. The assumption of these villagers is that migrants have knowledge about the medicines they bring. Based on their personal experience of using the medicines, migrants operate in their home villages like surrogate experts whose views are taken seriously by "patients."

My mother-in-law's case is not an isolated one. Many Haapulaar living in France have long been engaged in remitting medicine to their families back home. Along with other commodities, the travelers like me moving back and forth between home and host countries often carry both biomedical and the traditional healing products and objects. Medicine, cell phones, shoes, clothes, and money are among the many things people routinely carry home on behalf of migrants to their family members left behind. This circulation of medicine and many other material goods is far from being unidirectional. They travel both ways. On my way back, I was given medicinal plants and amulets to be distributed to family members in France. This is certainly a common practice for travelers between the Senegal River Valley villages and France.

In a survey conducted at the Foyer Aftam[2] and the Clos des Roses neighborhood in Compiègne, France, 21 out of 23 Haalpulaar migrants (11 women and 10 men) indicated that they send and carry prescription medicine to their communities.[3] Only two people said that they were not involved in such practices because of their potential harm to relatives. These two acknowledged, however, that they do share over-the-counter medicines when they return home. Some of the interviewees showed me several bags of pills, syrups, and ointments waiting to be sent home, leftovers of the interviewees' prescriptions. The French welfare system makes access to biomedicine very easy for the Haalpulaar migrants.

The migrants can help a patient at home to benefit from the generosity of the French health system with the complicity of family doctors. Those ill and in pain in Senegal will indicate to their relative(s) in France the symptoms of their illnesses. These are in turn repeated to a doctor in France as the migrant's own complaints. The doctor will prescribe medicine to the migrant.[4] After getting the medicines from the pharmacy for free, the migrant sends them to his relative back home. There are also cases in which the patient in Senegal will go to visit a doctor at a local hospital, get a prescription, and send it to relatives in France for purchase. The migrant goes to see his family doctor asking for a similar prescription under his name, with which he obtains the desired medicines for his relative from a French pharmacy without paying a penny.

Amad Sy, 43 years old with a primary level of education, works as an employee in a construction business. He was one of my interviewees who said that there are several people in his home village whose survival depends on the remittances of medicine from himself and other migrants from his village. He mentioned the case of his uncle, who has high blood pressure and to whom he sends some of his own pills (since he has himself a similar health condition) every two months.

Peggy Levitt (2001) has broadened our notion of migrants' remittances by adding to the obvious financial sendings an account of what she calls social remittances. The idea is that migrants not only send money to their home countries but are also vectors of social change through the ideas and practical knowledge they acquire during their stay in their host societies. The remittance of medicines by Haalpulaar migrants in France is a case in point. The migrants are transformed by their experiences in France and tend to be vectors of social change in their home communities in Senegal (Quiminal 1986). Haalpulaar migrants who have lived in France often behave as surrogate biomedical experts for their communities in Senegal based on the little knowledge about illness and medicine they have accumulated through their personal experience as patients in France. For many in the remotely located villages next to the river or deep in the highlands (*Ferlo*) of the Senegal River Valley, the migrants' medicine and expertise is highly appreciated. But traditional practices of healing are still predominantly the first option for these villagers. The migrants themselves, despite their stock of Western medicines, consult regularly with local healers, consume traditional medicine, wear talismans, and drink and bathe themselves with blessed water to prevent the evil eye or cure illnesses believed to be related to wind and spirits. After vacations at home, the migrants return to France with a provision of herbs, roots, concoctions, talismans, and blessed water for themselves and their families.

As with medicine, healers and patients are also in permanent motion between Senegal River Valley villages and France. The Barbes metro station in Paris hosts several African men handing out African healers' business cards every day. They claim to have the power to heal all illnesses, including cancer and HIV / AIDS. They also offer their services to solve social and economic problems (employment, promotion, love relations, etc.). African migrants, of course, are their most important clientele, but they receive a growing number of French nationals who consult them out of desperation. There are Senegalese traders who are bringing healing products from home and selling them in the open markets in France or during special religious or cultural events. During the religious celebrations of the 2009 edition of the *Daaka*[5] by the Haalpulaar migrants belonging to the Tijani Sufi order[6] there were two traders selling traditional medicine along with prayers beads, religious scarves, and the white hats which are markers of the Tijani religious identity.

The flow of patients back and forth between Senegal and France is frequent. The local patients may leave the Senegal River Valley villages for Dakar to get health care attention in one the capital's hospitals. But when there are complications, and the patient is wealthy or has a choice, the next step is to go to France. Retired migrants who return to Senegal to live in their rural homes often come back to France as patients in need of care. It is also common for migrants to go back to their villages of origin as patients of local healers. In most cases, these patients have tried the biomedicine in their host country without success. Migrants suffering from terminal illnesses are sent home by family members or village associations to seek traditional forms of treatment. Most of the Haalpulaar social networks in France include in their services to members assistance with repatriation in cases of illnesses that need the attention of traditional healers or *marabouts.*[7]

Some Haalpulaar believe that certain types of illnesses cannot be healed by Western medicine and the only choice left to a migrant who is suffering from a wind- or spirit-related illness is to go back home in search of traditional or religious forms of healing. These specific illnesses are believed even to worsen when the patient goes to see a doctor instead of a traditional healer or *marabout.* Migrants who have chronic diseases are believed to have committed the mistake of seeing a doctor or using biomedicine in a situation where recourse to traditional medicine would have been more appropriate. The wind- and spirit-related diseases do not accept, according to beliefs widely shared among the Haalpulaar, that the patient be subjected to any injection or transfusion. These common biomedical ways to administer medicine are believed to worsen the patient's situation.

However, despite these strong beliefs, Haalpulaar migrants do use, and in some cases abuse, biomedicine. Easy access to biomedical health care in France makes the Haalpulaar migrants more familiar with modern treatments of illnesses. The recourse to biomedicine has become as frequent as the recourse to the complex of traditional Haalpulaar healing practices comprising material and metaphysical, mystical and spiritual components.

The Haalpulaar migrants are known for maintaining very strong relations with their families and communities left behind. Therefore they maintain a strong sense of their religious and cultural identities. The circulation of people as both patients and healers, of knowledge, and of beliefs draws the suburbs of Paris and the northeast of Senegal together. Despite being in a highly modern and Western environment where people have a "rational" conception of illness and healing as material realities understood through a body of scientific knowledge and its correlated discourse and practices, the Haalpulaar migrants continue to invest in their traditional systems of understanding illness and healing that integrate material, metaphysical, and spiritual realities. This explains the simultaneous recourse by Haalpulaar in France to both biomedical and traditional health care systems, and the flows of medicines between France and Senegal.

Between Fascination and Mistrust

The attitude of Haalpulaar migrants toward what they call *Safaara tou-bakoobe* (Western medicine) is characterized by both fascination and mistrust. This ambivalence is made evident by the experiences narrated below of individual migrants during times when they needed medical attention. My cases focus mainly on male experiences because I collected my data in a local *foyer* (male migrants' dormitory) after a prayer for the dead ceremony attended only by men. My discussion with my informants started around the suspicious death of a Haalpulaar migrant who, as they said, "went to the hospital on his feet and by himself, and two days later was dead."

The death of Djiby, 59, was the predominant subject of discussion in Compiègne in 2005. He was a recent retiree who had worked for 25 years for a small factory in Compiègne. The common reaction toward the French health care system was that it deliberately uses black bodies as subjects on which to test some of its new medicines and practices without the consent of patients. Several similar death cases were evoked by Ali, 47, who strongly believes, like many Haaalpulaar migrants, that they are not a simple coincidence but part of a very well elaborated plan to exterminate retirees and to use black bodies as experimentation subjects. The following case sums up the lack of credit that some migrants give to biomedical diagnosis and treatment.

Ndiaye, 32, recently arrived in France. He did not go to a Western school. He works temporarily for a construction business. He has been granted asylum and is eligible for CMU (Couverture Medicale Universelle = Universal Medical Coverage), which is an insurance scheme that covers all his medical costs (including medical consultations and prescriptions). He felt that something was wrong with his body, and told me that he knew that he was ill. He went to see several physicians and medical specialists to have a thorough physical. He wanted "to make sure that there is no disease hiding in my body." All medical tests (blood and urine tests, scanners, radiographies, etc.) concluded that he was in good health. But Ndiaye was not convinced and insisted before his general physician that he thinks that there is something wrong with his body. He finally concluded that the biomedical diagnostic was not what he needed. "My disease," he said, "is unknown by the white men. I better turn to the traditional health practitioners and *marabouts*." He complained of stomachache and thought he might had been bewitched by some kin members who were jealous of his success at entering Europe and having been able to gain legal status.

Ndiaye's attitude is very common among the Haalpulaar migrants in France. Upon their arrival many were advised by family members who had already been there for a long period of time to have a physical. The underlying assumption here is that in Senegal access to biomedical health care is expensive and therefore very limited. Comparing France and Senegal, the migrants believed that the kind of health care attention you can get in France is better than what you can get in Senegalese hospitals and other health facilities. In many cases like Ndiaye's, migrants get their first physical in France. But even if one behavior of newcomers is to profit from the easy access to biomedical diagnostics and treatments, as indicated in the case of Ndiaye, they certainly do not believe that Western medicine can heal all their illnesses. Ndiaye contested the biomedical diagnosis he received by pointing out to me that the health professionals he visited could not find what he was suffering from.

Diamguel, 57, has no Western education. He worked as a janitor for the city council for 17 years and retired in 2002. He speaks of biomedical treatments in very flattering ways. "The white men's medicines are just magical," he said. "Every time I have some pain or feel ill and I go to see my physician, he always gives me very effective medicines that calm my pain and make me feel better." He also remarked, "Health care is in this country and not in Senegal." But when asked whether biomedicine is suitable to treat all diseases, Diamguel's response acknowledged the limits of the "white men's medicines" when it comes to addressing forms of illness unknown to them. According to him, biomedical personnel cannot treat diseases caused by *hendu* (wind), *badanal* (harm done by *marabouts*), or *cukugnagu* (witchcraft-related diseases). For each of these categories there is a corresponding traditional healer in Senegal. The illnesses of *hendu* are treated by traditional healers known as *jom ledde en*. *Badanal* is caused by *marabouts* who use Qur'anic scriptures, and it can only be undone by *marabouts* who have the same knowledge of the holy scriptures. *Cukugnagu* is healed by *fi birbaaji,* who are believed to be witches themselves. "If a person has one of these three forms of illness," Diamguel said, the doctor (biomedical physician) is unable to determine what he is suffering from. "It is why," he said, "our traditional ways are very important even in this country."

For Hamidou, 52, a worker in a local factory without any formal education, *"Safaara toubakoobe et safaara baleebe fof yiilete tan ko cellal"* ("biomedical or traditional, what matters to a patient is be healed"). He continues to say that,

> [i]t doesn't matter which treatment one is taking, going to the hospital or to the healer. In both cases what people are looking for is healing. Some diseases are cured better by our healers and others by Western medicine. When you are ill or one of your family members is ill, you just juggle between the healers, the *marabouts*, and the doctors until you or he gets better. In some cases, it is the combination of all of those three that is determinant.

Other migrants are very suspicious and very skeptical toward biomedical treatment. Salif, 63, worked as a dishwasher in a small restaurant in Compiègne. He retired in 1998 and returned to Senegal, where he lives with his family. He is convinced that as a migrant he was not given the proper medication by French doctors. He never accepted the flu vaccine given for free to retirees because, he said, "All retiree[s] I knew who have taken the flu vaccine died shortly after going back to their home villages." After returning home he was ill for a year and was convinced that the kind of disease he had could not be cured by biomedical treatment. He spent a considerable amount of money and time on traditional forms of treatment in Senegal. However, when his health deteriorated badly, he was forced by family members to go to France for treatment. When he arrived in France, his brother recalled, "He looked like a skeleton." His brother prefers biomedical treatments to traditional healing practices, and told him that being stubborn almost cost him his life. Salif said that many in the village did not understand his persistence in wanting to be healed by traditional practitioners and some mentioned to him that they wished they were in his place, being able to go to France for medical treatment at almost no cost.

Salif's experiences took place against the backdrop of an ongoing debate among Haalpulaar migrants on the unusually high death rate among retirees between 1995 and 2004. Many think that there is a conspiracy in the French health system to eliminate the African immigrants after their retirement so that they will not benefit from their pensions. Sall, 57, a recent retiree with a primary level of education, defended that point of view. He pointed out to me a number of suspicious deaths involving recently retired Haalpulaar who all died in very similar conditions after taking flu shots. He continued, "France needs us young and healthy; when we retire, we become a burden that they are not ready to support." There have also been a large number of medical malpractice instances involving Haalpulaar immigrants that reinforce this idea of being deliberately targeted and killed by French doctors. One wonders how much of this malpractice is the result of misunderstandings between Haalpulaar patients unable to express themselves in French and doctors who do not request translators and try to rely on their understanding of broken French or on patients' body language. But Sall's view of the matter is not unique. There have been some cases brought to court by migrants' associations that firmly believe these allegations. This atmosphere explains the reserve shown by many Haalpulaar immigrants toward the biomedical health system. What is at issue here is not the efficacy of biomedical forms of treatment, but rather the lack of trust that postcolonial subjects have toward a country that has a long history of domination and exploitation of their societies.

Kalidou, 58, lives with his family in Compiègne, on the edge of Paris. He did not have any formal education and speaks basic French. He retired in 2005 after working for 21 years for a small factory making plastic containers. Before eating his lunch and dinner, he takes a cocktail of biomedical pills because he has high blood pressure combined with diabetes. He pointed out to me that he survives by "eating drugs" and complained about the fact he has a lot of medicines to take in a daily basis. "Sometimes I wonder," he said, "if it is not better to have our herbs and medicinal concoctions." While many Haalpulaar migrants like Kalidou have embraced biomedical treatment, they are also, like him, very fearful of becoming dependent on the pills.

Women's attitudes toward biomedical treatment are as ambivalent as men's. One of the recurrent complaints among the Haalpulaar women in Compiègne is that some hospital staff and nurses abuse them when they are in delivery rooms. They argue that French doctors and nurses have no respect for African women who do not follow family planning. Athia, 44, stated that the French doctors and nurses in delivery rooms treat African women as "ignorant." They cannot understand why African women are not interested in family planning and the fact that they cannot speak French well reinforces the health professionals' prejudices about the irrationality of their choices.

Haalpulaar ambivalence toward biomedical care is most often present in cases where migrants think that afflictions come from metaphysical agents and they believe strongly that any biomedical intervention might worsen the illness. There is clearly a variation in the level of belief in the existence of metaphysical afflicting agents among Haalpulaar migrants. The bulk of the first generation, now in their fifties and without Western education, tend to hold more strongly to these beliefs, while the younger members of the first generation and members of the second generation tend simply to accommodate these beliefs without necessarily being convinced of their relevance. The choice of what form of treatment is appropriate depends on what is thought to be the nature of the illness. The combination of different forms of treatment is very common before determining whether an illness can be treated with traditional medicine or biomedicine.

In cases of suspicious deaths, what the Haalpulaar migrants oppose is not biomedicine as such but rather its (alleged) use by French health professionals to eliminate Haalpulaar retirees. Before retirement, the Haalpulaar do go to visit their doctors on a regular basis for host of health issues, which indicates their acceptance of the benefits of biomedical treatment. And so, despite the ambivalence that migrants feel about biomedicine, there is a general consensus, especially among the youth, about the need for hometown associations to intervene in improving Senegalese populations' access to biomedical treatment and medicine. What they want the villagers back home to benefit from is the *best* that biomedicine has to offer.

The orientation of migrants' interventions in health and education can be explained by a generational change in the leadership of hometown associations that took place in the mid-1980s. Between the 1960s and the early 1980s, Haalpulaar associations were led by a first generation that was entering their sixties with no formal education, while by the mid-1980s most hometown associations were led by the young generation, and these leaders had a high level of education. The old generation of leaders focused more on religious issues such as building mosques or cemetery fences and funding religious education (Kane 2000). The young generation is more open to the idea of intervening to improve home populations' access to education and health care. Initiatives for health caravans and community pharmacies to benefit villagers in the Senegal River Valley have come from the young generation of leaders who were able to find partners in their host societies. The following section will explore the experience of hometown associations and a federation of village associations in their attempt to fill the gap left by the Senegalese state after its disengagement from social sectors as dictated by the International Monetary Fund (IMF) and the World Bank.

Health Care Services in Postcolonial Senegal: Migrants' Associations Get on Board

After Senegal gained independence in 1960, national leaders encouraged very high expectations in the population. For Senegalese households, becoming independent meant being taken care of by their own government. The French welfare state model that was applied in Senegal improved the standard of living both in rural and urban areas. There were unprecedented efforts by the central government to build hospitals in the capital city and at least one regional hospital in each of the secondary cities, such as Thies, Louga, St. Louis, Kaolack, and others. The state built dispensaries, health centers, and health huts in rural areas. Access to Western-based health care was free and the price of medicine was kept low by state subsidies.

Despite this relative ease of access to health care, populations, especially in rural areas, were not enthusiastic about consulting biomedical health services. Many continued to consult local healers, whom they believed to be more effective that modern physicians. Belief in witchcraft and evil spirits still prevailed, and biomedical practices were unfamiliar and not always trusted. Recourse to Western medicine in rural areas had always been a last resort when local healers and religious priests declared they were defeated by a disease. In fact, the health care coverage provided by the state, despite its generosity, was far from being abused by the citizens. In the 1960s and 1970s, physicians toured villages to attract patients. There were awareness campaigns that attempted to convince illiterate populations to go to the biomedical physician first when they did not feel well.

The debt crisis of the 1980s resulted in the imposition of structural adjustment programs (SAPs) on many African countries, including Senegal, by the IMF and the World Bank. Dictated by liberal ideologies, the SAPs forged new economic structures in African states designed to reshape their priorities and commitments. The African states were asked to cut funding of social services, to cut jobs in the public sector, and to privatize state-owned businesses. The social sectors deemed non-productive were neglected in favor of the productive sectors: agriculture, industry, and commercial services. Therefore, funding for health care and education services was kept at marginal levels throughout the 1980s and 1990s. That meant that access to health care became a major hurdle for many households living on less than 1 USD a day. In the Senegal River Valley it was the migrants who had left the country who in the end intervened both as individuals and associations to provide access to social-sector services such as health care and education.

Health care costs are estimated to absorb an important part of household budgets in rural Senegal (see Wolf, chapter 3 in this volume). The migrants who come back to their home villages are also known, as I indicated earlier, to bring large amounts of medication they will be sharing with family members who suffer from similar diseases or who complain of similar pains. Biomedical practitioners in regional and local Senegalese hospitals condemn those practices, which they see as very risky, but many families say they have to fend for themselves to meet their medical needs and that the medicines sent by family members from France are welcomed. They trust that their family members in France are familiar with the medicines that they send home and therefore think it is not at all risky to take them. Family members in Europe also send money to support their kin, neighbors, and friends facing illness. The remittances of Senegalese migrants to the Matam region to which the Senegal River Valley belongs were estimated to total 7.3 billion FCFA in 2008 (Diop 2008). Many individual migrants state that the most important reason to send money to kin, neighbors, and friends is to pay for medical costs. People left behind are skilled at soliciting transfer payments from family members in France. Parents, wives, or children sometimes may report a fake illness to urge their family members abroad to send them money.

Aliou, 33, left his wife and two children in Senegal. He left school at the university level. He believes that his family is using the excuse of health care costs to obtain financial support for other reasons. He says,

I can't understand that my family members are getting ill one after the other. I send twice the amount I use to send to pay for hospital bills, transport tickets between the village and Dakar. First it was my mother, after it was my wife, and now my sister is in Dakar and is asking for help because her husband cannot pay for her medical bills. I can't know from here how ill they are. If someone tells you he or she is ill, you cannot refuse to help. But I wonder how long it will take me to start saying that I cannot support them all.

Abdou, 35, lives with his wife and his son in Compiègne. He has a Masters degree in management and works for a mobile telephone company. He had similar complaints as Aliou about the way his family members use health care as an excuse to ask him to send them money. In his case, he was asked to pay local healers and *marabouts* large sums of money for the treatment of his brother, who is mentally ill. Abdou complains that his brother's illness has ruined his life. His mother appears to have gone to see all the healers and *marabouts* she has heard about, and when they charge her, they take into account the fact that she has a son in France. Abdou estimates having spent about 8,000 euro so far on his brother's medical costs. Recently he asked his cousin to take his brother to the Fann Psychiatric Hospital in Dakar for treatment. After two weeks spent at Fann, his brother felt better and Abdou is convinced he spent all that money for nothing, putting the blame on his parents who will not listen to him and who turn to him to pay their debts to healers and *marabouts*.

There is clearly a social pressure on Haalpulaar migrants to redistribute part of their earnings in France to their family members left behind. The coverage of health costs is the excuse most often used by family members to obligate their relatives living abroad to send them money. Refusal to send money in such circumstances is seen as treason to the family and would put the immigrant in the position of losing face. By agreeing to send money, the immigrant earns some social capital and prestige within his family and community.

On the other hand, there are many Haalpulaar migrants like Amad Sy, 37, who choose to send medicine in order to avoid sending money to their relatives who request their help in facing health-related costs. The cases of Aliou and Abdou indicate some of the variation among Haalpulaar migrants with regard to sending money and their attitudes toward biomedicine. They are both part of the young generation that is very critical of the pressures people at home put on migrants to regularly send money to support family members facing adversities. They are also very critical of the recourse to traditional forms of healing. They encourage their family members to rely more on biomedical treatment. These attitudes are the result of these two individuals being exposed to Western schools that tend to undermine the credibility of traditional forms of healing while providing strong arguments for biomedical forms of healing.

The coverage of health care is not left in the hands of only individual immigrants. Groups of immigrants from the same village, region, or ethnic group organize collective action aimed at improving access to and quality of health care in their home community. I will turn now to some case studies of such collective action among Haalpulaar migrants in France. To appreciate the migrants' contributions, it is important to compare it with the role the Senegalese state has played in health care since the imposition of the structural adjustment plans.

Haalpulaar Migrants' Social Networks and Health Care at Home

The Pulaar saying, *"Celal ko afo galu"* ("Health is the first wealth") shows the importance that Haalpulaar place on health care. Among Haalpulaar migrants, the first priority of the social network (based on kinship, ethnicity, or home village) is to assist members in times of need or adversity. One of the recurrent objectives of these migrants' social networks is to give financial and moral support to members who face illness. As mentioned above, despite the easy access to health care and biomedicines that legal immigrants in France enjoy, many Haalpulaar migrants' associations include in the benefits offered to members assistance with repatriation in cases of terminal or mental illnesses that they believe necessitate the intervention of traditional healers.

Some migrants' associations extend help in accessing health care to their kin, neighbors, or friends left in their home villages. In France in 2004, I attended the meeting of the Burnaabe Association (the Burnaabe are a Haalpulaar social group specialized in pottery). The members gave some financial aid to family members seeking treatment in Dakar who did not have the means to pay their medical bills. Although coming from different villages in the Senegal River Valley on both the left and right side of the river, the participants in this association are all related through blood and marriage. The practices of endogamy and inter-village marriages make this group in France feel like a single family and reinforce the solidarity among the participants and the larger family left behind. Other social categories among the Haalpulaar all have similar forms of association that play major roles in helping the poor in communities of origin to obtain access to health care.

The devaluation of the franc CFA in francophone Africa in 1994 and the concurrent doubling of medicine prices has put poor families both in rural and urban areas in an even worse situation than before. Left on their own, families and local communities had to fend for themselves. I will examine now the contribution of migrants' village associations to solutions crafted by local populations in order to meet their needs for health care concerning reproductive health, public health, and disease prevention. I will look at two cases studies. The first is Thilogne Association Developpement (TAD), which is a village-based association present in several host countries. One of the major goals of the association is to provide health care to villagers left behind. The second case is Fouta Santé, which is a federation of most of the Senegal River Valley village associations in France. In cooperation with French hospitals and Médecins Sans Frontières (Doctors Without Borders), they organize health care missions to the region of Matam to treat common illnesses such as malaria, high and low blood pressure, diabetes, and the like.

Thilogne Association Developpement

In the Senegal River Valley, the migrants' associations have distinguished themselves since the early 1980s as important agencies in fostering the development of their local communities. Health care and education are the two sectors where their actions have been the most appreciated (Kane 2005). Lately, there is growing consciousness among migrants about their role as major players in the well-being of the people they left behind. Across France, there are hundreds of hometown associations from the Senegal River Valley primarily concerned with improving the living conditions of their rural villages and small towns.

In the context of the SAPs, the local populations have learned to turn more to their diasporic communities abroad than to the Senegalese government to deal with their economic and social problems. The hometown associations that were once more concerned about challenges facing migrants in the host country have progressively readjusted their goals to integrate the need to invest in infrastructure building as well as in social services in their communities of origin. Efforts over the last three decades have included building classrooms, health care facilities, and clean water distribution systems; and sending equipment, medicine, and books for community projects.

Thilogne Association Developpement (TAD) is one of the most dynamic hometown associations in France. Thilonge is a subdivision of the larger Matam region of Sengal and includes a number of different rural communities. The inclusion of the word "development" in the denomination of the migrants' associations is very common and indicates the spirit and fervor of its participants in wanting to bring progress to their local communities. Most of the leaders of hometown associations like TAD are in many way the "courtiers" of development, spending their time, money, and energy building partnerships with their host countries' organizations and public institutions interested in development issues.

TAD is truly a transnational hometown association with chapters in different countries around the world. The association is present in Africa (Senegal, Gabon, and Congo), in Europe (France and Italy), and in America (in several states including New York, Ohio, Kentucky, Tennessee, Colorado, and Michigan) (Kane 2000). TAD has two main objectives. The first objective is to protect and help migrants from Thilonge in their host countries by providing financial and moral support in times of need (social events such as birth, marriage, and death; or any adversity such as illness or legal problems). The second objective is to improve the living conditions in the home village by investing in community projects that make life better and more comfortable for the villagers. The association has built classrooms and whole schools to improve access to education. It has also helped rebuild a local health center and has sent ambulances, beds, and medical equipment that have improved the quality of health care services for the local community.

Demba, 42, a board member of TAD, explains the priorities of his village association in France as follows: "The state has stepped down in the domain of health care and education. Our people count on us to step in and address the basic needs in term of health care and education. Our strategy is to rely on our members' contributions and look for partners who want to help us in our efforts to address some issues of local development in our village of origin."

Demba's remarks are echoed by all the participants, who have repeatedly blamed the Senegalese government for not being able to take care of its citizens. During the TAD meetings at the Foyer d'Hauptpool in Paris in 2004, the speakers reiterated to the general assembly that they are the only hope for people left in their villages. Through the discourse of participants in hometown associations one can detect a sense of pride in being able to stand up for their rural communities. The sense of pride is even more salient when migrants return home, where they are welcomed as heroes. Samba, 47, who went back to Thilogne in 2008, talked about TAD members as development fighters. The local populations also claim that their only hope is their sons and daughters living in the diaspora.

TAD has been the main actor in taking care of the health care facilities in Thilogne. Since 1980, its total investments have amounted to more than 50,000 euro. This amount does not include the participation of TAD's partners, such as the Friends of Thilogne of Nancy, Médecins Sans Frontières (Doctors Without Borders), Nancy Hospital, and the Belgian Red Cross. These different partners helped the village association to provide a community pharmacy where the medicines are half the price of private pharmacies. Every year the community pharmacy receives generic medicines sent by TAD France. The medicines are the gift of the Nancy hospital and the Friends of Thilogne association based in the city of Nancy, France. This association brings together French citizens who admire the participation of TAD in improving local populations' health without much help from the Senegalese state. The Senegalese state has now recognized the important role migrants' associations play in the sectors of health and education. The government officials refer often to the migrants' associations as a good example of citizens' engagement for the development of their localities.

The community pharmacy helps the local population to get access to biomedicine at a very low cost. The money generated by the sale of medicine is reinvested in buying generic medicines to replace the stock. TAD continues to send shipments of generic drugs used to treat the most common diseases in the areas, such as malaria, high blood pressure, and diabetes.[8] The manager of the community pharmacy has been trained and is paid by TAD. The association also paid for the training and first few years' salary of a midwife's assistant (*matronne*), who between 2002 and 2005 was the only person helping to deliver babies in the hospital.

TAD has also sent two ambulances to Thilogne for the transport of patients. Before the arrival of the ambulances, patients used to take private mini-buses or bush-taxis to go to Ourosogui or Dakar. Between 1985 and 1998, more than 25 people died on the way to Ourosogui and Dakar. The number of people dying en route to the hospital has decreased significantly with the use of the ambulances between Thilogne and Dakar. The ambulance service is not free of charge for villagers, but the fee is very low. The money generated by the ambulances is used to pay for the driver and gas. TAD sends money every year to cover major repairs and maintenance. The ambulances render service to the surrounding villages; patients using cell phones can call in case of emergency. In 2002, TAD was given a third ambulance by the Belgian Red Cross. The leaders of TAD decided to give the ambulance to Kanel, a small city in the Senegal River Valley that was facing the same challenges Thilogne had before the arrival of the first ambulances.

Although the interventions of hometown associations like TAD in the Senegal River Valley remain impressive, they are faced by tremendous challenges regarding the management of their community projects at the local level. In 2008, the community pharmacy was almost brought into its knees when the local managers claimed there had been burglaries and 800,000 FCFA (2,000 USD) was stolen. This event affected the renewal of the stock of generic medicines and the increased dependency on medicine transfers from France. At the same time, the Health Committee in charge of supervising the community pharmacy as well as managing the money generated by the health services has been accused by TAD members of corruption. Six million FCFA (12,000 USD) disappeared during the renewal of the Health Committee in 2007. The outgoing Committee claimed to have left 6 million FCFA in the fund, and the new Committee claimed to have found not a penny. This situation is very frustrating for the members of TAD in France, who feel that they are funding community projects that end up being used by a few local politicians.

The organization of the Fouta Santé caravans seems to be a more compelling success story due to the fact that it is punctual interventions have been managed from start to finish by the migrants themselves.

Fouta Santé

Fouta Santé is a federation of hometown associations founded by Haalpulaar migrants originating from the Senegal River Valley and living in France. It includes more than 100 hometown associations like TAD which have in common a desire to intervene for good in their home communities. Fouta Santé gets its funding from the annual contributions of the hometown associations which are the members, and from fundraising campaigns in France targeting city and regional councils, public health institutions, local associations, and NGOs.

The board of Fouta Santé is chosen from the members sent by their hometown associations to the general assembly of the federation. Although in the beginning Fouta Santé targeted all the Senegal River Valley region, it has recently become associated with Matam, a newly designated region. As its name indicates (*santé* is French for "health"), the federation has only one goal: to improve access to biomedical health care in the Senegal River Valley. Mamoudou, 53, was one of the founding members and was the president of Fouta Santé for four years in the early 1990s. He explains the reasons that pushed them to create this kind of federal association.

> Each of our village associations was engaged in improving the living conditions of the population of their village of origin. Some village associations, like ALDA of Agnam, TAD of Thilogne, ADO of Ourosogui, were making remarkable efforts to help [the] local population to access to health care. They sent medicines and medical equipments regularly to their home villages. They built maternity homes, medical centers. Some of us who were active in those associations realized then we could do more if we combined our efforts. We got the word out and the idea was applauded by the different vil-

lage associations. Many of them [67] agreed to participate right away. Other village associations joined our federation later after realizing the difference we were making in the Senegal River Valley.

In the 1990s, Fouta Santé was very active in collecting medicine in France and sending it to local community pharmacies across the Senegal River Valley. It was only at the beginning of the 2000s that Fouta Santé started organizing the health caravans. The organization became Fouta Santé–Matam in December 2000 and was officially recognized as an association under the 1901 Law in France.

Since 2000, Fouta Santé–Matam has organized eight health caravans to the Senegal River Valley, providing health care to thousands of people who could not afford to pay for surgery or for very expensive types of medical treatments. To make these caravans successful, Fouta Santé leaders worked hard to find partners in France who were willing to give them financial, logistical, or professional support. They obtained much financial support from regional and city councils throughout France. Like all associations in France, they applied for subvention money, both at the regional and city levels. Most of this money is used to pay for airfare for a medical team composed of professional volunteers (surgeons, dentists, vision specialists, general practitioners, etc.). The money contributed by village associations that are members of Fouta Santé is used to pay for food and local transport for the medical team and the leaders of Fouta Santé who are accompanying them. The local populations in Ourosogui provide housing to the medical team and the members of Fouta Santé during the period of operation.

The medical team of the first caravan was composed of eight French medical specialists. They were joined by two Senegalese colleagues working at hospitals located in the country's capital. The team operated in a local hospital with very limited capacity, personnel, and medical equipment. The mission brought with it the material needed for surgical interventions. The trip lasted for eight days, during which the medical team worked around the clock to consult and operate on the most urgent cases. Between 2001 and 2004, the number of beneficiaries increased year by year due to the influx of patients coming from other parts of the country. The medical team increased its number of specialists in 2004, and the length of the stay went from eight days to two weeks.

From 2001 and 2004, the number of beneficiaries tripled, going from 1,278 to 3,637. The number of surgeries performed by the medical team quadrupled, from 97 to 436. The number of ophthalmological consultations went up from 289 in 2001 to 434 in 2005, while the number of ophthalmological surgeries rose from 55 to 224. The increased number of surgeries in ophthalmology is due to the large number of patients suffering from cataracts. The team cannot meet the high demand for surgery related to this specific disease. The caravans have tried to increase the medical teams and the duration of the caravan to serve as many patients as possible. Other medical units registered similar increases in both the number of consultations and surgeries. Ear, nose, and throat went up from 140 consultation and 5 surgeries in 2001 to 351 consultations and 15 surgeries in 2004. Gynecology consultations and surgeries went up from 205 and 10, respectively, in 2001, to 440 and 19, respectively, in 2004.

The impact of the health mission on medical services in the region goes beyond the two-week presence of the medical team. Every year the mission leaves medicines and medical equipment. They also transfer medical knowledge and techniques to the local staff, which ensures follow-up for patients in need of medical attention for longer periods of time. In 2005, 4,302 patients benefited from the Fouta Santé health caravan. The medical team performed a total of 453 surgeries, including 205 ophthalmological, 127 endoscopic, 47 abdominal/thoracic, 26 ear/nose/throat, 24 orthopedic, and 22 gynecological.

The last Fouta Santé health caravan that I studied, in 2006, recorded more patients consulted and treated than any previous year. The medical team included more specialists and the length of their stay was extended for three more days. As with the previous caravans, the Ourosogui hospital hosting the operations received medical supplies and equipment necessary for the follow-up of patients in need of prolonged care. Caravans have continued to occur every year since.

The health care mission organized by Fouta Santé has created an option for many people who are not fortunate enough to have a family member in Europe or in North America who can send money to cover medical costs. In fact, in local hospitals and medical centers, health care professionals advise their poor patients to wait for the Fouta Santé caravan to get medical attention for free. Some migrants also ask their family members to make use of the caravan in order to ease the burden of other health care costs that they bear alone. Some patients come from outside the region, especially from Bakel and southern Mauritania, seeking to benefit from the Fouta Santé caravan. The 2006 caravan was overwhelmed by a crowd of patients who obviously could not all be treated in a two-week period.

As mentioned above, the impact of the caravans goes beyond the actual presence of the medical team. The medical equipment and the medicines that the caravan brings with it are left behind in the hands of local health care professionals who are asked to use it for the treatment of the needy. However, many people have complained about the fact that after the caravan has left, nobody seems to care for the patients who did not have a chance to be treated during the stay of the medical team.

The health caravans are an attempt by Haalpulaar migrants in France, led by the young and well-educated, to let people at home benefit from the same health system they enjoy in their host country. They complement individual efforts by migrants to bring biomedical treatment to their families and communities more used to traditional treatments. This focus on biomedical treatment does not mean that the Haalpulaar migrants see their cultural healing practices as outdated, as is made clear by the hometown associations' provision of trips home for traditional healing in some cases.

Clearly, Fouta Santé health caravans are part of the movement of medicine, medical equipment, and health professionals from France to the Senegal River Valley. Unfortunately, the reverse movement of trained Senegalese health professionals is more common and more prolonged in time. The brain drain of health professionals is one of the major challenges to Senegal and to all of Africa. The French health professionals participating in the Fouta Santé caravans spend less than a month in Africa, while their Senegalese, Ghanaian, and Nigerian counterparts come to Europe to stay for their entire professional lives (Tall 2005; Manuh 2005).

The remittances of medicine as well as the organization of health interventions have become common practices in the Haalpulaar diaspora in France, as both individuals and social networks seek to improve health access for their families in Senegal. In the context of the application of the SAPs, the migrant sending communities in the Senegal River Valley turn more to their members abroad than to the state for help in accessing biomedical health services. The Haalpulaar migrants are answering the call by sending medicine, paying medical bills, organizing health caravans, sending medical equipment, and building medical facilities for their family members in Senegal. In the process of health delivery to rural populations, hometown associations and federations of hometown associations have become clearly important players that the local populations have learned to count on. It is nonetheless premature to think of these forms of interventions by migrants' organizations as more than a temporary coping mechanism; for they are far from real solutions to the deep crisis of African health systems.

The intervention of migrants and their organizations is not, however, just limited to helping their people access biomedical health care. They are simultaneously engaged in looking to the services of healers in their host countries, as well as supporting the transfer of patients believed to be inflicted with diseases that can only be cured by traditional medicine or prayers from Islamic clerics. Medicine therefore does not flow only in one direction, from France to the Senegal River Valley; the complete circuit also involves the sending of traditional medicine and prayers from home to host places.

The intervention of migrants and their associations in providing social services such as health care and education to their communities of origin has met with an ambivalent reception by the Senegalese state. On the one hand, these interventions point to the state's incapacity to provide for its people, which obviously degrades the image of the state in the eyes of its citizens. State officials have in the past used their authority to undermine some migrants' project that are seen as contrary to state priorities or planning. For example, certain migrants' associations have been denied the authorization to build hospitals or schools on the basis that the state has a tight territorial plan in terms of where to build health care facilities or schools according to population density and geographical situation. On the other hand, the state does not want to be seen as the only actor supposed to solve all the problems of its citizens. The initiatives of migrants and their associations are presented by government officials as examples of what responsible citizens should do to help themselves and the state to find solutions to the problems of rural communities. This attitude of less state and more citizen responsibility is of course one of the major principles of the neoliberal policies that supported the SAPs.

There is a growing recognition of the role of migrants and their associations in the development of places of origin. The French government recently introduced a co-development policy that ties together development cooperation and migration flow management. It has identified migrants and their associations as the major intermediaries between French cooperation agencies and local populations. Migrants and migrants' associations can get funding from French cooperation agencies to invest in development projects, creating jobs for the youth in major sending areas. The hope of the French government is to curb the migration flow from Senegal to France by creating jobs that will prevent youth from migrating.

The NGOs intervening in the health sector have also recognized the importance of hometown associations in areas with high rates of emigration. Some have developed partnerships to build health care facilities, health mutual schemes, and sensitization programs for communities of origin. The partnerships that migrants' associations like TAD and Fouta Santé are undertaking with French hospitals, associations, cooperation agencies, the Senegalese state, and local NGOs underscore their importance as stakeholders in any local, national, and global health policy targeting their communities of origin.

Notes

1. The Haalpulaar are a Fulani group living at the border area between Mali, Mauritania, and Senegal. Like their Soninke neighbors, they have been involved in transnational migration for a century.

2. The Foyer Aftam is a dormitory hosting male migrants who are single or who have left their wives behind.

3. This is a very recent survey taken May 10 –May 12, 2009. Twelve men were interviewed at the Foyer Aftam, a dormitory exclusively inhabited by male migrants, and 11 women were interviewed in the Clos des Roses neighborhood, which is predominantly inhabited by West African migrant families.

4. Migrants who have a social security card and who are members of a health mutual can get access to health care for free.

5. *Daaka* is a spiritual retreat of ten days organized by a small but rapidly growing branch of the Tijani Sufi order in Senegal. The retreat takes place every year at the outskirts of the holy city of Medina Gounass in the southeastern part of Senegal. The city was founded by Mamadou Seydou Ba, a Haalpulaar cleric who migrated from the Senegal River Valley in northern Senegal and created a new and fundamentalist branch of Tijani. Since 1992, a *Daaka* has also been organized in Mante-La-Jolie, a suburb of Paris with a high concentration of Haalpulaar migrants.

6. The Tijani or Tijaniyya Sufi order was created in the early nineteenth century by Cheikh Sidi Ahmed Tijani, an Algerian saint. The Sufi order spread rapidly in West Africa thanks to the Jihad of Omar Tall in the late nineteenth century.

7. *Marabouts* are religious clerics who use holy scripts for healing.

8. For infectious diseases, however, the local populations have to go to the local pharmacy to pay for antibiotic drugs. There are only a few antibiotic drugs sent by TAD and they are often about to expire.

References

Appadurai, Arjun, ed. 2001. *Globalization*. Durham, N.C.: Duke University Press.
Copeland-Carson, Jacqueline. 2004. *Creating Africa in America: Translocal Identity in an Emerging World City*. Philadelphia: University of Pennsylvania Press.
Diop, Momar Coumba, ed. 2008. *Le Senegal des migrations. Mobilité, identité et societies*. Paris: Karthala.
Geschiere, Peter, and Birgit Meyer, eds. 1999. *Globalization and Identity: Dialectics of Flow and Closure*. Oxford: Blackwell.
Kane, Abdoulaye. 2000. "Diasporas villageoise et développement local en Afrique: le cas de Thilogne Association Développement." *Hommes et Migrations* 1229: 96–107.
———. 2005. "Les diasporas africaines et la mondialisation." *Horizons Maghrébins* 53: 54–61.
Levitt, Peggy. 2001. *The Transnational Villagers*. Berkeley: University of California Press.
MacGaffey, Janet, and Rémy Bazenguissa-Ganga. 2000. *Congo-Paris: Transnational Traders on the Margins of the Law*. Bloomington: Indiana University Press.

Manuh, Takyiwaa., ed. 2005. *At Home in the World: International Migration and Development in Contemporary Ghana and West Africa*. Accra, Ghana: Sub Saharan Publishers.

Quiminal, Cathérine. 1986. *Gens d'ici, gens d'ailleurs*. Paris: Christian Bourgeois.

Tall, Serigne M. 2005. "The Remittances of Senegalese Migrants: A Tool for Development?" In *At Home in the World: International Migration and Development in Contemporary Ghana and West Africa*, ed. Takyiwaa Manuh, 153–170. Accra, Ghana: Sub Saharan Publishers.

EIGHT

Public Health or Public Threat?
Polio Eradication Campaigns, Islamic Revival, and the Materialization of State Power in Niger

Adeline Masquelier

In late 2003 rumors began circulating in the small provincial town of Dogondoutchi, Niger that the poliomyelitis vaccine administered to children was harmful. The vaccine, the rumor had it, caused sterility in children and had been developed by Western scientists to lower the world's Muslim population. When nurses dispatched to administer doses of Oral Polio Vaccine (OPV) to children under five tried to enter people's homes on National Vaccination Day, they were met with staunch resistance on the part of some parents who accused them of wanting to harm their progeny. In surrounding villages, similar scenarios ensued as health workers going house to house with polio drops tried to immunize the children targeted by the vaccination drive. Eager to cut short the emergence of a massive opposition to the WHO-sponsored campaign to eradicate polio, the *secrétaire général* of the Dogondoutchi prefecture dispatched police officers to a village where residents had denied health workers access to their children. There the officers promptly arrested two individuals who, by protesting the presence of health workers, had interfered with the drive. The two men were brought to Dogondoutchi under police escort. Once in the *secrétaire général's* office, they were lectured about the benefits of vaccination before eventually being released, but not before being charged a fine amounting to the cost of sending a health worker back to the village to resume inoculation. Despite concerted attempts by local public health officials to prevent further disruptions of the vaccination drive and alleviate parental concerns regarding the safety of the OPV, rumors that the vaccine was part of a Western plot to sterilize Muslim girls (and in some minds, boys as well) continued to hinder the success of the 2003 campaign. The vaccine was not safe, embattled residents reasoned, otherwise why weren't parents charged for it? After all, the government did not provide other free services anymore. In the eyes of suspicious parents the only reasonable explanation was that local officials were acting on behalf of impious Westerners eager to weaken the country's Muslim resurgence. While parental fears were largely articulated around the notion that the OPV caused infertility, a few individuals suspected the vaccine of inducing atheism. For yet others, it was the vaccine itself that struck children with polio. In some communities, polio campaigns were thwarted by alarmist claims that the vaccine passed on the AIDS virus and had been devised to deplete the world of its Muslim population.[1]

In elite liberal circles the prevailing view was that the failure of the campaign to wipe out polio in Niger was due to the influence that conservative Muslim clerics held over their followers. According to this logic, parents who had taken part in the boycott against polio immunization were following the dictates of religious leaders who were themselves influenced by prominent *malamai* (Muslim religious specialists) from neighboring Nigeria.[2] It was they, government officials acknowledged, who needed to be educated on the benefits of immunization before vaccinators could successfully embark on the next nationwide campaign.[3] In northern Nigeria, religious leaders had pressured public officials to halt the 2003 vaccination campaign amidst fears that the drive was part of a deliberate attempt to spread infertility (or HIV) among Muslims (Renne 2006, 2010). Government officials agreed to test the safety of the vaccine before resuming the campaign—a move that generated a *fracas médiatique* in the Western media. Teams of local medical experts undertook extensive investigations of vaccine factories in Indonesia, India, and South Africa before officially declaring that the vaccine was innocuous (Dugger and McNeill Jr. 2006).

In Niger the government took a firm stand against anti-vaccination advocates and refused to satisfy their demands that the vaccine be tested by local doctors. The OPV had been administered to millions of children over the last 40 years and was perfectly safe, health officials insisted in radio-transmitted and televised messages aimed at promoting the health benefits of vaccination. To stress the importance and safety of polio vaccination, President Mamadou Tandja himself traveled to southern Niger in 2004, urging residents to cooperate with campaign volunteers and give the vaccine to their children (Donnelly 2004).

For many Nigérien parents *"Vaccinons nos enfants!"* ("Let's vaccinate our children!") became a mantra of sorts, helping raise the overall polio vaccination coverage to 65 percent that year. For a small minority, however, the message of the president fell on deaf ears. In Dogondoutchi the followers of Malam Awal,[4] a charismatic and flamboyant Sufi preacher reputedly blessed with exceptional powers, remained unswayed by the presidential intervention—for reasons that will become clear below. When, in October and November 2004, immunization teams took to the road again with their iced vaccine carriers, the *'yan* Awaliyya (members of Awaliyya, Awal's newly founded Sufi order) refused once more to let their children be vaccinated against polio.[5]

In part because since the 2003 boycott of the vaccination drive in pre-dominantly Muslim northern Nigeria 18 once polio-free countries have had outbreaks traceable to that country, much has been written about the trou-bling resurgence of polio in the Muslim world and the supposedly backward ideologies that have brought the African continent to "the brink of reinfec-tion" (Kapp 2004: 709). If several northern Nigerian states became the "epi-center of an upsurge of the disease" (Kapp 2004: 709) in 2004 (with 521 of the 641 new cases registered by June 2006), it was, observers and news com-mentators claimed, because of the hostility and suspicion that Muslim leaders and their followers manifested toward Western health programs.[6] In other words, the failure of the WHO to stem the tide of the polio virus by 2005, as was originally planned, should be blamed on the ignorance and "supersti-tion" of victimized populations. "Fear and misinformation about the polio vaccine have become as deadly as any disease" Jonathan Majiyagbe, president of Rotary International (one of the partners in the polio eradication initia-tive), was quoted as saying in early 2004 after several northern Nigerian states refused to lift their ban against the vaccine despite repeated assurances that the drops contained no harmful substance (Kapp 2004: 709). "We must not allow these unfounded rumors to come between our children and their health," he declared.[7]

Although news analysts occasionally acknowledged the role that the media played in distorting facts or amplifying rumors related to the polio vac-cine, they rarely questioned the "geographies of blame" (Farmer 1992) whose outlines they unwittingly helped create by pathologizing local resistance to health campaigns. Through their problematic representations of "local knowl-edge" (Geertz 1983) as harmful, they characterized those who opposed the vaccination drive as "unsanitary subjects" (Briggs and Martini-Briggs 2003: 288) who, through their failure to internalize medical epistemologies and their refusal to defer to "enlightened" health professionals, were directly responsible for the spread of infectious diseases. In the West African case, noncompliance with WHO-mandated policies regarding polio prevention had quickly led to the resurgence of the polio virus, not only in areas where the disease was endemic but also in areas that had recently been declared polio-free.

Paradoxically, these unsanitary subjects were also seen as victims of politi-cal expediency and religiously divisive ideologies. Indeed, it was because they unquestioningly absorbed the supposed lies presented to them by unpro-gressive politicians or religious leaders looking to mobilize public support that they had become obstacles to the successful dissemination of preven-tive health care. In what follows I examine critically the resistance to recent polio vaccination campaigns spearheaded by Malam Awal in Dogondoutchi. I complicate the picture of ignorance and duplicity painted by the press to suggest ways that vaccination programs provide a privileged context for political critiques as well as the articulation of collective anxieties. Far from being an expression of obscurantism, the rumors that informed such resistance reveal a keen awareness of the workings of the state and of the power relations within which medical resources are embedded. By analyzing the politics and poetics of resistance to state-mandated vaccination, I hope to contribute to the discussion on the "social lives of medicines" (Whyte, van der Geest, and Hardon 2002: 13) and highlight how the production, distribution, and consumption of medicines are shaped by and shape relations between people in complex and fundamental ways.

With the decline of state-supported health care following the deployment of structural adjustment programs (SAPs), externally sponsored vaccination campaigns have become one of the primary conduits through which the state of Niger visibly asserts not only its authority (Rasmussen 1994) but also its materiality. To understand how and why communities resist "being a part of the public in 'public health'" (Fraser 1995: 57) in such contexts, we must address people's fear of external control by regulatory powers perceived as a threat to local practices of cultural reproduction (Ginsburg and Rapp 1995). These regulatory powers are part of what Foucault (1990) identified as biopower, that is, sets of techniques for producing disciplined bodies and achieving control over populations. At a time when the state is uniformly perceived as a vehicle for generating political deceptions and fraudulent deals, some Nigériens are suspicious of state-sponsored programs that loudly proclaim commitment to the national good. In this chapter I explore popular perceptions of state interference in the volatile context of polio eradication drives and consider how people's mistrust of state policies shaped their opposition to vertical health interventions. I evaluate the success of Malam Awal's controversial condemnation of the polio eradication campaign against popular perceptions of government inefficiency and corruption at a time when Nigériens have become both disillusioned by the vacuous promises of modern bureaucratic power and skeptical of any state-sponsored effort to contribute to public interest. I suggest that involvement in the preacher's Sufi order (and what that entails in terms of health care choices) was not a retreat into tradition so much as a means of facing the problems of the present in a country where—aside from generating discourses of state deficit—governmental inadequacies seem to have produced an abundance of regulatory procedures through which the state engages in active population surveillance. One of the most striking manifestations of these acts of surveillance is the state-sponsored vaccination campaign.

Malam Awal and the Rebirth of Sufism in Dogondoutchi

In the early 1990s, the liberalization of markets, politics, and media in Niger ushered in an era of religious revival that witnessed the rise of Izala,[8] a reformist movement originating in Nigeria bent on eradicating the supposedly wrongful innovations of local Muslim religious traditions, such as the celebration of the Prophet's birthday. Izala's popularity appeared to signal the decline of Sufism and of "traditionalist" *malamai,* who manipulated the words of the Qur'an in order to heal, protect, and empower—or conversely to bring defeat and disaster.[9] Izala reformists instructed local Muslims to educate themselves in Qur'anic matters and eschew the services of traditionalist *malamai*: the latter, they claimed, were charlatans who took advantage of people's gullibility and charged extravagant sums for the manufacture of medicines (amulets, etc.) and the performance of rituals that had no place in "true" Islam. Invoking God's assistance through prayer and visiting the local medical dispensary were the only avenues to health, reformist leaders insisted.

The 1997 arrival of Malam Awal in the Hausa-speaking town of Dogondoutchi changed all that. A well-known critic of Muslim reformists, the preacher had been invited to deliver anti-Izala sermons by traditionalist Muslim leaders hoping to curb the swift rise of reformist Islam. Claiming to have been sent by God, he quickly launched into aggressive diatribes against anti-Sufi reformism. Izala was not the only target of his incendiary sermons, however. The preacher also accused traditionalist *malamai* of greed, impiety, and ignorance. His opponents tried their best to silence him but to no avail. Awal's daily sermons attracted huge audiences. In a matter of weeks, the preacher found himself leading a large community of dedicated followers wary of both the righteous intolerance of Izala reformists and the greed of traditionalist *malamai* who allegedly filled their pockets at the expense of the poor.

Plans were drawn to build a mosque where disciples would assemble for prayer and instruction. Following his alleged confrontation with a spirit who had interfered with the construction of the mosque, Awal became the talk of the town: he could communicate with spirits, a gift he had received from God, his followers proclaimed (Masquelier 2009). Not only did he possess exceptional powers, but he seemed to be animated by blissful insight. In the eyes of his disciples there was no doubt that the preacher was endowed with divine grace. At a time of intensified debates over the democratization of Islamic knowledge and the legitimacy of Sufi practices, Awal provided incontrovertible evidence that religious authority should be rooted in the persona of a Muslim scholar who "spoke the truth." Countering Izala reformists' efforts to purify Islamic traditions, facilitate access to religious knowledge, and banish magical practices, he convinced many that ritual control of the occult was a vital and necessary dimension of Muslim authority: he presented himself as a great unifier sent by God to fight immorality and bring enlightenment to Muslim communities across Niger. Paradoxically, he stressed the value of moderate marriage expenditures and frugal lifestyles, thereby aligning himself with the reformists whose model of utilitarian moral economy he was initially invited to criticize.

The preacher's magnetic hold over the Awaliyya membership extended into the putatively secular domain of politics and public health. In tandem with the Muslim reformists he otherwise opposed, Awal condemned the secular orientation of the Nigérien state and accused local politicians of impiety and decadence. He denounced secular schools as dens of immorality and unconditionally opposed practices of birth control. In 2003, on the eve of a National Vaccination Day aimed at inoculating young children against polio, Awal instructed followers not to have their children vaccinated: the government could not be trusted. In view of the state's limited role in overseeing human welfare, health campaigns, he claimed, were a threat to children and part of a larger conspiracy through which Western powers attempted to sterilize the Prophet's followers. Awal's warnings that the polio vaccine was a contraceptive drug in disguise proved effective. When the vaccinators arrived to administer doses of OPV to the children, they were turned away by Awaliyya parents who would not be persuaded that the vaccine was harmless.

Despite efforts to combine the administration of OPV with the less controversial measles vaccination during the December 2004 public health campaign,[10] opposition to state-sponsored inoculation in the Awaliyya community remained strong. Health officials made it clear in their radio announcements that needles and syringes would be used only once, and that both vaccinations were free. Rather than helping melt resistance, however, the much advertised absence of fees and the health workers' determination to visit every village and enter every home (rather than meet patients at health facilities) heightened the suspicion of parents and strengthened their resolve not to let their children become casualties of the state's "nefarious" policies.[11]

Given the number of households visited during vaccination drives, health workers had little time to provide information to parents about the benefits (and possible side effects) of the vaccine. *Agents de santé* (health workers) would introduce themselves with a simple *"Salamu Alaikom. Polio!"* ("Greetings. Polio!"). They often had abrupt manners and did not greet people adequately upon entering their homes. Rather than appeal to parents' moral responsibility or stress the benefits of the vaccine, they simply asked how many children lived in the household and administered the vaccine to those present. After recording on paper the number and age of children present and scribbling the information on an entrance wall, they quickly moved to the next compound. The rushed nature of the procedure did little to allay people's suspicions that, as one man put it, "we weren't told everything."

When Malam Awal was summoned by local authorities to explain why he urged resistance to the campaign, he denied having ever forbidden anyone to have their children vaccinated or having spoken against the government, although he admitted to cautioning people against the potential threat of contaminated vaccines. It was all a big misunderstanding, he insisted, based on people's ignorance and their alarmist interpretation of rumors coming from Nigeria. Unlike religious leaders elsewhere in the country who were detained on grounds of inciting riots, Awal was allowed to leave after his interrogation. For health workers intent on promoting the benefits of vaccination to local residents, the preacher's relative immunity from prosecution meant that he would continue to spread malicious propaganda to bolster his position as guardian of "true" Islam. Local hospital employees were angry and frustrated by the administration's failure to silence him. According to a nurse, "Malam Awal threatened [local authorities], but they don't dare arrest him or even criticize him. He claims that no one can chase him out. He told the *sous-préfet* [local official] that the *dogon doutchi* [the rock formation after which the town is named] would crumble before he would leave town."

By the time of the 2003 polio eradication campaign numerous stories circulated that told of the fraud, trickery, and abuse in which Awal engaged. His prestige and popularity as a holy man had eroded considerably.[12] For a dwindling minority of committed *'yan* Awaliyya, however, he continued to embody virtue and personify religious authority—in direct opposition to the supposedly corrupt policies of the state. Despite assurances by the *secrétaire général* that anyone inciting disturbances during vaccination campaigns would be summoned to his office, the consensus among civil servants I spoke with was that little had been done to curb the preacher's damaging rhetoric. Despite his waning popularity, Malam Awal was a powerful man. Although local officials (with a few exceptions) did not share his vision of Islam as the remedy to the country's economic decline, and altogether resented his public interventions, they did not wish to antagonize him. Everyone in town knew that after accusing the preacher of embezzling public funds, the local tax collector was imprisoned for fraud. Malam Awal, on the other hand, had been mysteriously exonerated of any charges. Many people attributed this outcome to Awal's unique ability to manipulate the occult.[13]

Despite the skill with which the preacher captivated audiences with his erudition, his fiery delivery style, and his vivid narratives, not everyone believed that he possessed God-given powers. In the eyes of educated elites, Awal was an impostor who preyed on local residents by staging miracles and disseminating lies; he manipulated his followers so that they would work for him and support his extravagant lifestyle. Not only was he dishonest, his detractors insisted, but he had brought dissent to a community already fractured by religious disagreements. Countering the preacher's claims that he had restored harmony and cleansed the community of impiety, critics pointed to the number of divorces and family feuds provoked by his fractious rhetoric.

What infuriated local officials and health professionals was not the preacher's divisive religious message, however. Niger, they proudly insisted, was a secular country where everyone (including preachers such as Malam Awal) was free to practice the religion of his or her choice. Yet all the same, if religion was not a focus of state control, public health certainly was. This meant that when the health of Nigériens was at risk, no one, not even charismatic religious figures who promised salvation to their disciples, should thwart the government's efforts to protect its citizens. By urging his followers not to vaccinate their children against polio, Awal stepped into the realm of the secular and usurped state authority. His intervention had tragic consequences: several new cases of polio in town were later diagnosed, allegedly attributable to the refusal of 'yan Awaliyya to vaccinate their childen. "The day that God is finished with Malam Awal," a local official said to me, "his followers will be free of his tyranny."

Note that Awal's resistance to the Nigérien state is far from an isolated case. Izala reformists too have routinely defied the state to prevent the implementation of policies they perceive to be contrary to the teachings of Islam. They opposed the passing of the Family Code, a piece of domestic legislation designed to define the legal relationship between husbands and wives and between children and parents, on the ground that it was based on secular principles and therefore anti-Islamic. By mobilizing those who want Islam to play a larger role in the political life of the country, controversial legislations such as the Family Code have contributed to the development of an Islamic consciousness in Niger. In this regard Malam Awal's exhortation to his followers that they resist state-sponsored health programs must be assessed against the backdrop of rising Muslim opposition to state policies perceived to be challenging God's plan for humanity. Like other reformist projects that call for a return to the pristine Islam of Muhammad, Awal's vision of a new Muslim order cannot be defined as a strict rejection of modernity and Western values. It forges a middle path between Islam and modernity that responds to the aspirations of certain segments of society but rejects Western notions of authority, individuality, and accountability.

The Global Polio Eradication Initiative

Poliomyelitis is a highly infectious viral disease that leads to paralysis and muscle atrophy. It usually spreads through human-to-human contact, entering the body orally through the consumption of fecally contaminated water or food. Though it can strike at any age, it affects primarily children under the age of three. In 1988 close to 35,000 cases of polio were recorded in 125 different countries. That year, the World Health Assembly passed a resolution to eradicate the disease by 2000. A revised plan later called for the elimination of polio by 2005. This bold, unprecedented move known as the Global Polio Eradication Initiative (GPEI) involved more than 200 countries and some 20 million health workers and volunteers.[14] Thanks to an aggressive combination of information and vaccination campaigns sponsored by the World Health Organization (WHO) (in partnership with national governments, Rotary International, UNICEF, the U.S. Centers for Disease Prevention and Control, and various donors and humanitarian organizations) polio cases declined considerably worldwide. In 2001, some 575 million children received doses of the OPV (Bonu, Rani, and Razum 2004) as vaccinators systematically crisscrossed areas targeted by the worldwide drive. That year polio reached an all-time low, with fewer than 500 cases reported worldwide (Boustany 2005), and 134 countries received their certification of polio eradication (Diallo 2005a). In 2006 Niger and Egypt were removed from the endemic country list, reducing the number of endemic countries to a historic low of four (Issa 2006).[15]

Yet the ambitious goals of the GPEI remain elusive. In 2009 1,606 new cases were reported, most of them in Nigeria and the Indian subcontinent (Global Polio Eradication Initiative 2010). In West Africa several once polio-free countries experienced outbreaks of the disease, all allegedly traceable to Nigeria. As of May 2010 ten countries (Angola, Chad, Liberia, Mali, Mauritania, Nepal, Niger, Senegal, Sierra Leone, and Tajikistan) had reported cases of imported wild poliovirus (Global Polio Eradication Initiative 2010).

Everywhere on the African continent prevention through the implementation of health information campaigns and vaccination programs has been a major component of public health policies (Chilliot 2003: 427). In Niger upcoming vaccination campaigns are promoted through print, radio, and television advertisement designed to inform the public of the benefits of preventive health care. To ensure the success of the National Immunization Days of March and April 2006, health officials coordinating the country-wide effort publicly stated during the opening ceremony that the vaccine was "the only efficient weapon against polio,"[16] that it was safe, and that parents must cooperate with health workers, reiterating the content of earlier radio and television broadcasts. Parents who could not be home during the drive were enjoined to leave instructions so immunization could take place in their absence.

As an added bonus, children who received a dose of OPV would also be given vitamin A. In Niger vitamins are highly prized. They are believed to prevent a wide variety of illnesses, increase strength, and promote weight gain. In recent years they have become a popular means of dealing with a variety of health complaints ranging from "lack of blood" to headaches to tiredness. Like other pills obtainable through prescriptions, vitamins are part of a broader category of medicines popularly known as *kini* (from the French "quinine"). *Kini* are widely available from itinerant pill sellers who participate in the flourishing market of smuggled, fake, and illegally produced drugs—many of them manufactured in Nigeria. During the 2006 and subsequent polio vaccination campaigns, free medicated mosquito nets were provided as incentives for parents who had their children vaccinated. The initiative backfired. I was told by health workers that parents gratefully took the mosquito nets only to immediately re-sell them for a few thousand FCFA.[17] By erasing the ink on their vaccinated children's thumbs with chlorine, some mothers reportedly had their children inoculated several times to obtain additional mosquito nets. When health workers ran out of mosquito nets, parents refused to vaccinate their children unless assurances could be made that they would receive mosquito nets.[18] Suspicion and mistrust run in both directions: local residents have misgivings about health workers showing up on their doorstep (parents commonly tell their children that the "state nurse" will come and give them a shot when they misbehave); while health workers suspect parents of cheating, often assume they are unconcerned about their children's health, and do not hide their contempt for *broussards* ("bush people").

Notwithstanding efforts to stimulate widespread commitment to health prevention,[19] ensuring the successful reception of health programs among local populations can be a major challenge for medical teams, as the boycott of recent polio vaccination campaigns has shown. To account for the failure of such programs, anthropologists have invoked cultural differences: the models of medical prevention promoted by public health teams do not translate into (or even resonate with) local understandings and experiences of preventive medicine (see Fassin 1986; Jaffré 1996). In the case at hand, *'yan* Awaliyya resistance to the 2003 and 2004 vaccination drives in Dogondoutchi was not due to their lack of medical knowledge about vaccination.[20] Rather, it was motivated by a suspicion that the vaccine served a hidden, ugly purpose:[21] rather than protecting children, it harmed them, by ensuring that as adults they would not be able to reproduce. From this perspective, the vaccination boycott was prompted not so much by the campaign's failure to communicate adequately the purpose of disease prevention as by its failure to disentangle fact from fiction for Nigériens wary of their "deceptive" government.[22]

Medicine, Fakery, and the State

In Niger today it is no longer possible to deny that many facts are often fabricated or, conversely, that forgeries and falsifications have become so elaborate as to seem more "authentic" than the things, identities, and procedures they are modeled after. Over two decades after the imposition of the SAP mandated by international donors, the country is on the brink of bankruptcy and there is talk of widespread abuses of power, systemic illegality, and deepseated corruption. Reforms intended to liberalize the economy to concentrate effectiveness and enhance productivity in state institutions have promoted the "creation of shadow economic and administrative structures" (Hibou 1999: 95). Consequently, the "government no longer functions in a normal way" (Hibou 1999: 95). In the absence of clear rules, a climate of uncertainty has developed that fosters corruption and leads to "deviant forms of individual behavior and a general erosion of standards" (Hibou 1999: 95). Delays in the payment of salaries, endemic job insecurity, and growing financial obligations have encouraged civil servants to take part in the corrupt practices everyone else engages in for the sake of survival[23] (Bayart, Elis, and Hibou 1999; Blundo and Olivier de Sardan 2001a; Olivier de Sardan 1999). Within this regime of illegality, forged documents, fake drugs, and fraudulent transactions that circulate alongside the products and services they mimic so efficiently all promote the widespread use of deception and a range of what Migdal (1988) has described as "dirty tricks." As such, they help create a world in which the real and the imaginary are often interchangeable (Apter 1999; Comaroff and Comaroff 1999; de Boeck 1996; Piot 2010; Smith 2006). The state no longer exists as a unified political structure: it has become a "collective illusion, the reification of an idea that masks real power relations under the guise of public interest" (Aretxaga 2003: 400). At once remote and intimate, impotent yet paradoxically abusive in some of its incarnations, the state emerges not as the reality that stands behind the mask of political practice but as the mask itself, the mask which "prevents our seeing political practice as it is" (Abrams 1988: 58).

Contrary to what aid donors intended, neither economic nor administrative reforms (privatization, trade liberalization, and so on) have discouraged the existence of illegal forms of activity in much of Africa. Instead, these activities have become integrated into the "politics of the belly" (Bayart 1989), a system of semi-clandestine structures of economic, financial, and political powers that lie in the shadow of the official system enabling a few to prey upon those subordinated to them (Bastian 1999; Fisiy and Geschiere 2001; Geschiere 1995; Masquelier 2000; Sanders 2001; Shaw 1996; Weiss 1996). In Niger, government-sponsored health care offers a concrete instantiation of how the state participates in the informal economy through the creation of techniques of power and profiteering that have come to replace basic public services. Before it was refurbished as a regional hospital thanks to financing by the Belgian government a decade ago, the dispensary of Dogondoutchi was an empty and poorly managed facility that did not dispense much except arbitrary rules and prescriptions for medicines that few could afford to buy (Masquelier 2001). Patients with connections enjoyed resources and services not available to anyone else; these resources were part of shadowy social networks through which state employees routinely diverted public resources for private purposes. In late 1988 the building received a fresh coat of paint, no doubt to restore patient confidence in the well-being of the medical facility. Residents were not fooled by this attempt by the administration to mask the reality of increasing poverty and inequality, however. The dispensary's shiny exterior was simply a facade of prosperity behind which the state hid its inability to deliver anything but illusions to the people of Niger—unless they themselves participated in the politics of the belly.

"In the poorest country on earth, health can only be had at the expense of thousands of francs" notes Yacouba (2006: 1) in an article on the continued degradation of health services in Niger. He describes the regional hospital of the neighboring city of Maradi as a place where

> [t]here is nothing. No one to take care of you. And when hours after [you've arrived], you finally find someone to take care of you, the first thing you do is open your wallet[,] for even in emergency cases you must pay for everything! The real shock for us was when [my wounded colleague and I] were told that we had to go to a private clinic to get an X-ray; there is no X-ray machine in the Maradi hospital. Imagine for a moment: the hospital of this vast region is so impoverished that it must rely on the private sector for a simple X-ray. (Yacouba 2006: 1)[24]

Despite their impoverishment, state-controlled health facilities are central nodes in the landscape of deception that has developed to fill the void left by the retreat of the state.[25] Upon arriving at a health facility patients must first pay a "right of visit" bribe at the entrance, and they cannot hope to receive adequate care without distributing gifts (variously known as "gas money," "spice money," "tea money," or "kola money") to every attending nurse and physician (Blundo and Olivier de Sardan 2001a, 2001b). In Niamey, the country's capital, patients at major hospitals have been known to pay in advance for non-existent services or already occupied beds while individuals pretending to be doctors exhort huge sums from their families for operations that will never be performed. In one birthing center, the ambulance is largely used to pick up daily meals (reserved for employees) and for the director to run errands and drive her children to school. If, by chance, it is available for a medical emergency, patients' families have to pay for gas (Blundo and Olivier de Sardan 2001b). In the words of a Nigérien father, "Favoritism and the power of money have so completely changed the face of health care that it has become unrecognizable" (Olivier de Sardan, Bako-Arifari, and Moumouni 2005: 7).

Because in this "shadow state" (Reno 1995), nothing is what it seems,[26] ordinary citizens have learned to distrust state sponsored institutions and to rely, whenever possible, on personal relations or political networks that offer "far more effective instruments of public management" (Hibou 1999: 91; see also Bayart, Mbembe, and Toulabor 1992). Aside from routinely criticizing the poor quality of modern health care, they denounce the corruption of medical personnel, share stories about the dangers of fake drugs, and listen to rumors of what "really" happens to those who do not come back from the hospital. Aside from capturing the disenchantment of populations victimized by the degradation of health care services, such discourses on the costs and perils of state-sponsored medicine illuminate how Nigériens variously experience the power of the state (see Gupta 1995, 2005). They also remind us that despite the anemic state of its public institutions, the state is far from powerless.

Take the case of vaccines. Vaccines, because they are simultaneously promoted and criminalized, provide an especially fruitful locus for examining how the state comes to be constructed as predatory by ordinary citizens desirous to improve their prospects (and their health) but wary of the deceptive (and at times, coercive) tactics of public authorities. On the one hand, vaccination is a generally uncontested, even popular, mode of disease prevention.[27] By injecting a substance subcutaneously, the *allura* (needle) or *pikir* (from the French *piqûre*) participates in the indigenous logic dictating that to be efficacious, medicines must penetrate the corporeal envelope and interact with the foreign substance that is at the origin of the patient's affliction. I have heard people in Dogondoutchi say that because the medicine contained in the syringe circulates in the blood, it acts quickly on the agent of the disease. For this reason, shots are believed to be particularly efficacious in the treatment of conditions that result in a thickening, diminishing, or spoiling of the blood. They rapidly restore patients to their original strength by helping rejuvenate their blood (Chilliot 2003). Although their effects are not as immediate as injections, pills and other medicines absorbed orally (such as aspirin, vitamins, quinine, and so on) are similarly popular modes of treatment, as is attested by their ubiquitous presence on the tables of unlicensed street vendors.

For those who believe that the state is so corrupt that it can no longer be trusted to deliver even the most basic services, the loudly advertised availability of free vaccines invites suspicion. Because their experience of the state is routinely mediated by the culture of deception that has grown unhampered on the margins of licit official institutions, Dogondoutchi residents often cast doubt on the legitimacy of government-run projects. They complain that public officials routinely divert national resources for their own fraudulent use, leaving deserving citizens to fight for the crumbs. From this perspective, programs touted as serving the people are only instances of the "dirty tricks" through which the state surreptitiously extracts the wealth and vitality of its citizens, or worse, interferes with processes of social reproduction.[28] According to a local administrator, "the reason people were suspicious of the polio vaccine is that when you bring your sick child to the hospital, if you do not pay 5000 FCFA, they do not even look at him. They will let him die. But then you find out they've decided to vaccinate your child for free. So now you think that there must be something else, something else they are not telling you."

Other residents pointed out that the fact that health workers came all the way to people's homes, in stark contrast to their normal tendency to wait at the hospital, at least raised suspicions when it did not altogether confirm what *'yan* Awaliyya had known all along—namely that the central government, acting on behalf of foreign powers, was actively trying to eradicate not so much polio as the people themselves through systematic and well-funded sterilization programs. That vaccinators came not once but sometimes five times a year to inoculate children further puzzled parents. After all, some reasoned, why else would Nigérien authorities dissipate considerable funds to rid communities of a disease that afflicted comparatively so few children when so many more were dying every year of malaria, meningitis, and malnutrition? I was told a number of times that if the government really had the best interest of Nigérien children at heart, it would focus its attention on the devastating effects of malaria, diarrhea, and respiratory infections rather than invest funds on a disease that rarely killed anyone. By boycotting the polio campaign, *'yan* Awaliyya were not questioning the efficacy of oral vaccination, at least not explicitly. Rather, they were resisting the ways through which the means of

cure had allegedly been hijacked by state representatives to dole out deception, disease, and death. The fact that the vaccine was administered orally only
compounded people's suspicion of foul play. In the words of the director of
the Programme Élargi de Vaccination (Comprehensive Vaccination Program),
"People like shots. They never refuse shots. It's the OPV that makes them
uneasy."

Although many Dogondoutchi residents—including former members of
Awaliyya—found Awal's tactics questionable and even harmful, others shared
the 'yan Awaliyya's distrust of government-controlled health care. After all,
rumors of state-sponsored deceptions that maim or kill innocent victims
abound in this part of the world. In 2000 I heard from friends that a previous
state-sponsored meningitis vaccination campaign had resulted in the death of
many children because the real vaccines had been replaced with fake ones.[29]
An inquiry launched by the French government to identify the culprits responsible for the release of false vaccines during a meningitis epidemic in Niger in
1995 has traced the distribution of the pirated drugs all the way to the government of Nigeria[30] (Hibou 1999). More recently a wealthy trader with connections (but no pharmaceutical expertise) was accused of having sold 93 million
FCFA worth of vaccines to the Nigérien state and of having distributed kick-
backs amounting to 13 million FCFA (Keïta 2006). How could one verify the
integrity of vaccines, Keïta (2006) asked in his article, given the nepotism that
in recent history has shaped the sales and distribution of medicines—and just
about anything else—in Niger? Keïta's question was rhetorical, but it reminds
us that many of the medicines that circulate on the national market are pirated
drugs illegally manufactured or stolen from local hospitals. The fabrication of
fakery is big business, Keïta (2006: 2) suggested, before concluding that given
how much the state was willing to spend on medicine of dubious provenance,
it was not surprising that "Niger's budget continually showed a deficit."

It is worth noting that the suspicion surrounding state-sponsored vaccination programs is rooted in the widely shared assumption that the state is
there to provide for its citizens. People may not agree as to what they should
be entitled to, but they expect the state to do more for its citizens, especially
when it comes to health care. These claims about entitlement are grounded in
an expectation of free medical care inherited from the brief period of prosperity Niger experienced in the 1970s and early 1980s. Booming revenues from
uranium sales financed the expansion of medical, educational, and transport
infrastructure. When uranium prices went down due to environmental concerns about nuclear energy and the waning of the Cold War, the country was
forced to shrink its social services, notably its health infrastructure. In their
nostalgic allusion to the "good old times" Dogondoutchi elders often men-

tion the free services provided by a resourceful and responsible administration willing to cater to people's needs. During that time patients could also receive free health care—and food—at the local Catholic mission, where medical diagnosis and treatment were dispensed daily. The days when one could drop by the mission to receive free vitamins or powdered milk are long gone. Yet it is against such romanticized images of the services offered by mission and state facilities that the complex economy of vaccines (and other medicines) must be assessed if we are to understand the nature of people's disenchantment with state-sponsored health care.

Islam, Birth Spacing, and the State

If the Islamic revival that swept through Niger in the 1990s translated into the emergence of diverse religious configurations (such as the Izala reformist association and Awal's Sufi order), it is largely because through the public debates generated by Muslims of all stripes, a host of issues were voiced that spoke to people's experience of the economic crisis faced by the country. Today, Islam is the main instrument with which pious Nigériens can shape their opposition to the secular state. For those who denounce secularism as antithetical to the divine plan, the language of Islam is a means of voicing their appraisal of the moral worth of public officials who, as alleged pawns of foreign administrations, rarely do what is in the best interest of their constituency.[31] Unemployment, poverty, and the decline of the national economy, Izala preachers proclaim in their sermons, are a direct consequence of people's lack of morality and religious devotion. Since, from this perspective, corruption amounts to a sin perpetrated by "bad" Muslims (Sounaye 2005), only a return to "true" Islam will ensure society's salvation from further degradation. Nigériens, young and old, routinely draw upon this moralizing discourse to condemn state officials whom they see as acting against both the national interest and the precepts of the Qur'an (Masquelier 2007).

Although he came to epitomize for many the very sins he had initially been invited to rid the community of, Malam Awal continued to stress the virtues of pious comportment and religious education. In sermons that equated malfeasance to sin, he championed the rights of the poor and targeted "false" Muslims who, under the guise of encouraging almsgiving, used their social standing as *malamai* to extort from others resources they neither needed nor deserved. He promoted early marriages, vestmental modesty, and women's seclusion as the primary means of fighting moral decadence and sexual indiscipline. Like his Izala foes, Awal denounced the Family Code on the ground that the issues it addressed were already regulated by Islamic law and should not suffer human interference. If family law was against God's plan, so was birth spacing. God alone, the preacher claimed, decided how many children a couple produced; those who interfered with the divine plan were doomed to a hellish fate.

In the early 1990s when the state—pressured by international donors wishing to implement population control—cautiously started promoting birth spacing to ensure that more children would survive infancy, some Muslim religious leaders urged their followers to ignore these recommendations.[32] The Prophet Muhammad, they claimed, had instructed Muslims to have large families so that he would have a wider following than other prophets on Judgment Day. According to this logic, those who took the matter of reproduction into their own hands demonstrated that they did not trust God to provide for them.[33] Criticisms aside, programs aimed at edifying Muslim scholars on the benefits of birth spacing appear to have had an impact, at least in Dogondoutchi. According to a local health worker, "some in this town have seen the benefits of birth spacing. Their original hesitations are now resolved."[34] For a large number of Nigériens the use of contraceptives is nevertheless controversial. Although access to reproductive health services has expanded significantly nationwide in past decades, the use of modern methods of birth control remains low, especially in rural areas (Guengant and May 2001).

In keeping with Awal's dictates, members of the Awaliyya were steadfastly against birth control, arguing that the practice ran against God's wishes. As Mina, a follower of Awal, explained, "Birth spacing is against God's will. You must take the children that God gives you. After you die, [if you practiced birth control], the children whose birth you have prevented will [shame you]." State representatives who promoted birth spacing were not only "bad" Muslims, Malam Awal argued. They were also puppets of Western powers, especially the U.S. By encouraging Muslims to limit the size of their families, health workers promoting birth control helped the U.S. (by Awal's account, a morally bankrupt nation) control the fate of Islam. According to the preacher, vaccination programs through which anti-fertility drugs were covertly administered to young girls exemplified Western determination to weaken Muslim populations worldwide. These programs had to be resisted; the future of the Muslim community was at stake.

In this whole affair the role played by northern Nigerian resistors cannot be discounted. Northern Nigeria is a crucial source of inspiration for pious Nigériens seeking to Islamize their opposition to the state. Like other opponents of the polio vaccine, Malam Awal took his cues from his Nigerian counterparts, who since 2002 had forced the WHO to delay or cancel altogether several immunization drives. He most likely did not know that the resurgence of polio in Niger was attributed to cross-border movements originating in Nigeria. Although many people were aware that the rumors of a conspiracy behind the polio eradication campaign had originated in Nigeria, with the exception of health workers, they did not make a connection with reports that northern Nigeria was identified as the "epicenter" from which the virus spread to countries such as Niger.

The spread of the poliovirus and of rumors about vaccine safety is a reminder of the porousness of the Nigérien-Nigerian border arbitrarily drawn by France and Great Britain in the wake of the 1885 Berlin Conference. During the colonial period cross-border traffic continued unhampered in a region previously crisscrossed by Hausa merchants trading livestock, salt, textiles, foodstuff, and kola nuts. At independence, building crossing stations was not a priority for the newly created nations of Niger and Nigeria (Miles 1994). As a result, the border between the two countries "remains porous, patrolling haphazard, and smuggling a major economic activity for petroleum and taxed agricultural products" (Aker et al. 2010: 7). Interestingly, Malam Awal himself was a product of this particular geopolitical configuration: born in Goure, Niger, he grew up in northern Nigeria, where he attended school and worked as district chief and a judge before moving back to Niger and eventually settling in Dogondoutchi. Knowing that Nigériens valorize that which comes from Nigeria, he stressed his Nigerian roots.[35] After losing his popularity, he left for Nigeria again, returning only occasionally to Dogondoutchi. Awal, to paraphrase Behar (1996: 162), was a man "of the border": his life trajectory underscored his "nomadic" lifestyle and the fact that he was continually "between places."

Finally, I should note that although resistance to the polio eradication campaign in and around Dogondoutchi appears to have been largely prompted by Malam Awal's claims that the vaccine caused infertility in young girls, one cannot discount the role played by rumors in this affair. Recall that the OPV was rumored to cause not only infertility but also atheism, AIDS, and polio itself. It can be safely assumed that those who claimed to resist polio vaccination on the basis that the vaccine caused any of the last three conditions were not swayed by the preacher's damaging rhetoric but by more diffuse yet similarly ominous reports that the medicine poured down children's throats was "poison." Indeed not all those who boycotted the campaign followed the preacher's lead and called themselves members of the Awaliyya. Ascertaining whether these individuals opposed the vaccination because of Awal's claims or because they heard through the grapevine that the OPV was a threat to their children's health is a challenging task, however.[36] In all likelihood the various reports circulating about the alleged dangers of the OPV interfaced and spun off each other to create a tangled set of allegations that centered on the vaccine's harmful effects. From this perspective, it is not farfetched to consider whether Malam Awal himself might have been the victim of rumors designed to taint his reputation. This is not to say that the religious leader was not a major catalyst in this affair, but to suggest instead that once he had made public declarations about the risks associated with the OPV, he could no longer control how his statements would be interpreted. Awal was known to have enemies who on previous instances had spread noxious gossip to damage his public image. Regardless of the reasons invoked to justify resistance to government-sponsored vaccination programs, what emerges from this discussion is the critical role of medicine in crystallizing popular opposition to the state. By expressing skepticism about the OPV, parents in and around Dogondoutchi were not voicing doubts about the health benefits of vaccination so much as they were articulating possible motives behind the distribution of free health care. Their non-compliance exemplifies how medicines can become a "strategic point" (Whyte, van der Geest, and Hardon 2002: 76) around which to generate opposition to governmental policies perceived to be at odds with the moral basis of social reproduction in Nigérien communities.

On October 12 and 13, 2005, a meeting of Muslim religious specialists was held at the Imam Malick cultural center in Niamey under the aegis of the WHO and UNICEF. With the expert assistance of representatives from the Ministry of Public Health, the hundred or so attendees hailing from all eight regions of Niger exchanged views on the role of Islam in the vaccination controversy and ways that the Muslim community could become more actively involved in the process of disease eradication. With the Qur'an as the main source of reference, they considered carefully the problems encountered by health workers during vaccination drives and scrutinized the various methods used "to inform and sensitize local populations and encourage their participation in the fight against polio" (Issa and Gorel 2005). At the conclusion of the meeting, Muslim specialists unanimously supported the idea of putting together an Islamic guide on diseases linked to vaccination. "We have debated the problem of polio during two days [. . .] and we have agreed," Dr. Sambo Amadou noted before attributing the persistence of "pockets of resistance" to a lack of communication and information (Issa and Gorel 2005). "We think that Muslim specialists have understood that the vaccine is innocuous and has no impact on fertility, and that they will spread the message back home," he concluded (Issa and Gorel 2005).

Although the conference appears to have generated a productive exchange of ideas, it is far from clear how *malamai* such as Malam Awal, whose understanding of moral community is strikingly at odds with secular notions of citizenship and associational life, will be impacted by future efforts on the part of the government to encourage religious leaders' participation in the promotion of public health. As my analysis of the controversy surrounding polio eradication suggests, people's reluctance to heed the state's recommendation that all children under five be administered OPV cannot be satisfactorily explained by invoking what Dr. Amadou referred as "a lack of information." Even if, as his detractors claim, Malam Awal's motives were to deceive people, the preacher's unsettling message—and the subsequent rumors that fed off his revelations—nonetheless provides an effective critique of Western-based models of public health by exposing the cost of blindly embracing the technologies and trappings of modernity. Aside from reminding us that the body can become the site of powerful struggles for the control of social reproduction (Boddy 2007; Comaroff 1985; Foucault 1990; Ginsburg and Rapp 1995; Thomas 2003), the rumors of tainted vaccines illuminate how ordinary citizens come to imagine the workings of the state through the circulation of medicines in all their mysterious, coercive, and threatening dimensions. At another level, they also speak of the far-reaching ways in which the shift of human and financial resources spawned by the recent liberalization of the Nigérien economy has restructured the relation between health and citizenship, helping foster the perception in some quarters that state-sponsored treatments touted as life-saving medicines are nothing but tools for eliminating "undesirable" populations (see Kane this volume).

In Niger, *malamai*-led resistance to the 2003 and 2004 polio vaccination campaigns suggests that the transnational flow of medicines is complexly mediated by a range of competing social, moral, and economic practices that are themselves produced through the encounter between global and local forces. Understanding why certain public health interventions come to be resisted despite a general faith in biomedicine requires attending to the ways in which the implementation of neoliberal policies, the concomitant development of corruption, and the rise of diverse religious discourses have helped to "moralize" the economy of signs and practices through which Nigérien citizens resolutely negotiate their relationships to the state in an increasingly fickle and deceptive world.

Notes

1. Whether in Cameroon, Nigeria, India, or Pakistan, resistance to public health campaigns provides dramatic instantiations of how citizens express their

skepticism of the state's benevolence (Regis 2003; Nichter 1995; Renne 2010; Closser 2010). In Congo-Kinshasa, a polio vaccination program in the 1990s was boycotted by local populations after rumors spread that blood would be taken from children to be sent to Europe, where it would be used in transfusions to rejuvenate the ailing Mobutu (de Boeck 1998).

2. In 2004, a Muslim religious specialist of Nigerian origin living in a Nigérien village close to the border convinced some of his followers to resist state-sponsored vaccination. According to one health worker, the man "contaminated Niger with his ideas of conspiracy." Comments such as these index "concerns about national boundaries" (Nichter 1995: 619; Sontag 1988) and the importance of preserving local communities from outside threats, be they germs, false rumors, or tainted medicines.

3. In previous *campagnes de sensibilisation* (sensibilization campaigns), educational programs have generally targeted traditional healers, seen to be central nodes in the dissemination of information about disease and medicine.

4. *Malam* (teacher) is an honorific title bestowed on Muslim clerics and scholars.

5. Resistance to vaccination has a long history in the West as well. See Colgrove (2006).

6. According to a 20-year-old teacher from Kano, "The Western world has never wished Muslims well. Why should they expect us to believe that vaccines they make these days are not another frontier to wage war against Muslims?" (McKenzie 2003: 1).

7. For a critical analysis of the notion of "sanitary urgence" in the context of media-orchestrated health missions, see Hours (1987).

8. The full name of the anti-Sufi association colloquially known as Izala is *Jama'atu Izalat al Bid'a wa Iqamat al-Sunna* (Movement for Suppressing Innovations and Restoring the Sunna).

9. Although few Muslims in Niger follow the Sufi path, many are loosely identified as *'yan darika,* members of a Sufi order, because they ostensibly adhere to practices that—in the absence of a clearly defined sense of collective Sufi identity—can be loosely identified with Sufism, and also because they oppose Izala reformism.

10. Measles kills over 500 children every year in Niger. In December 2004, a nation-wide measles vaccination campaign targeted some 6 million children ranging in age from 9 months to 14 years (Diallo 2005b). Given the positive reception of the local population to measles vaccination drives, it was hoped that combining polio eradication with measles eradication would melt people's resistance to OPV.

11. Some residents of Zaria (in Nigeria) similarly resisted the polio vaccination initiative because, in addition to rumors of contamination by anti-fertility substances, they could not understand why, as one person put it, when "we are looking for medicine in the hospital to give to our children, we can't get it, but this one, they are following us to our houses to give it" (Renne 2006: 1862).

12. Many of Awal's followers became disillusioned by his greed, intolerance, and inability to live by the principles he championed and eventually left him.

13. Like other Muslim religious specialists who manufacture talismanic medicines, Malam Awal allegedly had the power to protect people from the corruption of others while helping them hide the frauds they themselves committed. His ser-

vices were sought by high-ranking civil servants who were particularly vulnerable to competitors' schemes as well as to accusations of corruption.

14. For a critical account of the historical and cultural underpinnings of eradication as a public health strategy, see Closser (2010).

15. The four countries that have "endemic polio" are Afghanistan, India, Nigeria, and Pakistan.

16. See *Journées nationales de vaccination* 2006.

17. Parents are frequently accused of selling mosquito nets they were given for free. I was not able to verify the accuracy of these accusations. These claims reveal the extent to which health workers have internalized the rhetoric of blame that paints those who resist the drive or fail to follow instructions as "backward," ignorant, and dishonest.

18. In certain areas vaccinated children were administered a *vermifuge* (dewormer) rather than given a mosquito net. The measure was not very popular; parents complained they were being "short-changed."

19. Ad hoc strategies have been developed to cultivate parental trust and enhance vaccination coverage. After the mosquito net distribution fiasco, a health worker told me that "next time" they would orchestrate things differently ("we'll take two cars, one to distribute the vaccines and one to distribute the mosquito nets") in an effort to minimize parental discontent.

20. When non-compliance is studied from the patient's perspective, a distinction emerges between patients acting out of ignorance and patients consciously resisting medication out of skepticism about the doctor or the treatment (Homedes and Ugalde 1993).

21. The Nigériens I spoke with would likely be surprised to learn that in the U.S. (alleged seat of the conspiracy to limit Muslim births), some parents opt not to vaccinate their children because of the supposed risks incurred (see Colgrove 2006; Kaufman 1967).

22. In Nigeria people have become adept at tricking the government back, using deceptive tactics as protection against abusive state policies. Families who resisted the vaccination drive erased the chalk marks on their doorways that signaled their lack of cooperation, or blackened their children's thumbs with the same ink used by vaccinators to identify immunized children (Dugger and McNeill Jr. 2006). In Niger, similar tricks were used to confuse health workers attempting to separate those who cooperated from those who did not.

23. As Blundo and Olivier de Sardan (2001a: 31) put it, "integrity is a luxury or a virtue that in the current context is inaccessible for most Beninois, Nigérien, or Senegalese citizens."

24. Many physicians appointed at public hospitals make money on the side by seeing patients at their private practice during working hours. There, patients pay for medical tests run with public equipment (Olivier de Sardan, Bako-Arifari, and Moumouni 2005).

25. For additional examples of how medical facilities elsewhere are part of this regime of dissimulation, see Hours (1985), Hunt (1999), Olivier de Sardan (2003), and Scheper-Hughes (1992).

26. The failure to distinguish the real from the fake in the context of health services is compounded by the fact that health workers rarely end up executing the tasks for which they were hired in the first place: "In health centers, employees at all levels accomplish tasks for which they have no competence or training.

Guards apply dressings, laborers give shots, orderlies are in charge of deliveries, nurses give prescriptions, and physicians are the administrators" (Olivier de Sardan 2003: 4).

27. On the popularity of injections in Africa, see White (2000); Whyte, van der Geest, and Hardon (2002); and Vaughan (1991).

28. Following Gupta (2005: 190), I wish to stress the importance of corruption discourse in popular representations of the Nigérien state, for "narratives of corruption help shape people's expectations of what states can and will do, and how bureaucrats will respond to the needs of citizens."

29. In 1996, families in Kano, Nigeria, accused the New York–based pharmaceutical manufacturer Pfizer of experimenting with the new antibiotic Trovan without fully informing the patients' parents of the risks their children incurred during treatment for meningitis. Eleven children who had taken part in the study subsequently died and scores more were disabled (Petryna 2005; Peterson this volume). When parents sued the company for wrongdoing in a U.S. federal court, the case was dismissed. A U.S. appeals court subsequently revived it, and in July 2009 Pfizer signed a 75 million USD agreement with Nigerian authorities to settle criminal and civil charges. Though Kano officials agreed to drop the charges in return for the settlement, the agreement does not affect charges filed against Pfizer by Nigeria's federal government, which is seeking 6 billion USD in compensation (Stephens 2009).

30. About 60,000 doses of the vaccine were used on children before doctors realized they were fake, and 2,500 children allegedly died as a result of the fakery.

31. For those for whom Islam is the ultimate system of value against which everything else is measured, members of the government are secular "fat cats" deputized by foreign administrations to do their "dirty work" (such as shrinking the Muslim population) in return for aid. Like the international bodies with whom they are conflated, agents of the state are primarily seen as ambitious, materialistic, and irreligious. Reformist preachers routinely criticize their secular ways modeled on foreign values, thereby reinforcing their identification with Western powers.

32. The Centre National de Santé Familiale (National Center for Family Health) was created in 1984 to introduce a policy of family planning aimed at guaranteeing the health of mothers and children through the implementation of birth spacing.

33. To those who argue that family planning produces well-spaced, healthy children who are adequately provided for by their parents, reformist Muslims and 'yan Awaliyya respond that this way of thinking is an insult to God. God alone provides for people, and Muslims everywhere must trust in His ability to care for His creatures. From this perspective, people experience hunger and want precisely because they don't obey God. Poverty is their punishment for doubting His powers.

34. Muslim religious specialists do not endorse the use of condoms as a mode of AIDS prevention, however. Condoms are not an appropriate means of fighting AIDS, they argue, because it hinders the realization of God's plan for His creatures.

35. West and Luedke (2006) similarly draw attention to Mozambican healers' tendency to claim to have been born across the border in Tanzania or to have received training somewhere else. Healers, they further remind us, cross material

as well as conceptual boundaries constantly: "So fundamental to the profile of the healer are transgressions of boundaries that one might conclude that the power of healing is in some profound way bound up with the act of crossing borders" (2006: 2).

36. After several rounds of vaccination within a year, some parents suffered from vaccination "fatigue." They denied the OPV to their children, believing the latter had had enough medicine against the disease.

References

Abrams, Phillip. 1988. "Notes on the Difficulty of Studying the State." *Journal of Historical Sociology* 1: 58–89.

Aker, Jenny C., Michael W. Klein, Stephen A. O'Connell, and Muzhe Yang. 2010. *Are Borders Barriers? The Impact of International and Internal Ethnic Borders on Agricultural Markets in West Africa.* CGD Working Paper 208. Washington, D.C.: Center for Global Development.

Apter, Andrew. 1999. "IBB = 419: Nigerian Democracy and the Politics of Illusion." In *Civil Society and the Political Imagination in Africa,* ed. John L. Comaroff and Jean Comaroff, 267–308. Chicago: University of Chicago Press.

Aretxaga, Begoña. 2003. "Maddening States." *Annual Review of Anthropology* 32: 393–410.

Bastian, Misty. 1999. "'Buried Beneath Six Feet of Crude Oil': State-Sponsored Death and the Absent Body of Ken Saro-Wiwa." In *Ken Saro-Wiwa: Writer and Political Activist,* ed. Craig W. McLuckie and Aubrey McPhail, 127–152. Boulder, Colo.: Lynne Rienner.

Bayart, Jean-François. 1989. *L'État en Afrique: La politique du ventre.* Paris: Fayard.

Bayart, Jean-François, Stephen Ellis, and Béatrice Hibou. 1999. *The Criminalization of the State in Africa.* Bloomington: Indiana University Press.

Bayart, Jean-François, Achille Mbembe, and Comi Toulabor. 1992. *Le politique par le bas en Afrique Noire: Contribution à une problématique de la démocratie.* Paris: Éditions Khartala.

Behar, Ruth. 1996. *The Vulnerable Observer: Anthropology That Breaks Your Heart.* Boston, Mass.: Beacon Press.

Blundo, Giorgio, and Jean-Pierre Olivier de Sardan. 2001a. "La corruption quotidienne en Afrique de l'Ouest." *Politique Africaine* 83: 8–37.

———. 2001b. "Sémiologie populaire de la corruption." *Politique Africaine* 83: 98–114.

Boddy, Janice. 2007. *Civilizing Women: British Crusades in Colonial Sudan.* Princeton: Princeton University Press.

Bonu, S., M. Rani, and O. Razum. 2004. "Global Public Health Mandates in a Diverse World: The Polio Eradication Initiative and the Expanded Programme on Immunization in Sub-Saharan Africa and South Asia." *Health Policy* 70 (3): 327–345.

Boustany, Nora. 2005. "Wealthy Muslim Nations Do Little to Stop Spread of Polio." *The Washington Post,* Aug. 17: A09.

Briggs, Charles L., with Clara Martini-Briggs. 2003. *Stories in the Time of Cholera: Racial Profiling during a Medical Nightmare.* Berkeley: University of California Press.

Chilliot, Laurent. 2003. "Médicament et prévention en milieu populaire songhay-zarma." In *Les maladies de passage: Transmissions, préventions, et hygiènes en Afrique de l'Ouest,* ed. Doris Bonnet and Yannick Jaffré, 427–464. Paris: Karthala.

Closser, Svea. 2010. *Chasing Polio in Pakistan: Why the World's Largest Public Health Initiative May Fail.* Nashville, Tenn.: Vanderbilt University Press.

Colgrove, James. 2006. *States of Immunity: The Politics of Vaccination in Twentieth-Century America.* Berkeley: University of California Press.

Comaroff, Jean. 1985. *Body of Power, Spirit of Resistance: The Culture and History of a South African People.* Chicago: University of Chicago.

Comaroff, Jean, and John L. Comaroff. 1999. "Occult Economies and the Violence of Extraction: Notes from the South African Postcolony." *American Ethnologist* 26 (3): 279–301.

de Boeck, Filip. 1996. "Postcolonialism, Power, and Identity: Local and Global Perspectives from Zaïre." In *Postcolonial Identities in Africa,* ed. Richard Werbner and Terence Ranger, 75–106. London: Zed Books.

———. 1998. "Beyond the Grave: History, Memory, and Death in Postcolonial Congo/Zaïre." In *Memory and the Postcolony: African Anthropology and the Critique of Power,* ed. Richard Werbner, 21–58. London: Zed.

Diallo, Mahamadou. 2005a. "Poliomyélite: La vaccination doit se poursuivre." *Le Républicain,* November 24. Electronic document: http://www.planetafrique.com/Republicain-Niger-new.com/.

———. 2005b. "Campagne de vaccination de masse: La rougeole, mieux vaut prévenir que guérir." *Le Républicain,* December 16. Electronic document: http://www.planetafrique.com/Republicain-Niger-new.com/.

Donnelly, John. 2004. "Headway Seen in Africa on Polio Immunizations: Progress Renews Hope for Eradication of Virus." *The Boston Globe,* Aug. 3: 7.

Dugger, Celia W., and Dona G. McNeill Jr. 2006. "Rumor, Fear, and Fatigue Hinder Final Push to End Polio." *The New York Times,* March 20. Electronic document: http://www/nytimes.com/2006/03/20/international/asia/20polio.html?ei=5088&en=96aebe4.

Farmer, Paul. 1992. *AIDS and Accusations: Haiti and the Geography of Blame.* Berkeley: University of California Press.

Fassin, Didier. 1986. "'La bonne mère': Pratiques rurales et urbaines de la rougeole chez les femmes Haalpulaaren du Sénégal." *Social Science and Medicine* 23: 121–123.

Fisiy, Cyprian F., and Peter Geschiere. 2001. "Witchcraft, Development, and Paranoia in Cameroon: Interactions between Popular, Academic, and State Discourse." In *Magical Interpretations, Material Realities: Modernity, Witchcraft, and the Occult in Postcolonial Africa,* ed. Henrietta L. Moore and Todd Sanders, 226–246. New York: Routledge.

Foucault, Michel. 1990. *The History of Sexuality, Volume 1.* New York: Vintage.

Fraser, Gertrude J. 1995. "Modern Bodies, Modern Minds: Midwifery and Reproductive Change in an African American Community." In *Conceiving the New World Order: The Global Politics of Reproduction,* ed. Faye D. Ginsburg and Rayna Rapp, 42–58. Berkeley: University of California Press.

Geertz, Clifford. 1983. *Local Knowledge: Further Essays in Interpretive Anthropology.* New York: Basic Books, Inc.

Geschiere, Peter. 1995. *Sorcellerie et politique en Afrique: La viande des autres.* Paris: Éditions Karthala.

Ginsburg, Faye D., and Rayna Rapp. 1995. *Conceiving the New World Order: The Global Politics of Reproduction.* Berkeley: University of California Press.

Global Polio Eradication Initiative. 2010. "Annual Report 2009." Electronic document: http://www.polioeradication.org/content/publications/annual report2009.asp, accessed May 05, 2010.

Guengant, Jean-Pierre, and John F. May. 2001. "Impact of the Proximate Determinants on the Future Course of Fertility in Sub-Saharan Africa." Paper presented at a workshop titled Prospects for Fertility Decline in High Fertility Countries. United Nations Secretariat, New York, July 9–11.

Gupta, Akhil. 1995. "Blurred Boundaries: The Discourse of Corruption, the Culture of Politics, and the Imagined State." *American Ethnologist* 22: 375–402.

———. 2005. "Narrating the State of Corruption." In *Corruption: Anthropological Perspectives,* ed. Dieter Haller and Cris Shore, 173–193. Ann Arbor, Mich.: Pluto.

Hibou, Béatrice. 1999. "The 'Social Capital' of the State as an Agent of Deception or the Ruses of Economic Intelligence." In *The Criminalization of the State in Africa,* ed. Jean-Francois Bayart, Béatrice Hibou, and Stephen Ellis, 69–113. Bloomington: Indiana University Press.

Homedes, Nuria, and Antonio Ugalde. 1993. "Patients' Compliance with Medical Treatments in the Third World: What Do We Know?" *Health Policy and Planning* 8 (4): 291–314.

Hours, Bernard. 1985. *L'état sorcier: Santé publique et société au Cameroun.* Paris: L'Harmattan.

———. 1987. "L'urgence comme politique." *Politique Africaine* 28: 89–95.

Hunt, Nancy Rose. 1999. *A Colonial Lexicon: Of Birth Ritual, Medicalization, and Mobility in the Congo.* Durham, N.C.: Duke University Press.

Issa, Oumarou. 2006. "Le poliovirus sauvage ne circule plus au Niger: L'heure est à la mobilisation pour la certification." *Le Républicain,* March 9. Electronic document: http://www.planetafrique.com/Republicain-Niger-new .com/.

Issa, Oumarou, and Alain Gorel. 2005. "Informer les religieux sur les bénéfices du vaccin contre la polio." *Le Républicain,* Sept. 22: 5.

Jaffré, Yannick. 1996. "Dissonnances entre les représentations sociales et médicales de la malnutrition dans un service de pédiatrie au Niger.» *Sciences Sociales et Santé* 14 (1): 41–71.

Journées nationales de vaccination. 2006. *Le Républicain,* Apr. 15: 1, 4.

Kapp, Clare. 2004. "Nigerian States Again Boycott Polio-Vaccination Drive." *The Lancet* 363 (9410): 709.

Kaufman, M. 1967. "The American Anti-Vaccinationists and their Arguments." *Bulletin of the History of Medicine* 41: 463–483.

Keïta, Oumarou. 2006. "Bonne gouvernance sous Tandja II: Un commerçant vend des vaccins à l'état nigérien." *Le Républicain,* Feb. 16. Electronic document: http://www.planetafrique.com/Republicain-Niger-new.com/.

Masquelier, Adeline. 2000. "Of Head Hunters and Cannibals: Migrancy, Labor, and Consumption in the Mawri Imagination." *Cultural Anthropology* 15 (1): 84–126.

———. 2001. "Behind the Dispensary's Prosperous Facade: Imagining the State in Rural Niger." *Public Culture* 13 (2): 267–291.

———. 2007. "Negotiating Futures: Youth, Islam, and the State in Niger." In *Islam and the State in Africa*, ed. René Otayek and Benjamin F. Soares, 243–262. New York: Palgrave.

———. 2009. *Women and Islamic Revival in a West African Town.* Bloomington: Indiana University Press.

McKenzie, Glenn. 2003. "Nigerian Muslims Skeptical of Polio Plan." *The Washington Post*, Oct. 25: 1. Electronic document: http://news.biafra nigeriaworld.com/archive/2003/oct/25/0043.html.

Migdal, Joel S. 1988. *Strong Societies and Weak States: State-Society Relations and State Capabilities in the Third World.* Princeton: Princeton University Press.

Miles, William F. S. 1994. *Hausaland Divided: Colonialism and Independence in Nigeria and Niger.* Ithaca, N.Y.: Cornell University Press.

Nichter, Mark. 1995. "Vaccinations in the Third World: A Consideration of Community Demand." *Social Science and Medicine* 41 (5): 617–632.

Olivier de Sardan, Jean-Pierre. 1999. "A Moral Economy of Corruption in Africa?" *The Journal of Modern African Studies* 37: 25–52.

———. 2003. "État, bureaucratie, et gouvernance en Afrique de l'Ouest franco-phone: Un diagnostic empirique, une perspective historique." Paper presented at CODESRIA, Dakar, Senegal.

Olivier de Sardan, Jean-Pierre, N. Bako-Arifari, and A. Moumouni. 2005. *La corruption dans la santé au Bénin et au Niger. Études et Travaux 40.* Niamey, Niger: LASDEL.

Petryna, Adriana. 2005. "Ethical Variability: Drug Development and Globalizing Clinical Trials." *American Ethnologist* 32 (2): 183–197.

Piot, Charles. 2010. *Nostalgia for the Future: West Africa after the Cold War.* Chicago: University of Chicago Press.

Rasmussen, Susan J. 1994. "Female Sexuality, Social Reproduction, and Medical Intervention: Kel Ewey Tuareg Perspectives." *Culture, Medicine, and Psychiatry* 18: 433–462.

Regis, Helen. 2003. *Fulbe Voices: Marriage, Islam, and Medicine in Northern Cameroon.* Boulder, Colo.: Westview Press.

Renne, Elisha. 2006. "Perspectives on Polio and Immunization in Northern Nigeria." *Social Science and Medicine* 63: 1857–1869.

———. 2010. *The Politics of Polio in Northern Nigeria.* Bloomington: Indiana University Press.

Reno, William. 1995. *Corruption and State Politics in Sierra Leone.* Cambridge: Cambridge University Press.

Sanders, Todd. 2001. "Save Our Skins: Structural Adjustment, Morality, and the Occult in Tanzania." In *Magical Interpretations, Material Realities: Modernity, Witchcraft, and the Occult in Postcolonial Africa*, ed. Henrietta L. Moore and Todd Sanders, 160–183. New York: Routledge.

Scheper-Hughes, Nancy. 1992. *Death Without Weeping: The Violence of Everyday Life in Brazil.* Berkeley: University of California Press.

Shaw, Rosalind. 1996. "The Politician and the Diviner: Divination and the Consumption of Power in Sierra Leone." *Journal of Religion in Africa* 26 (1): 30–55.

Smith, Daniel Jordan. 2006. *A Culture of Corruption: Everyday Deception and Popular Discontent in Nigeria.* Princeton: Princeton University Press.

Sontag, Susan. 1988. *Illness as Metaphor.* New York: Farrar, Straus & Giroux.

Sounaye, Abdoulaye. 2005. "Les politiques de l'islam au Niger dans l'ère de la démocratisation de 1991 à 2002." In *L'Islam politique au sud du Sahara: Identités, discours, et enjeux,* ed. Muriel Perez-Gomez, 503–525. Paris: Karthala.

Stephens, Joe. 2009 "Pfizer to Pay $75 Million to Settle Trovan-Testing Suit." *The Washington Post,* July 31. Electronic document: http://www.washing tonpost.com/wp-dyn/content/article/2009/07/30/AR2009073001847 .html.

Thomas, Lynn M. 2003. *The Politics of the Womb: Women, Reproduction, and the State in Kenya.* Berkeley: University of California Press.

Vaughan, Megan. 1991. *Curing Their Ills: Colonial Power and African Illness.* Stanford, Calif.: Stanford University Press.

Weiss, Brad. 1996. *The Making and Unmaking of the Haya Lived World: Consumption, Commoditization, and Everyday Practice.* Durham, N.C.: Duke University Press.

West, Harry G., and Tracy J. Luedke. 2006. "Introduction: Healing Divides: Therapeutic Border Work in Southeast Africa." In *Borders & Healers: Brokering Therapeutic Resources in Southeast Africa,* ed. Tracy J. Luedke and Harry G. West, 1–20. Bloomington: Indiana University Press.

White, Luise. 2000. *Speaking with Vampires: Rumor and History in Colonial Africa.* Berkeley: University of California Press.

Whyte, Susan Reynolds, Sjaak van der Geest, and Anita Hardon. 2002. *Social Lives of Medicines.* New York: Cambridge University Press.

Yacouba, Ibrahim. 2006. "C.H.R. de Maradi: Un hôpital "morbide" dépourvu de radio." *Le Républicain,* May 18. Electronic document: http://www .planetafrique.com/Republicain-Niger-new.com/.

NINE

School of Deliverance:
Healing, Exorcism, and Male Spirit Possession in the Ghanaian Presbyterian Diaspora

Adam Mohr

The political and social changes associated with globalization in the last two decades have resulted in radical shifts in the circulation of people, religious institutions, and healing practitioners between Africa and the African-born immigrants in the U.S. In particular, the large-scale immigration of Ghanaian Christians to the U.S. has led to the formation of a network of Ghanaian Presbyterian churches in North America. This network of churches has attempted to reproduce healing practices established at the Grace Deliverance Center in Ghana—the primary religious healing center of the Presbyterian Church of Ghana—through an annual healing and deliverance workshop held in New York. This school of deliverance is the principal mechanism by which the practices of deliverance—meant to free a person from illness or misfortune emanating from Satan—are taught to members of the Presbyterian Church's Prayer Teams, which are sub-church organizations responsible for the health and welfare of their congregations.

This essay addresses the attempts to reproduce religious healing across space and, in particular, the transformations that are necessarily contained within this process. In the U.S., Ghanaian women have increased earning capacities due to opportunities within the traditionally feminized health care industry. Ghanaian men frequently earn less money than their wives and have less control over their marriages and marital resources. Thus, the traditional power dynamic between men and women has become inverted within Ghanaian marriages in the U.S., resulting in a parallel transformation within gendered patterns of spirit possession. Among Ghanaian Presbyterians in the U.S., there is a high incidence of male spirit possession compared to its relative absence in Ghana, where spirit possession is limited to women.[1] Many Ghanaian Presbyterian men become spirit-possessed as a religious response to their social marginalization in the U.S., thereby transforming Ghanaian masculinity in both the material and spiritual realms.

Ghanaian Immigration and the
Ghanaian Christian Landscape in the U.S.

In the last 20 years there has been a significant increase in the number of African immigrants in the U.S. The U.S. Census estimates that by 2007 there were 1.4 million African-born immigrants residing in the country, compared to only 364,000 in 1990.[2] The number of African permanent residents admitted into the U.S. almost doubled from 66,422 in 2004 to 117,430 in 2006.[3]

Ghanaians comprise a large percentage of the total number of African immigrants. Between 2003 and 2006 the number of Ghanaians gaining permanent residency in the U.S. more than doubled.[4] In 2006, Ghana ranked fourth among African countries in its number of U.S. permanent residencies, after Ethiopia, Nigeria, and Egypt. But Ghana is only the twelfth most populous African state, while Ethiopia, Nigeria, and Egypt are numbers three, one, and two, respectively, in terms of population.[5] Therefore, a much larger percentage of the population of Ghana is immigrating to the U.S. than from any of the three largest African states.

Economic conditions in Ghana have fostered this large-scale emigration, beginning in the 1960s when the Ghanaian economy began to rapidly decline. With continued economic deterioration—such as low crop prices and high inflation—the pattern of large-scale emigration continued into the 1970s. The economic conditions only deteriorated further throughout the 1980s and into the 1990s, particularly due to the 1983 implementation of structural adjustment programs sponsored by the International Monetary Fund and the World Bank. While the economy began stabilizing by the turn of the twenty-first century, the pattern of large-scale Ghanaian emigration continued,[6] resulting in remittances sent from migrants back to Ghana that are now calculated in billions of U.S. dollars.[7]

This emigration pattern from Ghana to the U.S. has been enabled by immigration policies in the U.S. and Europe. Three immigration policies led to large-scale immigration to the U.S. by Africans, and by Ghanaians in particular. First, the 1965 U.S. Immigration Reform Act abolished country-of-origin quotas that had favored European immigrants, which increased opportunities for African immigration. Second, the Diversity Visa Program as part of the 1990 U.S. Immigration Act offered much greater opportunity to Africans. Third, the increased restrictions on immigration to Western Europe beginning in the 1980s, particularly between Africans and their former European colonizers, have led the U.S. to become the favored destination of African immigrants (Olupona and Gemignani 2007: 2). The closing of European borders included decreased immigration from Ghana to Great Britain. All these policies made it easier for Ghanaian immigrants to settle in the U.S. As a critical mass of Ghanaians immigrated to the U.S., most of whom were Christian, they established immigrant churches.

The majority of Ghanaian immigrants are from southern Ghana, where Christianity is the dominant religion. Since the 1980s Christian Ghanaian immigrants have been establishing congregations in the U.S. Many Ghanaian Pentecostal denominations, such as the Church of Pentecost, Assemblies of God, Apostolic Church, and Lighthouse Chapel International have formed branches in the U.S. The Church of Pentecost has the largest membership, both in Ghana (1.29 million) and in the diaspora (189,118), claiming nearly 12,000 members in over 70 congregations in the U.S. in 2005.[8]

A network of Ghanaian Presbyterian churches—some affiliated with the Presbyterian Church of Ghana (PCG) and others with the Presbyterian Church U.S.A (PC-USA)—have become established in the U.S. since the 1990s.[9] The congregations of the Ghanaian PC-USA and the Ghanaian Presbyterian Church Canada are members of the Conference of Ghanaian Presbyterian Churches, North America. As of 2007, there were nine member churches, located in the Bronx; Brooklyn; Columbus, Ohio; Houston; Langley, Maryland; Montreal; Philadelphia; Toronto; and Woodbridge, Virginia.[10] There are also three corresponding members—non-member churches that participate in the conference—which are affiliated with the PCG. These churches are located in the Bronx, Manhattan, and Worcester, Massachusetts.

More Pentecostal than the Pentecostals: Healing and Deliverance in the Philadelphia Ghanaian Presbyterian Church

In a survey conducted among four Ghanaian immigrant congregations in Philadelphia, I found the Ghanaian Presbyterian Church, called the United Ghanaian Community Church, to have the most robust religious healing practices. These findings were surprising considering that healing is one of the two practices, along with speaking in tongues, that most defines Pentecostalism (Wacker 2001: 65ff). The two largest Ghanaian Pentecostal churches in Philadelphia, the Assemblies of God and the Church of Pentecost, have a very different approach to healing and deliverance than the Presbyterian Church.

While healing and deliverance have become general features of Ghanaian Christianity within all denominations (see Bediako 2000: 312; Omenyo 2002), pastors, congregations, and denominations as a whole have responded to this phenomenon differently. Most believe that the Devil, acting through demons, is ultimately responsible for sickness or misfortune, although it is an individual's sin that enables the Devil to afflict them. Many Ghanaian Pentecostals believe that when a Christian is attacked by demons, leading to illness or misfortune, this attack should be combated by individual prayer (Asamoah-Gyadu 2005: 165–187). Some say that if you are a "true" Christian the Devil cannot harm you, and they see no need for deliverance practitioners. Both the Assemblies of God and Church of Pentecost in Philadelphia fall into this category.[11]

There are two aspects of the healing and deliverance ministry of the Ghanaian Presbyterian churches in the U.S. that set them apart from other Ghanaian churches in the diaspora. One, the Presbyterian churches have a separate group within the church that manages the health and welfare of church members. This group is called the Prayer Team. Two, the Prayer Teams are formally trained by Catechist Ebenezer Abboah-Offei, who established and currently manages the Grace Deliverance Center in Akropong, Ghana. These Prayer Teams study a deliverance manual written by Abboah-Offei in their home churches as well as receive training from Abboah-Offei during evangelism trips to the various Presbyterian churches in the U.S. Most influentially, however, the Prayer Teams participate in an annual deliverance workshop taught by Abboah-Offei in New York.

Before discussing the New York deliverance workshop in detail, I will give some particulars about the development of healing and deliverance within the PCG, which revolves around three organizations: the Bible Study and Prayer Group of the PCG, the Scripture Union (a para-church organization), and the PCG's Grace Deliverance Center. Abboah-Offei not only established this Deliverance Center, but also played leading roles in the formation of the Bible Study and Prayer Group, as well as the Scripture Union. The link between these institutions runs not only through Abboah-Offei's participation, but also through his kinship and marriage networks.

Healing and Deliverance within the Presbyterian Church of Ghana: The Emergence of Catechist Abboah-Offei

The first significant church to incorporate religious healing practices in Ghana was Faith Tabernacle Congregation, a Philadelphia-based divine healing church (Mohr 2011). Faith Tabernacle's rapid growth during the 1920s was paralleled by the expansion of Pentecostalism in the 1930s, which initially occurred within the extensive Faith Tabernacle network. Spiritual healing continued to be a predominant activity within early Pentecostalism in Ghana. With the success of Pentecostal churches in the 1940s and '50s, particularly of the Church of Pentecost (circa 1953) in the Presbyterian stronghold of

Ghana's Eastern Region, the PCG was forced to respond to the healing practices offered by these newer churches, which accounted for much of their success.[12]

In August 1963, the PCG decided to restore the New Testament ministry of healing (Omenyo 2002: 130). More than any single individual in the PCG, Reverend T. A. Kumi was most responsible for enacting this decision. Influenced by the charismatic revival in Scotland, Kumi introduced the healing ministry through seminars given at the Ramseyer Memorial Retreat Center, which later resulted in the formation of a number of prayer groups between 1962 and 1965.[13] These prayer groups were formally organized into the Bible Study and Prayer Group in March 1965, with 21 groups and 600 members.[14] The Bible Study and Prayer Group as an organization was composed of many members who had previously been associated with Scripture Union. As one Presbyterian pastor argued, the "Bible Study and Prayer Groups flourished because Scripture Union members were often in leadership positions."[15]

Scripture Union became the main para-church organization operating in Ghana's secondary schools by the late 1950s. Graduates with Scripture Union backgrounds had, by the late 1960s and early 1970s, formed groups in universities as well as town fellowships. Some of the members of Scripture Union fellowships introduced healing and deliverance into the prayer groups of their churches, including the PCG (Omenyo 2002: 96), whose Scripture Union group was called the Prayer Warriors.

Many of the Scripture Union Prayer Warriors had significant interactions with the Bible Study and Prayer Group of the PCG. This group included Edward Okyere, who in 1974 established the Warriors' Annual Retreat, a week-long gathering with a focus on fasting, prayer, healing, and deliverance (Barker and Boadi-Siaw 2005; Kumah 1994). Scripture Union's Warriors' Annual Retreat expanded by 1984 to include an annual deliverance workshop to formally teach healing and deliverance practices to the Prayer Teams that were by then developing in the mainline churches, such as the Anglican, Baptist, Catholic, Methodist, Presbyterian, and Evangelical Presbyterian.

One notable Presbyterian, Ebenezer Abboah-Offei, began participating in these deliverance workshops soon after they were established and by 2000 was formally teaching deliverance procedures in the Scripture Union deliverance workshop. Ebenezer Abboah-Offei was born in Akropong into the Presbyterian Church in 1957. While living in Asamankese in 1975, he became born-again as a result of joining Scripture Union in secondary school. At age 20, Abboah-Offei became president of the Asamankese Christian Fellowship and joined Joyful Way Incorporated, both Christian student organizations.

From 1979 to 1986, Abboah-Offei was president of the Scripture Union town fellowship in Asamankese. In 1987, he moved back to Akropong to teach agriculture at the Okuapemman secondary school.

In Akropong, Abboah-Offei rejoined his childhood congregation: Christ Presbyterian Church, the oldest continuously attended Presbyterian church in Ghana (founded c.1835). At Christ Church in 1987, Abboah-Offei became a leader in the Bible Study and Prayer Group. By 1989, Abboah-Offei was the Bible Study and Prayer Group president at Christ Church and soon became a church elder. During the early 1990s, Abboah-Offei was particularly influenced by the deliverance ministry of the Church of Pentecost's Owusu Tabiri, who led the church's most successful Prayer Camp in Sunyani until October 1995, when he established his own church. As Abboah-Offei became more involved in the healing and deliverance ministry throughout the late 1990s, he quit his teaching job to devote himself full-time to the Church.

As the Bible Study and Prayer Group began to grow within Christ Church and more and more people started flocking to the deliverance sessions, the leadership at Christ suggested that Abboah-Offei start a charismatic Presbyterian Church in Akropong. Thus, Grace Presbyterian Church opened on March 24, 1996 as both a church and a deliverance center: a place where, in addition to the two weekly deliverance services on Wednesdays and Saturdays, the afflicted could come for individual consultations offered Monday through Friday. By the summer of 2000, Abboah-Offei began offering a deliverance workshop at Grace, and in 2001 he was consecrated as a Catechist in the PCG.

The Bible Study and Prayer Group and Scripture Union are both organizations involved with healing and deliverance that predate the Grace Deliverance Center.[16] Catechist Abboah-Offei is linked with these two organizations through his participation since the 1970s. But in addition, the particular leaders who initiated healing and deliverance in the Bible Study and Prayer Group and in Scripture Union are linked to Abboah-Offei through kinship. T. A. Kumi, the primary person responsible for establishing the Bible Study and Prayer Group, is Abboah-Offei's great-uncle. While the beginnings of the Bible Study and Prayer Group in the 1960s predate Abboah-Offei's involvement (he was still a young boy), his relationship to his cousin Edward Okyere, who inaugurated Scripture Union's Warriors' Annual Retreat, did have an impact on his involvement. Eventually, Abboah-Offei became a leader in both organizations and opened the Grace Deliverance Center for the PCG. Subsequently, Abboah-Offei started teaching his own deliverance workshop in Akropong in 2000, with the New York workshop beginning in 2005.

Transnational Deliverance Workshop:
From Akropong to New York

Abboah-Offei's transnational healing ministry was also facilitated by a network of kinship ties between his wife Faustina and her aunt Paulina Atiemo, who is married to the Reverend Samuel Atiemo, Pastor of the Ghanaian Presbyterian Reformed Church in Brooklyn. Atiemo was the chief facilitator of the New York deliverance workshop as well as the 2006 President of the Conference of Ghanaian Presbyterian Churches, North America. Abboah-Offei and Atiemo had crossed paths before their marriages, however.

The two men knew each other from Asamankese, where Atiemo was born and Abboah-Offei went to secondary school. By the early 1970s, Atiemo was involved in a number of para-church organizations, including Scripture Union and Joyful Way Incorporated. Catechist Abboah-Offei was the Joyful Way prayer coordinator in Asamankese, and through this organization the two of them met. Abboah-Offei recalls that Atiemo was like a big brother to him, later financing and organizing his wedding. After Abboah Offei's marriage to Faustina, he and Atiemo got to know each other much better.

In October 1993, Atiemo moved to Brooklyn and established the Ghanaian Presbyterian Reformed Church. A year later, Atiemo visited his in-laws in London, where he discussed the slow growth of his Brooklyn church with Joseph Martinson, Paulina Atiemo's nephew and Faustina Abboah-Offei's brother. Martinson suggested that Atiemo contact Catechist Abboah-Offei and invite him to host a revival in order to boost membership. A few years later Atiemo contacted Abboah-Offei about coming to Brooklyn and holding a healing and deliverance revival. Unfortunately, Atiemo was not able to finance the trip.

But then, fortuitously, in 2001 the chairman of the Akropong Presbytery (the Church's governing body) wrote in a letter to Atiemo that he wanted Catechist Abboah-Offei to solicit funds for the Presbyterian University in Akropong through a series of healing services for the Ghanaian Presbyterian churches in North America. Eventually, in 2003, Abboah-Offei was sent to the U.S. to perform deliverance services and individual consultations for suffering Ghanaians as well as to solicit funds for the University.[17] During this trip, Abboah-Offei visited Ghanaian Presbyterian congregations in the Bronx, Brooklyn, and Manhattan; Chicago; Houston; Columbus, Ohio; Woodbridge, Maryland; and Worcester, Massachusetts. The trip was a success. Not only did the membership of the host churches increase, but numerous people were healed of various maladies.

After this U.S. evangelism trip in 2003, many of the U.S. Ghanaian Presbyterian churches invited the Catechist for return visits, and many non-Presbyterian charismatic congregations also invited him to conduct services. He traveled to the U.S. and Canada in 2004 and 2005, again to perform deliverance services and raise money for the Presbyterian University. Abboah-Offei decided to host a deliverance workshop in 2005, after performing services in several of the Presbyterian churches in North America. The primary goal of the workshop was to teach individual Prayer Teams how to minister to the afflicted within their own congregation.[18] The workshop was meant to create replicas of the Bible Study and Prayer Group of the PCG in the diaspora. This deliverance workshop in New York was the first attempt to fully replicate the deliverance course developed by Abboah-Offei and taught at Grace Deliverance Center in Ghana. As in Ghana, the Catechist was concerned with people consulting non-Christian healing practitioners for help and wanted to firmly establish a Christian alternative practice within the diasporic Ghanaian Presbyterian churches.[19] Abboah-Offei spoke with Reverend Atiemo, who was able to reserve space and make arrangements at the Presbyterian Retreat Center in Stony Point, New York.

In November 2005, Catechist Abboah-Offei offered a diaspora workshop for Ghanaian Presbyterian churches in New York. The timing of the New York workshop allowed the Catechist to also teach the Scripture Union deliverance course during the last week of December in Aburi/Kumasi, as well as his own deliverance course in Akropong, which began in mid-February. In 2005, members from the Prayer Teams from Brooklyn, the Bronx, Columbus, Houston, Manhattan, Montreal, Philadelphia, Toronto, Woodbridge, and Worcester attended, as well as various others who sought healing and deliverance through personal consultation with the Catechist.

Most of these suffering Ghanaians (non–Prayer Team members) came from greater New York, where buses connect Manhattan to Stony Point, although others came from much farther away. One person who attended the 2005 program flew from Houston for one night. Of the healings that occurred in 2005, most memorable was a woman with cancer who was prayed for. After she returned home from the retreat, her doctors could no longer detect the disease.[20] The large number of suffering people who came for deliverance required so much of Abboah-Offei's time that very little deliverance instruction was given to the Prayer Teams. Abboah-Offei and some of the other participating pastors decided to try to reduce the number of counselees by restricting the participation to Prayer Team members only, and only five from each church, in 2006. Therefore, in 2006, only Prayer Team members were invited to the deliverance workshop for training (although a few others were admitted for consultations).

Course Setting, Course Participants, and Course Structure

The Stony Point Center, one of three national conference centers of the PC-USA, is located on 32 acres of land in the Lower Hudson River Valley between New York City and West Point. Originally used as a missionary training center, in 1977 the Stony Point Center for Education and Mission was established by the PC-USA as a retreat and conference center for Christians all over the world (Flory 2000: 40). Stony Point aimed to become a global Christian village. This purpose was achieved when the members of the Conference of Ghanaian Presbyterian Churches in North America began meeting there annually in 2005 for deliverance workshops.

At the second deliverance workshop, in 2006, once again at least one member was present from each of the Prayer Teams representing Brooklyn, the Bronx, Columbus, Houston, Manhattan, Philadelphia, Toronto, Woodbridge, and Worcester.[21] In attendance were also several non–Prayer Team members who came for consultation, at least one visitor from Ghana, and an anthropologist (the author). Catechist Abboah-Offei was unable to attend the 2006 workshop due to exhaustion. In his place were his assistant, Samuel Asare, who works with the Catechist at the Grace Deliverance Center, and the host, Samuel Atiemo. There were approximately 80–100 adults attending the course throughout the week, although typically only half that number was present at any given time. More than 60 percent of the participants were women. The ages of the participants ranged from 23 to 66 and were fairly evenly distributed across the age range. Almost half of the participants had immigrated to North America in the 1990s, and over 70 percent had immigrated in either the 1990s or 2000s. Of the workshop participants, 50 percent worked in the health care industry, and over 70 percent had some post-secondary education either in Ghana or North America.[22]

The workshop took place from Sunday, November 26, 2006, to Saturday, December 2, 2006. The first Sunday was reserved for arrival and registration. The schedule from Monday through Friday followed the same pattern. Many of the Prayer Team members woke at 3:00 AM and prayed in groups until 6:00 AM, typically in one of the dorm rooms. From 6:00 AM–8:00 AM, all the participants gathered for praise and worship, which consisted of individual praying, group prayer, and singing and dancing. Group devotion occurred from 8:00 AM–9:00 AM when the participants would pray together about certain topics designated by a prayer leader. From 9:00 AM–12:00 PM various deliverance lectures/sermons were given by Samuel Asare or conference participants. At 12 PM there was a half-hour break, followed by another three-hour block of lectures/sermons. From 3:30 PM–6:00 PM there was group prayer, and from 6:00 PM–7:00 PM dinner, which was the only meal participants got during the day. The period of 7:00 PM–11:00 PM was allotted to lectures/sermons as well as individual consultations with Asare for participating members. By 11:00 PM the day was finished. This was the basic structure of the workshop from Monday through Friday, and on Saturday, December 2 the Prayer Teams left Stony Point to return to their home cities.

Diagnosis, Witchcraft Attacks, and Prayer Lines: Deliverance Replications in the Diaspora

The deliverance workshop has both a theoretical and practical component. While theories of disease, misfortune causation, spiritual attacks, and demonic possession are discussed during the lectures, which follow a booklet written by Catechist Abboah-Offei, there is a practical component as well. The practical component consists of teaching participants how to become deliverance counselors. This individual consultation procedure is taught to participants in two ways: through experiencing the process as a counselee and by participating as a counselor with one or more trained deliverance practitioners.

Individual consultation always begins with the counselee filling out a deliverance questionnaire in order to diagnosis his or her affliction. The questionnaire administered by Abboah-Offei has seven sections which ask particular questions about a person's past. Section 1 asks personal information, such as name, clan, occupation, and marital status. Section 2 asks the counselee to describe the affliction, its duration, and actions taken to alleviate it thus far. Section 3 asks questions pertaining to family background, such as whether one's parents had worshiped in Aladura churches (indigenous churches considered illegitimate and spiritually dangerous), whether one's family members had visited "native doctors" or ancestral shrines, and whether there are ancestral stools in the family or curses laid upon its members. Section 4 asks questions similar to section 3, but with respect to the afflicted individual, not to his or her family.[23] Section 5 asks about unusual phenomena experienced, such as hallucinations, hearing strange voices, or having voices inside one's head. Section 6 asks questions about antisocial behavior, such as excessive hatred, anger, or sexual disorders. Finally, Section 7 asks about unusual phenomena experienced in dreams, such as being abused, losing money, or talking with dead friends/family. Answers to Sections 1 and 3–7 should give an indication of what is causing the affliction indicated in Section 2 if the individual's problem has a spiritual cause.

The questionnaire is examined by a counselor, who attempts to diagnose the problem based on the data collected. The counselor meets with the counselee to discuss the problem, prays with him or her, and (hopefully) delivers that person from his or her (potentially) demonic affliction. One way to determine if the disorder has a demonic etiology is for a counselor to pray with and lay hands on the afflicted individual. If the demons begin to show themselves, through a process called manifestation, then the disorder is spiritual. Meyer, in her study of several Christian groups in Eweland, argued that this practice functions as a Christianized oracle (1999: 159).

This questionnaire was filled out by all participants attending the deliverance workshop in New York. Every evening several people met with Samuel Asare and Samuel Atiemo to participate in counseling sessions as counselors and counselees during the allotted time for "clinic," as the counselor training segment was called. The counseling sessions occurred in private rooms off the main conference center. In standard practice, this consultation would take place privately, with only the counselee and one or more trained deliverance counselors from the Prayer Team present. The workshop consultations in New York were held with slightly larger groups in order to train participants to become counselors.

During the course of the workshop, deliverance practices were also performed during public deliverance services. On two separate occasions participants in the workshop were attacked by demonic spirits: one with epileptic seizures and another through a near accident. Subverting the afflicting agents required the prayer efforts of all the workshop participants.

On the morning of November 28, 2006, Samuel Asare gave the morning lecture at Stony Point. Asare announced that during the previous night one of the participants had fallen ill, and he gave some background on the case. Kofi Acheampong (pseudonym) had been attending prayer meetings at his home church to receive healing for his epilepsy. The Prayer Team at his home church suggested that Acheampong come to Stony Point and be seen by Catechist Abboah-Offei for relief from his condition. For reasons unknown, Acheampong left his medication in Texas—which greatly angered Asare, whose theology and practice of healing is incorporative of biomedicine.[24]

During the first night at Stony Point, Acheampong had mild seizures. The Houston Prayer Team prayed vigorously for him to recover. When the seizures ceased, the Prayer Team members thought he had recovered. Sometime in the middle of the second night Acheampong had more serious seizures, began to bleed, and was rushed to the hospital. Many people at the workshop believed he was bewitched.

After explaining this course of events, Asare led the group of 60–80 participants in a prayer line praying against witchcraft, which was the diagnosed afflicting agent responsible for Acheampong's seizures. A prayer line involves a series of prayer topics that all the individuals involved pray about out loud at their own pace, following prompts read by a leader. The series of prayer topics that constitute the witchcraft prayer line are found within Abboah-Offei's deliverance manual. For example, the sixth entry in the witchcraft prayer line in the book reads, "break all witchcraft alliances, links and communication networks and bum all gadgets with the fire of God" (Abboah-Offei 2006: 105). Once the prayer topic was read by Asare, everyone prayed about this issue individually, in varying tones and pitches, simultaneously. Each of these prayer topics would last for between five and ten minutes. When the volume of prayers would begin to decrease, the next prayer topic would be read out loud by the leader. This prayer line against witchcraft attacks lasted for almost two hours.[25] The following night another spiritual attack occurred.

During the night of November 28, a pregnant woman named Mary Anim (pseudonym) fell asleep in her room. She had put a towel over a lamp in order to create a dimmed light in the room. Early in the morning she awoke to a fire alarm. The towel was smoking. Mary responded by rushing the lamp and towel outside. Once outside, the towel immediately caught fire. The following morning, November 29, Samuel Asare interpreted this event.

Unlike in the previous case, Asare did not interpret this event as a direct witchcraft attack. The event was interpreted as the replication of a specific biblical demonic attack recounted in Revelations 12:1–4. This biblical passage tells of a pregnant woman confronted by a red dragon that meant to consume the pregnant woman's child. It was represented pictorially for the course participants (figure 1). Asare reported: "If it had not been for God, a baby and its mother would have been swallowed by a great red dragon." The biblical red dragon which attacked the pregnant woman the previous night, argued Asare, was the Devil and acted as the accomplice of witches, which are malevolent agents believed to feed on children and unborn babies.[26] This interpretation by Asare was followed by a deliverance lesson about shedding demonic bondage and was finished with a prayer line against demonic altars. Demonic altars are structures on which sacrifices are made, where curses are enacted and where demons or witches consume victims (Abboah-Offei 2006: 37–38). Destroying the power emanating from the altar—considered the source of the afflicting power—through prayer was meant to free Anim from the danger posed to her and to her baby by the Devil and by witches.

Samuel Asare indicated on the morning after Mary Anim's incident that the target of the Devil and/or witches was not only the woman and child, who were nearly consumed by a fire, but all participants in the course. One message consistently reiterated during the lectures was that participation in the deliverance ministry abounds with demonic confrontation. Samuel Asare stated: "You will not achieve your goals on a silver platter. You have to struggle. Whenever there is something good coming, you will be confronted by the Evil One." These statements were most visibly realized by the spiritual attacks on Kofi Acheampong and Mary Anim.

But during the course of the lectures as well as the praise and worship sessions there were other signs of demonic possession, referred to as manifestation.[27] During the course of preaching, praying, singing, or dancing many people were prayed for or had hands laid on them. If a person was possessed, the demons would resist expulsion and thereby cause various kinds of unnatural (or more precisely supernatural) movements or utterances by their host. Some people's eyes rolled back in their heads. Others fell over. Some screamed and jumped. Others get violent, attacking the people praying for / with them. Many collapse to the ground and often vomit different types of objects and substances. This often violent process of expelling demons from Christian bodies and replacing them with the Holy Spirit was performed throughout the week.

A number of beliefs and practices with respect to healing and deliverance have been replicated in the Ghanaian Presbyterian diaspora.[28] Prayer Teams at individual churches in the U.S. and Canada have been trained through a course taught at the Grace Deliverance Center by Catechist Abboah-Offei. Through this course, the Bible Study and Prayer Group of the PCG has been replicated through the Prayer Teams in the diaspora. The questionnaire (or diagnostic tool) is the same, which suggests that the same range of afflicting agents affect Christians in Ghana as in America. The individual counseling session has also been replicated transnationally, used not only during the deliverance workshop, but also by the Prayer Teams of the various Ghanaian Presbyterian churches. The methods of laying on hands, anointing with oil, and prayer are the same in Ghana and in the U.S. When a specific attack occurs, a diagnosis is determined and intercessors gather and read prayer lines against the specific afflicting agent.

The afflicting agents also are the same in Ghana and the U.S., as was demonstrated in the cases of Kofi Acheampong and Mary Anim. In the Ghanaian Presbyterian community in both countries, witchcraft attacks on pregnant women are common (figure 2), and witches are interpreted as the Devil or working in conjunction with the Devil (Meyer 1992). As Samuel Asare discussed in one of his Stony Point lectures, a number of afflictions listed on the questionnaires he examined were obvious witchcraft attacks.[29] The afflicting

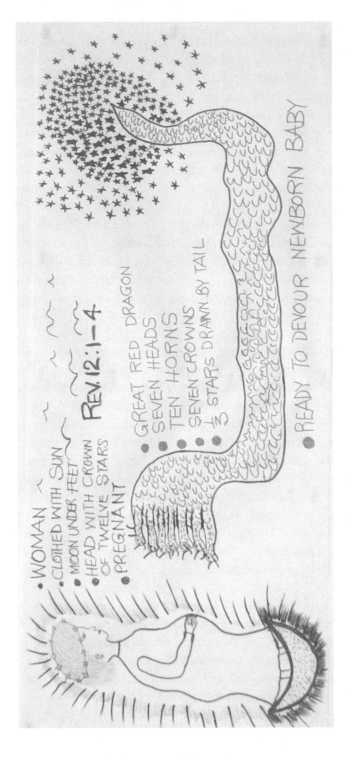

Fig. 9.1. Pictorial representation of the demonic attack on a pregnant woman that occurred the night of Nov. 27, 2006 during the deliverance workshop in New York. Depicted in this drawing by Samuel Asare is the great red dragon from Revelations 12:1–4, believed to be the Devil and working in conjunction with witches to consume the unborn child.

agents, such as witches, were however almost always located in Ghana and not outside.[30] Interestingly, in Ghana itself, people are rarely afflicted by agents outside of the country. But, when Americans suffer from the same causes, they are presumably being afflicted from afar.

Yet, although aspects of Abboah-Offei's deliverance ministry have been replicated within the Ghanaian Presbyterian churches in North America, particularly through the medium of the Stony Point deliverance workshop, influences in Ghanaian and American societies are different and changes have occurred in both places. One significant difference between Ghana and the diaspora is the high percentage of male spirit possession found in the U.S. In the following section I will describe the shifting relationships between Ghanaian men and women in America which have resulted in male spirit possession within this Christian community, a phenomenon almost never observed in Ghana.

Female Economic Empowerment and Male Spirit Possession: Deliverance Ruptures in the Diaspora

The immigration of Ghanaians to the U.S. has altered many types of social relationships, but none so much as gender. Immigration frequently alters gender relationships, most commonly by enhancing women's status because of higher demand for immigrant women in the U.S. labor market and their relative ease of entry. This in turn raises women's status relative to their home countries, while concurrently decreasing men's status (Mahler 1999; Pessar 1995, 1999; Zentgraf 2002). This shift in power frequently extends to the religious sphere within immigrant congregations (Boddy 1995; Kim and Kim 2001). The altering of relations between men and women in both the economic and religious spheres holds true for the Ghanaian Presbyterians in the U.S., where many Ghanaian women earn more money than their husbands and many Ghanaian men become spirit-possessed.

During a visit to the Grace Deliverance Center in Ghana in February 2007 I observed a noticeable division of labor within the deliverance ministry. The men in Abboah-Offei's Deliverance Team, comprised of over 60 male and female members, performed the ritualized aspects of the ministry. Other male members of the Team served as counselors during individual consultation. Men also physically interacted with spiritually possessed individuals, through the laying of hands or restraining them. By contrast, assisting the afflicted in filling out their questionnaires was the exclusive domain of the female workers. Woman also participated as intercessors, praying in groups with men for the afflicted.

While most of the interactive deliverance workers were men, the great majority of spirit-possessed individuals were women.[31] Both men and women visited Grace Deliverance Center for help with a variety of problems. But only women became possessed and experienced demonic manifestation. At Akropong, I witnessed over 25 demonic possession cases. They took place during public deliverance services preached by Catechist Abboah-Offei, during private deliverance consultations at Grace, and during private consultations by people seeking help who came directly to Abboah-Offei's home. Every person possessed by a demon was a woman.

Female spirit possession has been interpreted in a variety of ways by anthropologists. Some have postulated that female spirit possession is a result of biochemical reactions to nutritional deficiency (Kehoe and Giletti 1981); others have viewed it as an acting out of subconscious childhood traumas (Obeyesekere 1990); still others have characterized possession as an effort by women to alleviate their subordinate status in society by attaining certain goals (Lewis 1971). Many feminist scholars envision female spirit possession as a form of subordinate or subaltern discourse (Boddy 1988; Morsy 1991; Ong 1988). This interpretation holds true for female spirit possession within the context of Christian therapeutics in Ghana.

Meyer (1999) argues that female spirit possession in the context of Ghanaian deliverance expresses the tension between society and the individual. This tension is found within women's attempts to maintain Christian conjugal families within a patriarchal Ghanaian society where many conjugal resources are drawn toward the matrilineage (see Soothill 2007: 83–86).[32] Many women attempt to sever these kinship obligations through conversion to Christianity, which demonizes non-Christian rites that reinforce matrilineal ties (Engelke 2004; Meyer 1998). The attempt to break with the matrilineage rarely achieves success, thereby producing a stressful situation in which many women become possessed by matrilineally-associated spirits. Witches are one prime example of a matrilineally-associated afflicting agent, believed to harm only those within the witch's own family. Tensions between the matrilineage and the conjugal family are expressed through female spirit possession.

Tensions are not only found between a woman's conjugal family and her extended family. These tensions also exist between husbands and wives in Ghana over resource allocation. Most married Ghanaian women live in their husband's home following patrilocal residence patterns. The division of labor within Ghanaian homes dictates that the men predominantly work outside the home while the women care for the home and children and are responsible for food preparation.[33] Within most households in Ghana, there is a separation

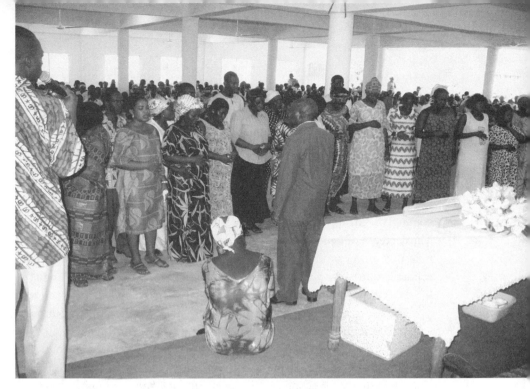

Fig. 9.2. Pregnant women praying against the power of demons and witches that want to harm their unborn children at Grace Deliverance Center, Akropong, Ghana on Feb. 10, 2007. Notice the division of labor between men and women. The man in the grey suit leads this prayer line. The man with the microphone repeats the prayer for the audience. Behind the single row of pregnant women, who are essentially laying hands on their unborn babies, are male deliverance workers prepared to subdue any of the women in case demonic possession occurs. PHOTO: MOHR.

of finances between husbands and wives wherein each is responsible for some of their own expenses and the expenses connected with their children. Many of the resources earned by a man are allocated to his matrilineage and are not invested in the conjugal family. Many women must subsidize the insufficient resources they receive from their husbands with agricultural work and petty trade. In many instances, women rely on their paternal or maternal families for shelter and assistance in times of need.

Historically, the farther the distance from the base of the matrilineage, the more Ghanaian women have had to rely on the conjugal family for support, which compounds the hardship for women (Allman and Tashjian 2000: xxxiii). This was particularly the case in the first half of the twentieth century, when many Ghanaian married couples migrated to cocoa farms, sometimes great distances from home villages and towns. This generation of female Ghanaian migrants consistently struggled to secure independence. On the cocoa farms

women were responsible for running the domestic sphere as well as for providing labor on their husbands' farms. Women, however, did not reap direct
benefits from the wealth produced by those farms.

While this sketch of conjugal relationships in both the colonial and postcolonial eras is meant to give the reader a sense of the prevailing structures
that individuals work within, I want to point out that variations do occur
across different regions, ages, and classes. Recent research has shown that
sharing financial responsibility within conjugal relationships is much more
common in Ghana today, particularly among Pentecostals (Soothill 2007: 200).
The decrease of gendered division of labor within Ghanaian marriages is significantly more common, however, among Ghanaian immigrants in the U.S.,
primarily due to economic earning opportunities for Ghanaian women in the
U.S. health care industry.

The more recent immigration of Ghanaians to the U.S. has produced a
very different division of labor within conjugal Ghanaian families, even while
a small minority of Ghanaian immigrant families follows the general pattern of men working outside the home and women caring for the home.
The opportunity for economic advancement by Ghanaian women has been
enabled by their greater earning potential within health care and social work
fields generally, and nursing specifically.[34] I refer to these professions together
as the health care industry. The U.S. is currently experiencing a high demand
for skilled work in traditionally feminized sectors such as the health care
industry, where positions are increasingly filled by skilled female immigrants
(Kofman 2004). Many Ghanaian Christian women have found employment
in the U.S. within the health care industry. Nearly all informants give cultural
and economic, not religious, reasons for their participation in the health care
industry. Ghanaian women's participation in the U.S. workforce as nurses is
due to job availability as well as their propensity to care for the elderly, injured,
or mentally retarded as younger family members must do in Ghana.

The predominance of Ghanaian women within the health care industry
is supported by the survey data collected during the New York deliverance
workshop in 2006. Twenty of the 30 female respondents worked in some
capacity within the health care industry. Of these 20 women, 9 were nurses,
nurses' assistants, or nursing students. In contrast, the employment trend
among Ghanaian men was to work in the transportation or machinery industries, as cab drivers, truck technicians, and machine operators. These professions accounted for 7 of 18 male responses. The average earning potential in
the nursing industry—particularly for nurses (RNs) and nurse practitioners
(LPNs)—is greater than that of various transportation/machinery professions,
although some men did have higher-paying jobs in areas such as accounting
and insurance.[35] A few men also worked in the health care industry.[36] In many

of these households, the wife's income is greater than her husband's, and in the majority, the spouses' two incomes are at least close to equivalent. This has served to elevate women's status and increase their autonomy, but has also led to a great deal of marital conflict as husbands and wives adjust to a new gendered division of labor.

A few key areas within home life cause most tension in the Ghanaian Christian diaspora.[37] With Ghanaian wives working the same hours and making the same money as their husbands, many Ghanaian men in the U.S. are expected to participate in the domestic sphere. Most are not eager to do so. Disagreements revolve around creating and maintaining joint bank accounts, and deciding who gets to spend the money, and how.[38] Manuh noted that many Ghanaian women in Toronto alleged their husbands tended to treat the joint accounts as their own and made withdrawals without their knowledge and consent, for the benefit of themselves and their extended families in Ghana (1999: 87). Conflict between the needs of the conjugal family and those of the extended families on both sides are frequent areas of dispute. Many Ghanaian women in the U.S. have much more power within these areas of conflict due to their financial autonomy.

These disputes often lead to the dissolution of marriages, and many informants suggested that the divorce rate in the U.S. is much higher than in Ghana.[39] If physical altercations occur and the state intervenes in the U.S., it is the husbands who are expelled from the home, while in Ghana men have ownership over a couple's shared residence and if altercations occur it is almost always the women who are forced to leave. For immigrant families who are separated from their extended family in Ghana, there are no elders present to assist in settling marital disputes, although Christian pastors and church marital committees are increasingly playing that role.[40]

Consequently, many Ghanaian men in the diaspora feel emasculated and marginalized by the economic independence of women and by their own participation in domestic duties such as child rearing, food preparation, and cleaning. This decrease in men's authority within marriage, combined with increased expectations by extended family for greater financial support from their higher-paying overseas jobs, have led many immigrant men to exhibit a traditionally feminine religious response to their marginalization, namely, spirit possession.[41] While men get possessed less frequently and less violently than women in the U.S., they are possessed far more frequently than in Ghana. It is not uncommon to hear among Ghanaian Presbyterians, as Manuh observed for Ghanaians in Toronto (1999: 85), that in the U.S. Ghanaian men have become women and women have become men. Female economic independence and male spirit possession have transformed understandings and practices of Ghanaian masculinity in the Ghanaian Presbyterian diaspora.[42]

One example occurred at the Ghanaian Presbyterian church in Philadelphia, during a week-long healing revival held by Abboah-Offei in April 2006. A male member of the church, David Frimpong (pseudonym), had been experiencing chronic illness and misfortune since immigrating to the U.S. in 1996. Frimpong had frequent stomach pains and was once taken to the emergency room, where doctors could not diagnose the cause of his pain. His first child was born premature and almost died. Frimpong continually performed poorly in school and at work due to poor concentration. In the course of one year, he bought six different cars and each one successively broke down. His marriage was under duress; Frimpong and his wife argued frequently over managing their finances and dividing household duties. Convinced that there was a spiritual cause to his sickness and misfortune, Frimpong came for deliverance during a week-long healing and deliverance program at the Philadelphia church hosted by Catechist Abboah-Offei.

Frimpong met with Abboah-Offei briefly for a one-on-one consultation on the morning of April 25, 2006. He filled out the deliverance questionnaire and discussed his situation briefly with the Catechist, who rendered a diagnosis: Frimpong's disorder was spiritual and originated from within his extended family. His sister-in-law had become jealous that her husband had financially facilitated Frimpong's immigration to the U.S. As a result of her jealousy, she placed Frimpong on the altar of an *aduruyefo* in order to harm or kill him. An *aduruyefo* is an Akan religious practitioner known to either help or harm people with spiritual medicine.[43] After revealing this diagnosis, Abboah-Offei instructed Frimpong to return to the deliverance service that evening.

During the middle of the service, Abboah-Offei led a prayer in which he called for the spirit of failure to be broken in the name of Jesus. The Catechist signaled to two Prayer Team members and Samuel Asare to usher Frimpong from a pew toward the rear of the sanctuary into the central isle. Abboah-Offei began to shout "break, break, break that darkness hovering around you!" Frimpong's face became contorted as he slowly fell backwards, throwing his hands in the air and shouting; he became possessed, after which he lost consciousness and was lowered to the floor by the Prayer Team members. He lay on the floor for about ten minutes while being tended to by two of the Prayer Team members. Then he slowly moved back to his seat, but remained visibly dazed for the rest of the service.

A similar set of events occurred four days later on April 29 when Frimpong returned for the evening service. He recalled praying in the audience, which was followed by the experience of something moving inside him that held him down and burned. This burning sensation was particularly strong in his stomach. He could barely stand upright and held onto the pew tightly. Eventually,

Frimpong stumbled into the aisle and fell down possessed, flailing his arms and foaming at the mouth. Abboah-Offei approached Frimpong lying on the ground, laid hands on him and ordered the demonic bondage emanating from the *aduruyefo* to be broken. In Frimpong's own words, Abboah-Offei breathed the Holy Spirit into him, which expelled the demons.[44] Such an example of male spirit possession in the context of deliverance is rarely, if ever, seen in Ghana.

Research in the Ghanaian Presbyterian Church in Philadelphia from 2005 through 2008 and at the 2006 and 2007 Stony Point deliverance workshops indicated that 25 percent of all possession cases over that time were men. One informant suggested that men in the diaspora no longer have their pride, given the shift in power between men and women. With no pride or authority to protect, men are highly susceptible to seeking redress through spiritual means. It is common for men to suggest that female spirit possession in Ghana is a sign of spiritual weakness, one that reflects their place in Ghanaian patriarchal society.[45] I would argue that spirit possession is a sign of marginalization, in both Ghana and the diaspora, within relationships between individuals to their conjugal family, their kin, and the larger society.

In this chapter I have outlined the process by which healing and deliverance practices have become established in the Ghanaian Presbyterian Churches through the U.S. Prayer Teams trained in the U.S. by Catechist Ebenezer Abboah-Offei, who manages the Grace Deliverance Center in Ghana. Training in these practices has been disseminated through annual deliverance workshops in New York since 2005, in which Prayer Teams study both theoretical and practical components of Christian healing and deliverance.

From observing deliverance practices both in Ghana and the U.S., I have found various continuities as well as ruptures to have taken place within this transnational migration of people, ideas, and practices. The Bible Study and Prayer Group of the PCG has been replicated in the diaspora as the Prayer Teams within the Ghanaian Presbyterian churches of North America. The same deliverance course materials written by Abboah-Offei are used both in Ghana and the U.S. The same types of afflicting agents, particularly witches, affect Ghanaians both at home and in the diaspora. These agents have the potential to cause various types of sickness as well as misfortune. Witches located in Ghana continue their attempts to destroy unborn children in the diaspora. But changes have also occurred within these Christian healing practices as they are introduced in the diaspora.

The most notable difference within deliverance practices in the U.S. is the high proportion of spiritually possessed men. Gender relations within Ghanaian conjugal families have shifted in the diaspora due to the increased economic independence of Ghanaian women enabled by the opportunities within the traditionally feminized health care industry. In contrast to the migrations to the cocoa farms in the early twentieth century, which made Ghanaian women more economically dependent on their husbands, immigration to the U.S. in the twenty-first century is increasing Ghanaian women's economic independence and power within their conjugal families. This shift toward female empowerment within their marriages has left many Ghanaian men feeling emasculated, shifting ideas and practices of masculinity. This feminization of men extends from the domestic sphere, where they participate in child rearing, food preparation and household chores, to the religious sphere, where many men become possessed by afflicting spirits.

Notes

1. See Meyer (1999) for a treatment of female spirit possession in Ghanaian Christianity. Male spirit possession in Africa is rare, but certain cases have been discussed (Colleyn 1999; Lewis 1971).

2. U.S. Census Bureau 2005, American Community Survey, Tables GCT-T1-R, B05006; Terrazas (2009). By 2007, the African-born population constituted 3.7% of the total foreign-born population in the U.S.

3. U.S. Homeland Security, Office of Immigration Statistics, Table 10: Persons Obtaining Leal Permanent Resident Status by Broad Class of Admission and Region and Country of Birth: Fiscal Year 2006.

4. 4,410 in 2003 versus 9,367 in 2006 (U.S. Homeland Security, Office of Immigration Statistics, Table 3: Persons Obtaining Legal Permanent Resident Status by Region and Country of Birth: Fiscal Years 1997 to 2006).

5. The population of Ghana is nearly 23 million people (CIA Factbook, www.cia.gov/library/the-world-factbook/.) Also, U.S. Department of Homeland Security, Office of Immigration Statistics, Table 11: Persons Obtaining Legal Permanent Resident Status by Region and Country of Birth.

6. In 1995, Peil estimated that 20% of Ghanaian citizens lived outside of Ghana (1995: 349). More conservative estimates were given between 10% and 15% in 2004 (Wong 2006: 357).

7. The Bank of Ghana estimated the number of remittances at 1 billion USD in 2005, although since up to 65% of total remittances are unregistered, the figure could have been as high as 3 billion USD (Mazzucato, van den Boom, and Nsowah-Nuamah 2005).

8. Church of Pentecost, Summary Statistics, 2005. I refer to both the Ghanaian-born immigrant community and Ghanaian Christian communities in North America as a "diaspora," agreeing with Akyeampong (2000: 204–213), who follows Clifford's (1994: 308) general definition of diaspora as a group having collective homes away from home with alternative public spheres and forms of community consciousness that maintain identifications outside of the national time/space. I also follow van Dijk (2004), who refers to Ghanaian Pentecostals in the Netherlands as the Ghanaian Pentecostal diaspora.

9. The first Ghanaian Presbyterian community in the diaspora was established among Ghanaian students in London. In October 1961, the PCG sent the

Rev. F. W. K. Akuffo to London to cater to the spiritual needs of the more than 3,000 Ghanaian students residing there. In November 1961, Akoffo was installed as an Assistant Minister of the Oxendon Church in London and Chaplain to the Ghanaian students in London (PCG, Reports for 1961: 84). There continue to be Ghanaian Presbyterian churches in greater London, although as of 2007 none had developed Prayer Teams (interview with Ebenezer Abboah-Offei, February 12, 2007).

10. These include the Ebenezer Presbyterian Church (Woodbridge), Ghanaian Presbyterian Church (Maryland), Ghanaian Presbyterian Church (Montreal), Ghanaian Presbyterian Church (Toronto), Ghanaian Presbyterian Reformed Church (Brooklyn), PCG Missions (Bronx), Ramseyer Presbyterian Faith Fellowship (Columbus), Trinity Presbyterian Faith Fellowship (Houston), and the United Ghanaian Community Church (Philadelphia).

11. Some recent evidence suggests that the Church of Pentecost's approach to healing and deliverance is shifting in the diaspora. In November 2007, Prophetess Boateng from the Church of Pentecost's Edumfa Prayer Camp in Cape Coast conducted healing and deliverance services at several Church of Pentecost branches in North America, including Philadelphia. Her focus was on prayer and repentance, in order to cast out the demons resulting from sin that were causing much illness and misfortune to church members in the diaspora. Edumfa was the Church of Pentecost's first prayer camp, established by Maame Grace Mensah in 1959 (Onyinah 2002).

12. The Church of Pentecost in the Eastern Region had approximately double the number of congregations and members present any other region in Ghana by 1970 (Minutes, Church of Pentecost Church Council, March 1970, in Larbi 2001: 192f). The 1966 Synod report of the PCG claimed that by that year the Church of Pentecost had more adult members than the Presbyterian Church (Report on "Prayer Groups and Sects," PCG, Minutes of the 37th Synod, 1966: 41–54).

13. By the 1960s, Pentecostal practices such as healing and speaking in tongues became established in mainline churches in Europe and North America. This movement is referred to as the charismatic revival or renewal (Harrell 1975). There was much interaction during the early 1960s between Kumi and other Pentecostal groups such as the Church of Pentecost, which used the Presbyterian-owned Ramseyer Memorial Retreat Center to hold the Church of Pentecost annual convention in 1963 (PCG, Minutes of the 34th Synod, 1963: 51).

14. Report on "Prayer Groups and Sects," PCG, Minutes of the 37th Synod, 1966: 47.

15. Reverend Appiah, quoted in Barker and Boadi-Siaw (2005: 154).

16. The Grace Deliverance Center is the flagship deliverance center of the PCG. Five other centers operate within the PCG, located in: Atibie (Kwahu) led by Reverend Nana Ntim Gyakari; Jejemireja (Brong Ahafo) led by Brother Daniel Ansu; Gilgal Prayer Center in Boma (Brong Ahafo); Miremano (Brong Ahafo) led by Brother Andrew Kye; and Chirapatre in Kumasi (Asante) led by Brother Fred Darko (PCG website, http://www.pc-ghana.org/evanglism.html).

17. This was only one of two instances where resources flowed from the U.S. to Ghana. The other was when I, at the request of Abboah-Offei, collected money from the Ghanaian Presbyterian congregation in Philadelphia in order to purchase a projector for Grace Deliverance Center.

18. Abboah-Offei did not create the individual Prayer Teams, however. This was done locally at each church in coordination with its pastor.

19. Statistics taken at Grace Deliverance Center show that of the 15,000 Christians who have undergone consultation, 75% had previously consulted some other form of religious healing practitioner outside the Church.

20. Interview with Catechist Ebenezer Abboah-Offei, February 15, 2007.

21. There are two Ghanaian Presbyterian Churches in the Bronx, one affiliated with the PC-USA called the PCG Mission, and one with the PCG called PCG. Both churches had Prayer Team members in attendance.

22. Twenty-five of 50 respondents reported working in some form of the health care field. Responses included: drug abuse therapist, mental retardation worker, nurse's assistant (CNA), nurse's aide, health care provider at nursing home, home health assistant, home health aide for the elderly, nurse (RN), nurse practitioner (LPN), pharmacy technician, extended care provider, physical therapy assistant, mental health care provider, and pre-operative clinic coordinator.

23. This category includes Aladura churches, native doctors, dwarfs, *mallam* (Muslim healers), and usage of concoctions/talismans/charms.

24. Abboah-Offei's healing ministry, as almost all churches in Ghana today are, is strongly incorporative of biomedicine. This distinction, to incorporate as opposed to not incorporate biomedicine, is important to Ghanaians involved in deliverance because abstaining from biomedicine is a practice affiliated with certain forms of traditional healing, particularly healing cults. Faith Taberancle, however, is a church that has always abstained from using biomedicine.

25. Importantly, Asare interrupted the prayer line once to make sure that everyone understood that they were praying against supernatural witches, and not real people, such as aunties or grandmothers.

26. It is common for several spiritual agents to be involved with someone's illness or misfortune within this deliverance system.

27. Abboah-Offei writes that manifestations are signs of the presence of a spirit/demon, which occur in various forms during the process of deliverance. There are 62 signs listed, some of which include climbing on objects, removal of clothes, hitting head on floor, screaming, fainting, hissing, snarling, and spitting (2006: 27–29).

28. These observations are based on research in Philadelphia from July 2005 through July 2007, at the New York Deliverance Workshops in November 2006 and 2007, and at Grace Deliverance Center in February 2007.

29. Samuel Asare lecture, November 28, 2006.

30. The one exception was an accusation against Haitians and Puerto Ricans for using "black magic"—probably referring to Vodun and Santerismo—in order to beat out Ghanaian Christians for jobs. Abboah-Offei led this discussion in Philadelphia in April 2006.

31. Meyer observed this division of gendered labor in deliverance practices in Agbelengor and the Evangelical PCG in her research in Eweland (1999: 160).

32. A matrilineage is a genealogically defined group of kin who trace descent and membership through mothers.

33. Opportunities for most women to earn relatively high levels of income are restricted due to low educational attainment and fewer employment opportunities than men (Manuh 1999: 82).

34. African female migrants were more than twice as likely to report working in the health care industry than other foreign-born women in the U.S. in 2007 (Terrazas 2009: 5). In the same year, 28% of all African immigrant women worked in the health care profession.

35. The average yearly salary in Philadelphia within the nursing industry ranged from $27,000 for a nurse's assistant (CNA) to $40,000 for a nurse practitioner (LNP) to $63,000 for a nurse (RN). On the other hand, the male-oriented jobs ranged from $32,000 for taxi and light truck drivers to $40,000 for heavy truck drivers (www.swz.salary.com).

36. Four of the 19 men worked in the health care industry: a nurse, a preoperative clinic coordinator, a mental health care worker, and a nurse's assistant.

37. With the increasing rise of Christianity in Ghana, a greater emphasis on the conjugal family has corresponded to increases in marital tension and spousal abuse (Soothill 2007: 205–208).

38. Some men contended that because they immigrated first and later brought their wives over, they were entitled to control their wages and demanded that women hand over their checks to them (Manuh 1999: 87, 2003: 103).

39. Similar situations were found among Ghanaians in Toronto in the late 1990s (Manuh 2003: 104), as well as among Nigerians in the U.S. (Gemignani 2007: 139).

40. On May 12, 2007, the Session of the UGCC in Philadelphia established a "Family Life Committee" responsible for family, marriage, and parental counseling. The three members of the Family Life Committee were also the leading members of the Prayer Team.

41. Nearly 60% of remittances sent to Ghana were by men in 1999. On average, Ghanaian remitters sent 474 USD over a 12-month span. Most senders were children (38%) and siblings (23%) of household heads, not spouses (6%) (Mazzucato, van den Boom, and Nsowah-Nuamah 2005: 140–141). Remittances, therefore, were sent to Ghana primarily by men to members of their matrilineage.

42. This is not to suggest that gender relationships and ideas of masculinity are not changing in Ghana, but to say that changes are occurring more rapidly and in different ways among Ghanaian immigrants in the U.S. For example, see Cornwall (2003) for a discussion of shifting masculinities in southwestern Nigeria.

43. The earliest written accounts of this practitioner are listed as *odu'yefo* (Rattray 1927: 40), or as *oduyefo* or *oduruyefo* (Christaller 1933: 101). The etymology of *aduruyefo* comes from *aduru*—meaning medicine, drug, powder, or poison—and *ayefo,* which is a maker, author, mischief-maker, or mischievous enemy (Christaller 1933: 101, 587). This maker of medicine harnessed an ambivalent power which could be used to either cure or inflict harm. This general definition and etymology applies today.

44. Interview with David Frimpong, April 8, 2007. Abboah-Offei literally took large breaths of air and expelled them into Frimpong's mouth.

45. Meyer also found the same thing. In fact, this line of research was inspired by her work on female spirit possession within the three churches she studied in Eweland (1999).

References

Abboah-Offei, Ebenezer. 2006. *Church Leaders Training Manual: Practical Theology Resource in the School of Deliverance.* Akropong, Ghana: Grace Deliverance Team.

Akyeampong, Emmanuel. 2000. "Africans in the Diaspora: The Diaspora and Africa." *African Affairs* 99: 183–215.

Allman, Jean, and Victoria Tashjian. 2000. *"I Will Not Eat Stone": A Women's History of Colonial Asante*. Portsmouth, N.H.: Heinemann.

Asamoah-Gyadu, J. Kwabena. 2005. *African Charismatics: Current Developments within Independent Indigenous Pentecostalism in Ghana*. Leiden, the Netherlands: Brill.

Barker, Peter, and Samuel Boadi-Siaw. 2005. *Changed by the Word: The Story of Scripture Union Ghana*. Bangalore, India: Bangalore Offset Printers.

Bediako, Kwame. 2000. "Africa and Christianity on the Threshold of the Third Millenium: The Religious Dimension." *African Affairs* 99: 303–323.

Boddy, Janice. 1988. "Spirits and Selves in Northern Sudan: Cultural Therapeutics of Possession and Trance." *American Ethnologist* 15 (1): 4–27.

———. 1995. "Managing Tradition: Superstition and the Making of National Identity among Sudanese Women Refugees." In *The Pursuit of Certainty: Religious and Cultural Formulations,* ed. Wendy James, 15–44. London: Routledge.

Christaller, Johann G. 1933 [1881]. *Dictionary of the Asante and Fante Language Called Tshi (Twi)*. Basel, Germany: Basel Evangelical Missionary Society.

Church of Pentecost. 2005. *The Church of Pentecost, Summary Statistics Worldwide*. Accra, Ghana: Church of Pentecost Statistics and Records Department.

Clifford, James. 1994. "Diasporas." *Cultural Anthropology* 9 (3): 305–306.

Colleyn, Jean-Paul. 1999. "Horse, Hunter, and Messenger: The Possessed Men of the Nya Cult in Mali." In *Spirit Possession: Modernity and Power in Africa,* ed. Heike Behrend and Ute Luig, 68–78. Madison: University of Wisconsin Press.

Cornwall, Andrea A. 2003. "To Be a Man is More Than a Day's Work: Shifting Ideals of Masculinity in Ado-Odo, Southwestern Nigeria." In *Men and Masculinities in Modern Africa,* ed. Lisa A. Linsay and Stephen F. Miescher, 230–248. Portsmouth, N.H.: Heinemann.

Engelke, Matthew. 2004. "Discontinuity and the Discourse of Conversion." *Journal of Religion in Africa* 34 (1–2): 82–109.

Flory, Margaret. 2000. *Dear House, Mission Becomes You: Gilmore Sloane House Stony Point Center Stony Point, New York 1949–1999*. Louisville, Ky.: Bridge Resources.

Gemignani, Regina. 2007. "Gender, Identity, and Power in African Immigrant Evangelical Churches." In *African Immigrant Religions in America,* ed. Jacob K. Olupona and Regina Gemignani, 133–157. New York: New York University Press.

Harrell, David E. 1975. *All Things are Possible: The Healing and Charismatic Revivals in Modern America*. Bloomington: Indiana University Press.

Kehoe, Alice B., and Dody H. Giletti. 1981. "Women's Preponderance in Possession Cults: the Calcium Deficiency Hypothesis Extended." *American Anthropologist* 83 (3): 549–561.

Kim, Kwang Chug, and Shin Kim. 2001. "Ethnic Role of Korean Immigrant Churches in the United States." In *Korean Americans and Their Religions: Pilgrims and Missionaries from a Different Shore,* ed. Ho Youn Kwon, Kwang Chun Kim, and R. Stephen Warner, 71–94. University Park, Pa.: Pennsylvania State University Press.

Kofman, Eleonore. 2004. "Gendered Global Migrations: Diversity and Stratification." *International Feminist Journal of Politics* 6 (4): 643–665.

Kumah, Paulina, ed. 1994. *20 Years of Spiritual Warfare.* Accra, Ghana: Scripture Union Prayer Warriors Ministry.

Larbi, Emmanuel K. 2001. *Pentecostalism: The Eddies of Ghanaian Christianity.* Accra, Ghana: Blessed Publications.

Lewis, I. M. 1971. *Ecstatic Religion: An Anthropological Study of Spirit Possession and Shamanism.* Harmondsworth, U.K.: Penguin.

Mahler, Sarah J. 1999. "Engendering Transnational Migration: A Case Study of Salvadorans." *American Behavioral Scientist* 42 (4): 690–719.

Manuh, Takyiwaa. 1999. "'This Place is Not Ghana': Gender and Rights Discourse among Ghanaian Men and Women in Toronto." *Ghana Studies* 2: 77–95.

———. 2003. "Ghanaian Migrants in Toronto, Canada: Care of Kin and Gender Relations." *Ghana Studies* 6: 91–107.

Mazzucato, Valentina, Bart van den Boom, and Nicholas N. N. Nsowah-Nuamah. 2005. "Origin and Destination of Remittances in Ghana." In *At Home in the World? International Migration and Development in Contemporary Ghana and West Africa,* ed. Takyiwaa Manuh, 139–152. Accra, Ghana: Sub-Saharan Publishers.

Meyer, Birgit. 1992. "'If You Are a Devil You Are a Witch and, If You Are a Witch You Are a Devil.' The Integration of 'Pagan' Ideas into the Conceptual Universe of Ewe Christians in Southeastern Ghana." *The Journal of Religion in Africa* 22 (2): 98–132.

———. 1998. "'Make a Complete Break with the Past.' Memory and Post-Colonial Modernity in Ghanaian Pentecostal Discourse." *The Journal of Religion in Africa* 28 (3): 316–349.

———. 1999. *Translating the Devil: Religion and Modernity among the Ewe in Ghana.* Trenton, N.J.: Africa World Press.

Mohr, Adam. Forthcoming. "Capitalism, Chaos, and Christian Healing: Faith Tabernacle Congregation in Southern Colonial Ghana, 1918–1926." *The Journal of African History* 51 (1): 3–83.

Morsy, Soheir A. 1991. "Spirit Possession in Egyptian Ethnomedicine: Origins, Comparison, and Historical Specificity." In *Women's Medicine: The Zar-Bori Cult in Africa and Beyond,* ed. I. M. Lewis, Ahmed Al-Safi, and Sayyid Hurreiz, 189–208. Edinburgh: Edinburgh University Press.

Obeyesekere, Gananath. 1990. *The Work of Culture: Symbolic Transformation in Psychoanalysis and Anthropology.* Chicago: University of Chicago Press.

Olupona, Jacob K., and Regina Gemignani. 2007. "Introduction." In *African Immigrant Religions in America,* ed. Jacob K. Olupona and Regina Gemignani, 1–26. New York: New York University Press.

Omenyo, Cephas. 2002. *Pentecost Outside Pentecostalism: A Study of the Development of the Charismatic Renewal in the Mainline Churches in Ghana.* Zoetermeer, the Netherlands: Uitgeverij Boekencentrum.

Ong, Aihwa. 1988. "The Production of Possession: Spirits and the Multinational Corporation in Malaysia." *American Ethnologist* 15 (1): 28–42.

Onyinah, Opoku. 2002. "Akan Witchcraft and the Concept of Exorcism in the Church of Pentecost." PhD diss., University of Birmingham.

Peil, Margaret. 1995. "Ghanaians Abroad." *African Affairs* 94: 345–367.

Pessar, Patricia R. 1995. "On the Homefront and in the Workplace: Integrating Immigrant Women into Feminist Discourse." *Anthropological Quarterly* 68 (1): 37–47.

———. 1999. "Engendering Migration Studies: The Case of New Immigrants in the United States." *American Behavioral Scientist* 42 (4): 577–600.

PCG. 1962. *Reports for 1961.* Akropong: PCG Press.

Rattray, Robert S. 1927. *Religion and Art in Ashanti.* Oxford: Clarendon Press.

Soothill, Jane E. 2007. *Gender, Social Change, and Spiritual Power: Charismatic Christianity in Ghana.* Leiden, the Netherlands: Brill.

Terrazas, Aaron. 2009. "African Immigrants in the Unites States." MPI: Migration Information Source. Electronic document: http://www.migrationinformation.org/U.S.focus/display.cfm?id=719.

van Dijk, Rijk. 2004. "Negotiating Marriage: Questions of Morality and Legitimacy in the Ghanaian Pentecostal diaspora." *Journal of Religion in Africa* 34 (4): 438–467.

Wacker, Grant. 2001. *Heaven Below: Early Pentecostals and American Culture.* Cambridge, Mass.: Harvard University Press.

Wong, Madeline. 2006. "The Gendered Politics of Remittances in Ghanaian Transnational Families." *Economic Geography* 82 (4): 355–381.

Zentgraf, Kristine. 2002. "Immigration and Women's Empowerment: Salvadorans in Los Angeles." *Gender and Society* 16 (5): 625–646.

PART 3

Moving Through the Gaps

TEN

It's Just Like the Internet:
Transnational Healing Practices between Somaliland and the Somali Diaspora

Marja Tiilikainen

At the airport of Addis Ababa, Ethiopia, in the summer of 2005, I became acquainted with Faadumo. Both of us had traveled the same route all the way from Finland, and we both were on the way to Hargeysa in northern Somalia—Faadumo was going to visit her family and I was going to do my first fieldwork in the area. Faadumo was a young woman with a neat appearance. Her head was uncovered, and she was wearing a long jean skirt. As we approached Hargeysa, she covered herself with a black veil. Faadumo seemed to take interest in my study and told me that her mother knew a lot about traditional healing practices. At that time I did not yet foresee that Faadumo would become one of my key informants. Her multifaceted and even tragic story gradually came to light over several meetings in Somalia and Finland. Faadumo was divorced and had a teenage son who had been raised by Faadumo's mother in Hargeysa. She was in regular contact with the child by telephone, the internet, and annual visits. In recent years she had tried to bring the child to Finland, but the Finnish authorities did not believe that she was the biological mother. In Finland Faadumo had suffered from various symptoms and illnesses, such as stomach pain and loss of appetite. She had also become increasingly mistrustful of other people and had started to isolate herself at home. According to a Finnish doctor, Faadumo was depressed, but according to an Islamic scholar and healer (*sheikh*) in Hargeysa, these symptoms were caused by witchcraft. One of the aims of Faadumo's trip was to verify this diagnosis and, if necessary, try the sheikh's treatment, which she had earlier refused.

Faadumo's journey to Hargeysa raises interesting questions concerning her personal experiences, but also concerning African migrants' illness experiences and their health-seeking behavior in a broader sense. A vast body of research has emerged around migration and health. It has been emphasized that the categorization of illnesses, the needs of immigrant patients and the healing practices they are accustomed to often differ from those used in

Western health care services (Henry 1999). In Finnish health care, migrants are often seen as a challenging and "difficult" patient group, and health care staff often express a need to know more about migrant patients' cultural understandings related to health and illness in order to ease clinical encounters with them. However, these high-level Finnish doctors and nurses may not be aware that their patients are simultaneously relying on treatments from other sources. Faadumo is one of those migrants who seek treatment in a country of origin for an illness that cannot be treated in Finland and other Western countries.

It is well known that patients in general search for various alternative or supplementary therapies in addition to biomedical treatments (e.g., Kleinman 1980; Johannessen et al. 1994; Lindqvist 2002). In the case of migrants, the search for a remedy crosses borders not only between different health care sectors but also between nation-states (Dyck 1995; Kangas 2002; Messias 2002). For instance, according to a study by Grace Xueqin Ma (1999), simultaneous use of Western and traditional Chinese health practices is very common among Chinese immigrants in the U.S., and 32 percent of them travel to China or Taiwan for care. The concept of "medical pluralism" has expanded in meaning as health care sectors are internationally broadening in the context of globalization. Traveling and keeping in contact with people across the world has become part of everyday life, enabling easy, cheap, and quick transnational medical consultations. Hence, today's medical pluralism is a broader and more complex phenomenon than before.

The aim of this chapter is to highlight how transnationalism organizes the practices of healing among Somalis in exile. What are the reasons that Somali families in the diaspora search for treatments in Somaliland? What kinds of treatment and medication are sought after and used? What are the means of transnational communication, consultation, and healing? And, moreover, what is the impact of globalization and migrants returning "home" for local, "traditional" healing methods?

The chapter is based on 14 weeks of fieldwork carried out in northern Somalia, often referred to as Somaliland, in the summers of 2005 and 2006 as part of my post-doctoral research.[1] In addition, a few interviews were conducted in Helsinki and London. The study belongs to the fields of comparative religion and medical anthropology. The fieldwork in Somaliland was mainly concentrated in the Hargeysa area. The data was gathered by ethnographic methods and consists of taped interviews and discussions, photographs, videotapes, and field notes. It includes observations and interviews of several local healers (about 15) and patients from the diaspora (about 30 illness cases). I also attended healing rituals and visited hospitals, including mental wards and traditional pharmacies. As my Somali language skills are rudimentary, I employed Somali field assistants and friends, one male and several female, to help with Somali language interviews and field contacts. Except for one healer, all names in this article are pseudonyms. The secessionist Republic of Somaliland, which occupies the northwestern part of Somalia that used to be a British colony, has been self-governing for years but has not been internationally recognized. In this chapter, I mainly refer to Somaliland because it was my field site. In general, however, the findings of the study also apply to Somalis who live in or originate from other regions of Somalia.

The Somali Diaspora, Illness, and Transnational Ties

Transnational dimensions in health, illness, and healing are part of a larger phenomenon that has been described by the concepts of transnationalism and diaspora. Recent research has highlighted the importance of transnational networks for migrants living in today's globalized world: at the same time as migrants are integrating into receiving countries, they remain connected to the countries and relatives they have left behind (Wahlbeck 1999b; Levitt 2001). The phenomenon of transnationalism is not new, but in the era of globalization the linkages between migrants and their homelands are more intense than before: the ease of communication and transportation makes it possible to keep in touch more frequently and quickly than before. Today, it is increasingly common to live in a social world that stretches between places and communities in two or even more nation-states (Vertovec 2001; Bryceson and Vuorela 2002; Levitt 2004). The concept of diaspora was previously connected to the exile of the Jews, but the meaning has been extended to include the experiences of many displaced communities. The definition of diaspora often includes the idea of forced migration (Safran 1991; Cohen 1997). Diaspora can be seen as a type of transnationalism; the term has been regarded as particularly suitable for describing the relationships between refugees and their previous home countries (Wahlbeck 1999a).

Transnational social fields emerge when migrants maintain economic, social, cultural, religious, or political connections with other migrants, and with their families and collective groups in two or more localities (Vertovec 2001: 575). The intensity and frequency of transnational contacts varies between different groups and individuals and over time (Levitt 2001, 2004). These contacts are maintained through, for example, visits, sending money and other items, telephone calls, and other virtual means of communication such as the internet and faxes. Transnational networks often form an important resource for welfare (Clifford 1997: 256f).

We can describe the Somali diaspora using a set of terms defined by William Safran (1991: 83f): Somalis are dispersed from their country of origin to several foreign countries; they retain a collective memory of Somalia; Somali migrants often feel that they are not fully accepted in their resettlement countries; exiled Somalis usually regard Somalia as their ideal home to which they wish to be able to return; they are committed to the rebuilding of the homeland; and they continue to maintain relationships to the homeland that importantly define their ethnocommunal consciousness and solidarity.

The civil war in Somalia was the result of a complex historical development (see, e.g., Besteman and Cassanelli 1996; Samatar 2001). The events that finally caused the civil war to erupt started in northern Somalia. In 1988 the Somali National Movement (SNM), a principal opposition to the regime of General Maxamed Siyad Barre, moved from its base in Ethiopia to northern Somalia (Somaliland) and launched an offensive against oppressive government forces. The government responded by bombing the northern cities—including destroying the city of Hargeysa by aerial bombardment—poisoning wells, and planting hundreds of thousands of land mines. As many as 60,000 civilians were killed by the Somali government between 1988 and 1990 (Geshekter 1997: 79; Rebuilding Somaliland 2005: 13). In 1988 some 650,000 Somalis from northern Somalia fled to Ethiopia, and foreign aid to the Somali government was frozen due to reports of human rights abuses (Human Development Report Somalia 2001: 214). Upheavals in the north reverberated into the south. The Somali state collapsed in January of 1991 when Maxamed Siyad Barre fled the country. Somalia fell into anarchy, and the mass flight of Somalis began—over one million are estimated to have fled to neighboring countries and outside Africa (Human Development Report Somalia 2001: 58).

Today, Somalis are living all over the world. In Europe Somalis have settled particularly in the United Kingdom, where a community of Somali seamen had been living since the nineteenth century (Jordan et al. 2004). The United Kingdom, as well as Italy and France, also have historical and colonial ties to the Somali-inhabited area in the Horn of Africa. Large Somali communities also live in Canada and the United States. Somali families started entering Finland in 1990 as asylum seekers. Since the beginning of the 1990s, the number of Somalis in Finland has increased, mainly as a result of family reunifications and children born in Finland. At the end of 2010 there were some 13,000 native Somali speakers in Finland, women constituting almost half of them. The Somali population in Finland is young: in 2010 about 39 percent were under 15 years of age (Statistics Finland 20011). The majority of the Somali population lives in the metropolitan Helsinki area. Most Somalis in Finland originate from southern Somalia, which continues to be politically unstable, rather than from Somaliland, which began to stabilize in the mid-1990s.

The Somalis who have ended up as asylum seekers outside of Africa are a heterogeneous group and comprise people from diverse educational backgrounds, classes, and areas. However, the majority have been relatively well-educated and skilled people from cities (Samatar 2001: 23). Educationally, Somali refugees in Finland range from illiterate adults (especially women) to adults with university degrees (Tiilikainen 2003: 53; Alitolppa-Niitamo 2004: 30). The unemployment rate among Somalis has remained high, even though in recent years the situation has improved. For Somali men, who by custom should be responsible for maintaining their families, unemployment and living on social welfare has been very hard to endure. In 2011 there were some 165,500 foreign citizens living in Finland, very few compared to other European countries. Relative to other immigrants in Finland, Somalis have experienced a great deal of discrimination and racism. One reason for this is that the arrival of the Somalis coincided with an economic depression which left many Finns unemployed (Jaakkola 1999). This increased fears that Finns would have to share social welfare benefits with the newly arrived refugees. Moreover, the visible position of Somalis as the largest refugee group, the largest Muslim group, and the largest immigrant group of African origin in Finland has tended to draw negative attitudes toward them. The media coverage of Somalis has often been problem-centered.

Many Somalis in the diaspora support the reconstruction of their home country in various ways, often through Somali organizations (Kleist 2007). Somalis in Finland are also actively involved, for instance, in political life, development co-operation projects, and construction businesses back in Somalia. Remittances from abroad have been crucial for the survival of many households during the prolonged conflicts in the Horn of Africa (Horst 2003; Hansen 2004; Lindley 2009). The role of immigrants and refugees in assisting their families and supporting the rebuilding of their (previous) home countries is often stressed, but giving help and support is not a one-way road. The Somali mothers in my previous study (Tiilikainen 2003) described the importance of transnational family networks in dealing with problems such as the difficulty of bringing up children: they might frequently ask for advice from a grandmother in another country or even send a child all the way to the Horn of Africa to be brought up there by relatives.

Somalis in exile may also benefit from relatives and contacts back in Somalia when searching for treatment and cures. Transnational health care includes not only people who cross borders while they search for suitable treatment, but also the transfer of advice, treatments, and medicines. Border-crossings may be made through personal travel, but can also happen in suitcases; memory; or in virtual space and time, through telephone calls, faxes, and the internet. Medicines and other medical supplies move from Western countries to Somalia and vice versa—but the type of medicines moving in each direction is different: family members in Somalia receive European medicines and vitamins that are considered effective, whereas on the way back to Europe and other Western countries suitcases are filled with such things as camel milk, herbal medication, and cassettes with Qur'anic recitations against evil spirits.

In my PhD research (Tiilikainen 2003), I approached Somali immigrant women's painful experiences through the concept of social suffering (e.g., Kleinman, Das, and Lock 1997). The trauma and distress experienced by Somalis—in my study particularly Somali women—had two faces: on one hand, the political violence of the civil war, and on the other hand, discrimination, losses, and worries experienced in exile. Somali women frequently complained about various bodily symptoms such as pain, tiredness, and "stress," which they linked to their histories and experiences as refugees and immigrants. Hence, Somali immigrants are vulnerable due to accumulated suffering, and, according to my interpretation, traumatic memories and everyday worries are present in women's symptoms and ill health (see also Tiilikainen 2001, 2005).

Somali cultural concepts related to the etiology (origins), definition, and treatment of illness differ from medical concepts and practices in Finland and other Western countries. In Somali culture, mental distress in particular is often connected to spirits, witchcraft, and the evil eye (Pelizzari 1997; Lewis 1998: 107–132; Rousseau et al. 1998; Carroll 2004; Tiilikainen 2003). Several studies have shown, on the one hand, high rates of mental disorder among Somali refugees and, on the other, a low level of service use among them (Silveira and Ebrahim 1995; Bhui et al. 2003; McCrone et al. 2005: 351). Differing illness explanations make the utilization of Western mental health services by Somali immigrants problematic (Mölsä and Tiilikainen 2007; Mölsä, Hjelde, and Tiilikainen 2010) and hence may serve as one of the starting points for approaching an understanding of their transnational healing practices.

Looking for Treatment in Somalia

HEALTH SERVICES IN SOMALILAND

Somalia is one of the poorest countries of the world and has for the past 20 years been devastated by fights, famine, and government collapse. Somalis are Sunni Muslims, and Islam lays the grounds for basic ideas regarding health, illness, suffering, and healing. Public health services were weak even before the civil war and were mainly concentrated in cities. At that time, and still today, there was only one mental health hospital in the whole country, in the northern city of Berbera. In addition, there were and are psychiatric wards in connection to the general hospitals of Mogadishu and Hargeysa. The civil war ruined the infrastructure of the Somali state, and public health services were driven into crisis.

While Somaliland has been relatively stable compared to southern Somalia since the middle of the 1990s and is struggling toward democratic governance, the scars of the civil war are still visible. Roads, sanitation and sewage systems, and access to clean water are urgently needed. Beggars, street children, and mentally ill people who suffer from traumatic experiences of the war or excessive use of narcotic *khat* leaves are a common sight on the streets of Hargeysa. Due to a lack of international recognition and a fragile security and peace, international companies and organizations have been reluctant to invest and channel resources into Somaliland. Postwar conditions and needs, extreme poverty, and lack of government control have contributed to growing entrepreneurship in the health sector. In Somaliland, educated heath care staff often choose to work in private clinics where they have access to better salaries. Private services, however, are in many cases too expensive for ordinary patients. In addition to private clinics run by medical doctors, there are numerous clinics run by religious and other healers. Some of these healers are well known and may even work in conjunction with medical doctors.

Folk healers continue to have an important role in the overall health care system in Somalia. Different healers use different techniques to diagnose and treat patients, depending on their religious interpretations and inherited and learned skills (e.g., Antoniotto 1984; Serkkola 1994). According to Leendert Slikkerveer (1990), Somali treatments can be divided into: (1) treatments which deal with supernatural and social agents and relationships and, (2) natural treatments and remedies such as the treatment of wounds and fractures, herbal medication, and cupping. The first group of healers may have expertise in spirits and spirit possession cults such as *saar* (also spelled *zar*, about which see, e.g., Lewis, Al-Safi, and Hurreiz 1991), or they may be religious healers. Somali Islam has traditionally been Sufist, but during recent decades and particularly during the civil war the influence of Sunni political Islamist groups has intensified (Menkhaus 2002). New Islamic awareness and knowledge have resulted in redefined and reshaped religious practices and, moreover, have affected the explanations for illnesses and "proper" ways of healing. According to my observations and interviews, Islamic clinics known as *cilaaj*, which claim to concentrate on "pure" Islamic healing methods, such as herbal medication and exorcising *jinn* by reciting the Qur'an, have become increasingly popular, whereas *saar* rituals, which are nowadays often seen as non-Islamic, are arranged much more seldom than before (see Tiilikainen 2010a).

My data has concentrated on those Somalis who return to Somaliland from the diaspora in order to consult Islamic and other traditional healers. According to my interviews, Somali migrants may also consult and visit local medical doctors and hospitals, but the majority seem to turn to healers. Some of the healers' clinics in Somaliland have become very popular since the war and attract many patients from the diaspora.

It is very difficult to know how many of those Somalis who visit Somaliland, particularly in summer, actually visit healers' clinics and homes. I usually asked the healers for the number of their patients who come from the diaspora each year. The answers cannot be considered very accurate, as healers do not usually have systematic patient registers, and I noticed that they are prone to exaggerate the numbers. One of the most popular healers, Sheikh Mahamud Rage,[2] whose clinic is situated around 40 kilometers outside Hargeysa, asked his assistant to draw up statistics of Somali patients from the diaspora. According to the records, handwritten in thick books, between July 4, 2005 and August 1, 2006, the sheikh had 991 patients from abroad (see table 10.1).

As Sheikh Rage receives around 100 patients a day and works five days a week, the total number of patients in a week is around 500. The time given to each patient varies greatly: sometimes a few minutes are enough for the diagnosis; sometimes the diagnosis and treatment may take up to 15 minutes or even longer. If he worked an entire year in the same way, it would mean 26,000 patients in 52 weeks. In practice, the number of patients is probably smaller, especially during Ramadan. Moreover, the number of patients is not evenly distributed throughout the year, for there is a peak in the summer. Hence, this is a very rough estimation, but based on these numbers we can calculate that 3.8 percent of all his patients might come from outside Somaliland. About half of those come from the neighboring countries of Djibouti and Ethiopia. The relatively high number of people from Djibouti can partly be explained by the fact that people there like to escape the hottest season in Djibouti by visiting the more temperate Somaliland. The third largest group of outsider patients is Somalis from the United Kingdom. The statistics also show that other patients come quite evenly from all over the world.

REASONS TO "GO HOME"

Why do Somalis from the diaspora visit and consult healers in Somaliland? What are they looking for in a poor country with poor health facilities?

Table 10.1. Sheikh Rage's patients from the diaspora according to country, July 4, 2005–August 1, 2006.

Djibouti	347	Kenya	17
Ethiopia	211	Finland	14
United Kingdom	118	Australia	13
Arab countries	42	Kuwait	13
United States	39	Belgium	11
Yemen	30	Holland	11
South Africa	27	Denmark	10
Canada	26	Germany	9
Sweden	24	Qatar	6
France	17	Turkey	6
		Total	**991**

Ahmed, whom I met at a Sheikh Abdi's clinic in July 2005 told me about his experiences:

> I have had this problem since 1990. Mostly I have pain in my head, and also I have something, I don't know, circling around my body. All over the body. When I checked with some of the sheikhs [in the U.S.], they told me this problem is not a medical problem, but that this is a religious problem, and Islam knows more than what doctors know. So, they urged me strongly to read the Qur'an, they give me more advice and how to protect yourself from devils and similar things. [. . .] So, I tried my best, I read the Qur'an. But still I was feeling so strongly, this is a psychic problem. [. . .] There is somebody I can't see that was fighting inside me. Circling, and trying to change my attention. I was doing a very tough work, I was working two jobs when I got sick. You have to pay attention, to focus on what you are doing, yeah? This took away, changed my focus, I could not concentrate. I was feeling bad headaches and pain in the stomach. [. . .] The only way you can fight against it is when you listen to the Qur'an. As soon as I listen to the Qur'an, my attention comes back. So I am always very close to the Qur'an, I read it myself a lot.

> The doctors did not find anything. Most of the time they ask you if you have any stress about the home or from work. Some of them

give you the advice to go home, to take a vacation, a long vacation, or to change jobs, or ask what is wrong with your house and about family problems or something like that. But I told them, everything is all right. And then I have this problem. But they [the doctors in the U.S.] could not find anything wrong. But one day they gave me 20 tablets, not sure what kind of tablet. And I used that, while I had bad headaches. And I got some sleep, just to rest. But I never had any other tablets. Usually every year, I checked myself twice, a full check-up, to see if anything was wrong with my stomach or. [. . .] Because the pain was growing, growing a lot, and sometimes I stayed at home because I couldn't go to work. [. . .]

When I heard that they have the medical place here, I came to the doctor [in Hargeysa]. And, in fact he showed me what is wrong with me. I realized what is wrong. I realized the problem is not a medical problem, they told me this problem is the *jinn*. You know, a *jinni* is an ancient creature, right? The *jinn* go into a human being through some reason. My case was a spell, it [a *jinni*] enters with a spell. They gave me something to drink, and he [the *jinni*] sat in there. So, anything I do, he [the *jinni*] controls. The Qur'an is the only way to stop him.

And this is the first time in 15 years that I know what is wrong with me. If you don't know what is wrong with you, but you are feeling sick, this is another sickness, right? So, when I came here, I discovered the problem. And, actually, most of my problem left now that I know the problem. [. . .] Still I am feeling something now, but I can say, 80 percent of what I was feeling is already gone. I am feeling very good now, and more healthy than when I came here. Really, I can control myself very well, everything. So, Alhamdulilah, I continue now to read the Qur'an and take whatever medicine they have here. So I am very much hoping I am at the end soon.

Ahmed had arrived from the U.S. in March and had visited Sheikh Abdi's place regularly since then. His treatment included listening to the recitation of the Qur'an, herbal medicine to clean the stomach from the influence of witchcraft and the *jinn,* and cupping.

Based on my data, Ahmed's case is not unusual among patients returning from the diaspora. It typifies one of seven reasons I identified that Somalis in the diaspora may return home for treatment. People in this first category return because *despite continuous, vague symptoms, a doctor in the resettlement country was not able to give them a diagnosis or prescribe proper treatment.*

In another category are those returning Somalis who have been diagnosed in the diaspora, but *the patient or his/her family does not accept/trust the diagnosis, treatment, or medication.* In particular, Somali families seem to find psychiatric and neurological diagnoses such as schizophrenia, psychosis, depression, autism, and epilepsy difficult to accept. Symptoms related to these conditions have traditionally been understood in the framework of spirits, the evil eye, and witchcraft. For example, I saw a father who brought his 17-year-old son from Denmark to a sheikh. The father said that according to Danish doctors the boy suffered from schizophrenia, and he had also been in a mental hospital for half a year. The father wanted to hear the sheikh's opinion and make sure that the boy did not have *jinn* or any other problem that could be cured easily. The father explained: "Now he gets injections. When he gets the medication, he acts like a normal person. But afterwards the symptoms come back again. The Danish doctors said that he has to use the medicine continuously. But I do not want my son to live only with the help of medication." In this case, the sheikh did not find *jinn,* but urged the family to continue with the medication, along with careful observation of religious rules. According to a doctor who works at the mental hospital of Berbera, Somali families do not trust European psychiatric medicines, but believe that the patients are being poisoned.

Faadumo also falls into this second category of patients. According to Faadumo's psychiatrist in Finland, she had depression. The doctor prescribed medication for her, but she only accepted sleeping pills. In the summer of 2005, Faadumo visited Sheikh Abdi's *cilaaj* for the third time, and he repeated the witchcraft diagnosis. The sheikh had told her the same thing twice before and had given her herbal medication to take back to Finland. Faadumo told me that earlier she did not believe in the sheikh or his medicine, and she had lied to her mother that she had taken the medication. But gradually, when her condition became worse, she started to think about the sheikh's words. This time she decided to try the sheikh's treatment and medication—at least it would give her and her mother certainty and peace of mind. For over a month Faadumo came to a sheikh's clinic almost every morning to listen to a Qur'an recitation in a separate women's room. In addition, she was given herbal medication which made her vomit—the aim was to purify the stomach from the poison that a witch had given to her.

The third group of Somalis who visit healers in Somaliland are those who accept the diagnosis and use the medicines given by a Western doctor, but *search for an alternative treatment in order to restore their health or stop taking (chemical) medicines regularly.* For instance, I interviewed a 60-year-old woman,

Dahabo, who lives in Finland. She had had diabetes for about five years and had been given insulin injections twice a day. But when I met her in Hargeysa, she had not used insulin for the last 20 days she had been there. Dahabo explained: "I wanted to try to see if I can stop it altogether because I used it many years. And when I injected so frequently, the skin on my legs and stomach became so sore. I wanted to try to see if I can manage without insulin. I stopped it immediately when I came (to Somaliland)." Back in Finland Dahabo said that during her six-month stay in Hargeysa she had tested her blood sugar regularly, and in the entire time needed to take insulin about ten times. She had not used any other medication, but drank camel milk daily.

Another example from this category is Hibo from the U.K. For two to three years she had not been feeling well; she suffered from a hyperactive thyroid, symptoms of arthritis, stomach problems (gastritis), and also consti-pation and hemorrhoids, followed by anemia. In the U.K. she used medica-tion for her ailments. But when she came to Hargeysa, she felt much better and stopped all the medication, except the medication for her thyroid. She believed that her improved condition largely resulted from the organic food in Somalia. In addition, Hibo visited a Sufi healer, who arranged a healing ritual and prayed for her.

According to a pharmacist (herbalist), one group of Somalis coming from abroad are "old people" who want to visit traditional healers, because "they know these things existed and were useful before they left." He told me about a customer who came from the United Kingdom for a one-month vacation. The main purpose of the visit was to take certain herbal medicines. The phar-macist explained that Somalis may want to avoid chemical medication because they are afraid of possible side effects.

The fourth group among those who search for transnational healing in Somaliland are migrants who *have problems with the medication or treatment given by a medical doctor*—either it does not help them, or it is too expensive. For instance, one mother told me how her son had been suffering from skin problems since he was 5 years old. When he was 13 years old, sheikhs in Hargeysa read him the Qur'an, and a mixture of olive oil and herbs was mas-saged into his skin. Since that treatment, the boy has had no problems. I also met a woman from Canada who visited traditional healers in Hargeysa in order to cure her infertility when she could no longer afford hormonal treat-ments in Canada.

The fifth category consists of those *whose problems are seen to be tied to the Western lifestyle*. The problems are typically connected to drug and alcohol abuse, and some of those affected may have been in jail or a mental hospital.

In these cases the family may decide to take the patient back to Somaliland, hoping that he or she recovers and gets rid of the bad habits "at home," in the midst of his/her own culture and religion. Among these returned people are also adolescents who, according to their custodians, have become too Westernized. They are commonly called *dhaqan celis*—those who are returned to culture. For instance, I had a discussion with a male patient in the mental ward of the Hargeysa hospital. He had lived ten years in England and had abused drugs and alcohol. Finally, he became "mad" and homeless. A relative took him back to Somaliland. As his condition did not improve, after approximately half a year he was taken to the mental ward. A mental hospital is usually the last resort when families have no other place to bring their mentally ill family members. Before that, the family has usually tried several healers. If no help is found, a violent patient may end up in chains at home or in the mental ward/hospital, where proper resources and medication are not available.

Ill migrants also return to Somaliland when doctors *tell them that they have an incurable disease that may be terminal and offer them no hope.* In these cases migrants may wish to get well in Somaliland by a miracle, Allah so willing; or alternatively, die and be buried in Somaliland.

Finally, Somaliland healers may also be visited for the *prevention of illnesses and protection from harmful agents, in the style of a "check-up."* For example, in women's *sitaat* rituals, where the Prophet and those women who are closely related to him are praised by special religious songs and hymns, a blessing is received (see Kapteijns and Ali 1996). These events are usually arranged during pregnancy, but some *sitaat* groups gather regularly two or three times a week. Nowadays it is common to arrange a ritual when a visiting Somali woman is about to go back to a country of resettlement. The *sitaat* is usually videotaped, and the woman can bring the video with her to the diaspora for continuous remembrance and blessing (see Tiilikainen 2010b).

According to some healers, patients who come from abroad differ from their local clients: in contrast to local Somalilanders, Somalis from the diaspora have often been so "poisoned" by drugs, alcohol, and medications that their bodies have to be cleansed first. Moreover, witchcraft cases from abroad have been more serious and difficult to treat than those whose origin is in Somaliland. Some healers also complained that Somalis from the diaspora often do not have enough time for the treatment, but come and visit the healers very close to their departure from Somaliand.

Earlier research has shown that women in particular are believed to be prone to spirit possession (e.g., Boddy 1989; Lewis, Al-Safi, and Hurreiz 1991; cf. Kane, this volume). According to my interviews and observations in Somaliland, this is the case even now—most patients who are seen to be suffering from the evil eye, witchcraft, and spirits are women. Moreover, the majority of the patients from the diaspora who come to visit sheikhs and other healers for these reasons or on suspicion of these complaints are women. Men are more likely to suffer from drug and alcohol abuse and violent behavior that may have led to homelessness, jail, or a mental hospital in a resettlement country—most young or even older Somalis who have been taken back by their relatives to be treated for these types of problems are men.

Transnational Contacts with Healers in Somaliland

A visit to a healer may be the main reason for a trip to Somaliland, but it is more common to combine health-related activities with a vacation trip. Some Somalis travel quite regularly, for example once a year, between Europe and Somaliland. Most Somalis in the diaspora, however, cannot afford frequent travel, and have to save money over several years to make a journey. In addition, the movement of asylum seekers and refugees across nation-state borders is often regulated. For instance, a long stay in Somalia during the citizenship application process is not a positive signal for the Finnish authorities. Another restricting factor is that a person traveling with an alien passport loses social benefits from the state during the time she or he stays outside Finland.

Healers in Somaliland usually stress that it is desirable that an afflicted person come to the country personally and be physically present during the healing act. Close relatives in Somaliland, in particular mothers, play an important role in choosing a healer and arranging communication with him or her. Healers are at least partly chosen by familiarity and reputation. In addition, patients and their families may visit several healers, depending on the end results and the opinions and recommendations of other people. If an ill person himself or herself cannot travel to Somaliland, a relative may visit a healer, describe the symptoms, and carry the medication across the borders. Medicine may be something that a patient eats or drinks (e.g., honey, camel milk, herbal medicine, or *cashar*—holy water over which a sheikh has recited the Qur'an), spreads on the skin (e.g., a mixture of oil and herbs), burns (e.g., incense, words from the Qur'an), or listens to (e.g., a recitation of the Qur'an). Medicine may also have a protecting power: for instance, a sheikh may write a prayer which a patient carries around in a tiny package or keeps at home. Due to the lack of an official postal system, it is complicated, unreliable, and expensive to send items from Somalia, and hence, it is a common practice to give extra packages and bags to anybody who is known to be traveling into/out of the country.

Due to financial and other factors, traveling to Somalia is not always possible, and patients need to rely on virtual connections. This may also be necessary in acute and severe cases. Virtual contact with the healers before, during, and after the treatment can be made through telephone calls, email messages, faxes, and even internet-based means. Once I witnessed a telephone call from Norway: a daughter of a Somali family had fallen ill, and by phone the sheikh diagnosed *jinn* based on the symptoms described by her father. He promised to recite the Qur'an for her and thus try to expel the *jinn* through his mobile telephone the same evening. Before that he asked the father to send him detailed information about the case by email.

In addition to physical and virtual connections, a spiritual connection between healers and patients is possible. Because many healers deal with the relationship between God, spirits, and a patient, it is not surprising that heal-ing is possible without the patient—God and spirits are part of today's global-ized world, and they can easily transcend borders. One precondition usually is, however, that the patient sends money to the healer in Somalia. In these cases, family members in Somaliland may represent the patient and take part in a ritual.[3] Afterward, video cassettes or taped recordings may be sent to the person abroad to enable her or him to take part virtually and receive blessings and possible messages from the participants.

At least some migrants seem to keep contact with healers even after they have returned to Europe. A Somali woman in London told me that after treat-ment in Somaliland, she had decided to send 100–200 USD yearly to the healer, who then would slaughter animals and pray for her on the commemoration day of a popular Sufi sheikh. The woman was afraid that if she failed to send the money, she would fall seriously ill or things would not go as well as they were at the moment. After her arrival from Somaliland, she had become very ill, and she had found it hard to believe in the healer. After a successful opera-tion, however, she said that perhaps the prayers and the healer's connection with the spirits and the Sufi sheikhs had helped her after all—and who knows what would have happened without the treatment and subsequent efforts of the healer in Somaliland.

Local Healers in a Global World

Healers in Somaliland face the same problems as other Somalis who want to travel abroad: with a Somali passport it is very difficult to get entry visas for Europe and other Western countries. Hence, journeys are often restricted to other neighboring African countries, or Arab countries such as Yemen, the United Arab Emirates, and Saudi Arabia. Nonetheless, healers are not isolated, but have access to a global flow of information through television, the internet, and personal contacts. Importantly, patients coming from abroad may also be a resource and part of the process of building healers' personal transnational networks. Satisfied patients from abroad may bring further contacts, equipment, gifts, money, and new patients to healers in Somaliland, or perhaps even arrange an invitation and visa to enter Europe or the U.S. A foreign telephone number on the wall of a healer's clinic not only enforces the image of a powerful healer, but is also an indicator of a transnational relationship between healer and patient.

According to my observations of healers in Somaliland, it is very difficult to draw clear lines between "traditional" and "nontraditional" healing practices. I will give three examples. Sheikh Ibrahim has a small clinic where he receives patients daily, in particular women who suffer from various gynecological problems. The walls of the waiting hall are covered with anatomical pictures, and the bookshelves beside his table are filled with Arabic religious books, books on herbal medicine, and English-language medical books (even though Sheikh Ibrahim speaks very little English). A Qur'an recitation cassette is played aloud all day. Ibrahim has a computer where he keeps the patient register, and through the internet he looks for medical information and keeps in contact with patients and colleagues abroad. He writes prescriptions on a sheet of paper printed with his name. Ibrahim would like to combine religious and modern medical knowledge, but he has studied medicine only from pictures, the internet, and by talking to some medical doctors. His diagnoses have a solid basis in Somali cultural and religious understandings, as he mostly tells patients that they suffer from *jinn,* the evil eye, or witchcraft; however, he may also draw an anatomical picture where he points out, for instance, where exactly a *jinni* has blocked a tube. The treatment is always *cashar* (holy water) combined with some herbs.

Sheikh Mursal has practiced as a healer for over 30 years. He used to be a bonesetter and an herbalist, trained by other traditional healers. Through experience he learned more about human anatomy and started to perform more complicated procedures. Today, Mursal has a small, crowded hospital in a house partially in ruins at the center of Hargeysa, where he performs brain surgeries and saves the legs and arms of patients that other doctors wanted to amputate by transplanting animal bones into the human body. Before the operations, he sends the patient to be X-rayed. The conditions under which he gives anesthesia and operates on patients are very simple. Sheikh Mursal has never studied medicine.

The third example is a female healer, Nasra, who heals with the help of spirits whom she calls *nuuraani.* She calls herself a doctor. Her healing practice is extremely interesting to observe, as she mixes different elements stemming from Somali culture, Islam, and modern medicine. In making a diagnosis, Nasra might, for example, use eggs to check whether the person suffers from witchcraft, open the Qur'an and list a patient's symptoms and illnesses by reading an Arabic text (even though I believe she does not know Arabic), feel the patient's pulse, take urine and blood samples, and measure blood pressure. Modern equipment and techniques are, however, interpreted within a traditional framework and in a way that underlines her magical powers. For example, Nasra says that her spiritual helpers brought her the blood pressure meter she uses as well as a popular massage device.[4] Moreover, the blood and urine samples are sent to a "spiritual laboratory," where her spirits examine them and give her the results the following day.

Different healers have different resources. It is already common to have mobile phones, but the poorest healers who do not have so many patients (at least not from abroad) may not be able to afford one. In addition, a new generation of healers who have a better education than the older sheikhs and other healers usually have better access to and more interest in modern technology, which may help them to develop their practice and also attract patients from the diaspora. The arrival of transnational patients in Somaliland probably also motivates healers to develop their practices to better serve this client group.

Spirits, the evil eye, and witchcraft are part of a Somali healer's worldview, even though distances, interpretations, and metaphors are changing as a result of globalization and modernization. A sheikh described the nature of *jinn:*

> This *jinni* [a *dabayl,* or cyclone *jinni*] makes himself wind, it is a thousand kilometers long. The wind that you see in the ground is his feet, and the head is up in the clouds. Then it enters into a human body, the wind comes down, and a *jinni* opens like an antenna, a *jinni* makes himself at home in the body. Then it stays there and is like a space station. *Jinn* can come and go as they want. [. . .] Every country, every region, a *jinni* is everywhere. It is inside the person, it does not have a [flight] ticket. It goes wherever you go. A *jinni* is faster than the internet, it can be everywhere in one second. I do not know how to describe how fast it is. A *jinni* is like living electricity, it can penetrate this wall, it can penetrate seas, mountains, everywhere, like electricity, just as simple as living electricity. And it has a brain, a mind, a heart, life, a soul. We cannot see *jinn* because nobody can see electricity. Like mobile phones, like the internet. In only a second they can circumnavigate the world. And they even have a very powerful mental recorder. Through that he can record every place that he crossed: I saw people like that, I saw towns, have you ever visited

London? He can say, now I can go, and bring you. In an instant he can give you all. [. . .] They work just like the internet.

Hence, Somali healers and their illness explanations do not necessarily contradict the concepts of modernity, but are given new life and significance through new conditions and interpretations. The flexibility and adaptability of healers, their worldview, and the language they use reproduce and renew Somali healing culture and keep it alive.

Discussion

The transnational life world opens up new approaches to understanding African migrants' illness experiences and illness behavior. Somali illness explanations such as spirits, the evil eye, or witchcraft fall outside the domain of Western medical doctors and encourage migrants to engage in transnational health-seeking behavior. In trying to understand the meaning of different explanatory models and transnational health behavior, the observations of Hanne Mogensen (2005) from Uganda are interesting. According to Mogensen, Ugandan patients and their relatives "move back and forth between different diagnoses because each calls for different responses and responsibilities" (2005: 229). Hence, patients' agency is displayed in the way they choose a suitable explanatory model in different social contexts that will result in a desirable response in a particular field. Following Mogensen's notion, Somali patients in a Finnish or other Western clinic know "the rules of the game": complaints of headache, stomach pain, and sleeplessness will probably lead to examinations and prescriptions that are available within the time-space of the Finnish health unit (cf. Mogensen 2005: 231). Somali expressions of illness and distress, instead, signify a way to be and act inter-subjectively. Illness carries meaningful social relationships and moral duties in relation to the past, present, and future. For example, before a patient can be healed from problems caused by spirits, relatives need to take responsibility for arranging and participating in the treatment.

Somalis in the diaspora also travel to Somaliland for alternative treatments and medications, or when they wish to find a cure for serious illnesses or incurable conditions. Traveling home to a socially, culturally, and religiously familiar environment is itself often experienced as therapeutic and healing. Western health services, particularly mental health services, may raise mistrust and dissatisfaction among Somali migrants, whereas Somali healing and returning home includes a strong element of hope. In addition, healing in Somalia touches upon questions of cultural and religious identities. For example, some patients who had gone through long treatment periods in sheikhs' clinics described how they had learned a lot about Islam and how they had become stronger as persons through the treatment (see Tiilikainen and Koehn 2011). Hence, illness and treatment in Somalia ideally construct morally, culturally, and religiously conscious persons who are aware of their roots. Indeed, healing may be a meaningful acculturation process for Somali patients who have lived for years in the diaspora. Moreover, the healing process strengthens the unity of the family and serves as a reminder of the importance of close family ties. Neither the patient's age, social status, nor education directly correspond to whether she or he chooses to travel for treatment to Somalia or not, or what kind of a healer she or he visits. The younger or sicker the patient is, the larger the role of the family in making decisions about the treatment. However, one general trend seems to be that in line with the general Islamization process in Somalia, many families seem to prefer healers whom they believe heal with "pure" Islamic methods.

Transnational health care is an important resource for Somali migrants. Healers in Somaliland, together with their treatments and medications, provide migrants with significant explanations, certainties, and alternatives, in particular in the field of mental illness and chronic disease where Western medical diagnoses may be difficult to accept. Physical border crossings, however, may be restricted by practical, financial, and political factors, and hence, virtual homecomings, advice, and treatments become important as well. But transnational health care may also have negative consequences for patients. Medical treatment in Somalia does not correspond to the level of medical treatment in Finland. Patients who travel to Somalia may stop taking vital medication prescribed by a Finnish doctor, or they may run out of medicine and not be able to find the same medication in Somalia. Hence, the transnational realities of many Somali and other migrant families pose a challenge for health care providers in migrant receiving countries (Koehn and Tiilikainen 2007). Even though the number of migrants who do return home for treatment is not very large, the phenomenon reflects the areas and problems in the encounters between migrants and health care services that need to be considered.

Somali diagnoses tie Somalis in the diaspora to their country of origin. This may be seen not only as a positive, but potentially also as a negative dimension of transnational connectedness. For instance, in Faadumo's case it was her mother who was convinced about witchcraft being a reason behind Faadumo's illness. She continuously reminded her daughter of this by telephone while she was in Finland and insisted that she follow the sheikh's instructions. Thus, partly because of her mother, Faadumo could not reject the idea of being bewitched, which may have affected her capacity to accept and get relief from the treatments available in Finland. Traveling between Europe or the U.S. and Somalia because of illness and treatment, sometimes repeatedly, is also a dispersing experience which may have consequences for the whole family in the diaspora. If a mother has fallen ill and returns to Somalia for treatment, under-aged children may travel with her if the father cannot take care of them alone. If the visit is extended for several months, or even years, the children may forget the Finnish language and will certainly fall behind at school.

Once someone has returned to Somalia, it is not always clear that a reverse return—back to Finland or another Western country—is at all possible. Psychologist Hussein Bulhan, who works in Hargeysa, has stated that sometimes families are not willing to allow people who have been returned and treated in Somaliland to travel back even though they had become healthy: families do not seem to believe that an adolescent or an adult who used to abuse alcohol and drugs or who had been suffering from severe mental distress can recover. Without a passport, money, or the support of relatives it is very difficult to return to Europe. One of the young patients of Hussein Bulhan finally felt desperate enough to commit suicide.

And what happened to Faadumo? After the treatment in Somaliland she did not fully recover, but did feel a little better. The next visit to Somaliland was not for another year and a half. On that visit Faadumo stayed almost half a year with her mother and son. She did not visit the sheikh, but she met a nice man, fell in love, and got married. Now she is pregnant and back in Finland. She is happy and is waiting for her husband to get permission to move to Finland. Instead of poison she has a new life growing in her stomach. Was this all thanks to the sheikh's treatment—or simply that Faadumo found meaning in her life again?

Flows also change the landscape.[5] Transnational networks are a resource not only for Somali migrants, but also for Somali healers, whose travel outside Somalia is restricted. Local healers learn from their mobile patients. Patients from abroad open up new possibilities and horizons to healers, and change their healing practices, together with larger processes of Islamization, globalization, and modernity. Healers have an important role in providing services in the postwar Somaliland context. Those healers who manage to attract patients from the diaspora not only prosper personally, but also have an impact on the image of Somali healers in general. Patients who arrive from the diaspora and who rely on local healers often believe them to possess a secret healing power derived from ancient cultural or religious knowledge. The continuity of Somali healing, however, is profoundly intertwined with healers' ability to change their practices and adapt to changing conditions and needs in local and global worlds.

Notes

1. This study was part of a wider research project called "Changes in the Population, Changes in Distress—Challenges for Finnish Health Care," under the Health Services Research Programme (TERTTU) by the Academy of Finland (2004–2007). The study, including my fieldwork in Somaliland, has been funded by the Academy of Finland, the Ella and Georg Ehrnrooth Foundation and the Nordic Africa Institute. I am grateful for all the help and support provided by my assistants, friends, and informants in Somaliland. I also want to acknowledge Professor Janice Boddy, who carefully read and commented the manuscript.

2. Here I uniquely use a real name.

3. Somali migrants may also arrange wedding parties or celebrations after childbirth in Somalia, even though the couple or parents of the newborn baby themselves physically stay in Finland.

4. When asked for the first time, however, Nasra said that she received the equipment as a gift from England.

5. I thank Professor Susan Reynolds Whyte for this remark.

References

Alitolppa-Niitamo, Anne. 2004. *The Icebreakers: Somali-Speaking Youth in Metropolitan Helsinki with a Focus on the Context of Formal Education.* Helsinki: The Family Federation of Finland, The Population Research Institute.

Antoniotto, Albert. 1984. "Traditional Medicine in Somalia: An Anthropological Approach to the Concepts Concerning Disease." In *Proceedings of the Second International Congress of Somali Studies,* ed. Thomas Labahn, 155–169. Hamburg, Germany: Helmut Buske Verlag.

Besteman, Catherine, and Lee V. Cassanelli, eds. 1996. *The Struggle for Land in Southern Somalia: The War Behind the War.* Boulder, Colo.: Westview Press.

Bhui, Kamaldeep, Abdisalama Abdi, Mahad Abdi, Stephen Pereira, Mohammed Dualeh, David Robertson, Ganesh Sathyamoorthy, and Hellena Ismail. 2003. "Traumatic Events, Migration Characteristics, and Psychiatric Symptoms among Somali Refugees." *Social Psychiatry and Psychiatric Epidemiology* 38: 35–43.

Boddy, Janice. 1989. *Wombs and Alien Spirits: Women, Men, and the Zār Cult in Northern Sudan.* Madison: The University of Wisconsin Press.

Bryceson, Deborah Fahy, and Ulla Vuorela. 2002. "Transnational Families in the Twenty-first Century." In *The Transnational Family: New European Frontiers and Global Networks,* eds. Deborah Bryceson and Ulla Vuorela, 3–30. Oxford: Berg.

Carroll, Jennifer K. 2004. "Murug, Waali, and Gini: Expressions of Distress in Refugees from Somalia." *The Primary Care Companion to the Journal of Clinical Psychiatry* 6 (3): 119–125.

Clifford, James. 1997. *Routes: Travel and Translation in the Late Twentieth Century.* Cambridge, Mass.: Harvard University Press.

Cohen, Robin. 1997. *Global Diasporas: An Introduction.* London: UCL Press.

Dyck, Isabel. 1995. "Putting Chronic Illness 'In Place': Women Immigrants' Accounts of their Health." *Geoforum* 26 (3): 247–260.

Geshekter, Charles. 1997. "The Death of Somalia in Historical Perspective." In *Mending Rips in the Sky: Options for Somali Communities in the 21st Century,* eds. Hussein M. Adam and Richard Ford, 65–98. Lawrenceville, N.J.: The Red Sea Press.

Hansen, Peter. 2004. *Migrant Remittances as a Development Tool: The Case of Somaliland.* Migration Policy Research, Working Papers Series No. 3. Copenhagen: Denmark Department of Migration Policy, Research, and Communications.

Henry, Rebecca R. 1999. "Measles, Hmong, and Metaphor: Culture Change and Illness Management under Conditions of Immigration." *Medical Anthropology Quarterly* 13 (1): 32–50.

Horst, Cindy. 2003. "Transnational Nomads: How Somalis Cope with Refugee Life in the Dadaab Camps of Kenya." PhD diss., University of Amsterdam.

Human Development Report Somalia. 2001. Nairobi, Kenya: United Nations Development Program, Somalia Country Office, Nairobi.

Jaakkola, Magdalena. 1999. *Maahanmuutto ja etniset asenteet. Suomalaisten suhtautuminen maahanmuuttajiin 1989–1999.* Työpoliittinen tutkimus 213. Helsinki: Edita.

Johannessen, Helle, Laila Launsø, Søren Gosvig Olesen, and Frants Staugård, eds. 1994. *Studies in Alternative Therapy 1; Contributions from the Nordic Countries.* Odense, Denmark: Odense University Press.

Jordan, Glenn, with Akli Ahmed and Abdi Arwo. 2004. *Somali Elders: Portraits from Wales.* Cardiff, Wales: Butetown History & Arts Centre.

Kangas, Beth. 2002. "Therapeutic Itineraries in a Global World: Yemenis and Their Search for Biomedical Treatment Abroad." *Medical Anthropology* 21 (1): 35–78.

Kapteijns, Lidwien, with Mariam Omar Ali. 1996. "Sittaat: Somali Women's Songs for the 'Mothers of the Believers.'" In *The Marabout and the Muse: New Approaches to Islam in African Literature,* ed. Kenneth W. Harrow, 124–141. Portsmouth, N.H.: Heinemann.

Kleinman, Arthur. 1980. *Patients and Healers in the Context of Culture.* Berkeley: University of California Press.

Kleinman, Arthur, Veena Das, and Margaret Lock. 1997. "Introduction." In *Social Suffering,* eds. Arthur Kleinman, Veena Das, and Margaret Lock, ix–xxv. Berkeley: University of California Press.

Kleist, Nauja. 2007. "Spaces of Recognition: An Analysis of Somali-Danish Associational Engagement and Diasporic Mobilization." PhD diss., Sociologisk Institut, Københavns Universitet.

Koehn, Peter, and Marja Tiilikainen. 2007. "Transmigration and Transnational Health Care: Connecting Finland and Somaliland." *Siirtolaisuus—Migration* 2007 (1): 2–9.

Levitt, Peggy. 2001. *The Transnational Villagers.* Berkeley: University of California Press.

———. 2004. "Transnational Migrants: When 'Home' Means More Than One Country." Migration Information Source, Migration Policy Institute. Electronic document: http://www.migrationinformation.org/Feature/display.cfm?ID=261.

Lewis, I. M. 1998. *Saints and Somalis: Popular Islam in a Clan-based Society.* London: Haan Associates.

Lewis, I. M., Ahmed Al-Safi, and Sayyid Hurreiz, eds. 1991. *Women's Medicine: The Zar-Bori Cult in Africa and Beyond.* Edinburgh: Edinburgh University Press for the International African Institute.

Lindley, Anna. 2009. "The Early-Morning Phonecall: Remittances from a Refugee Diaspora Perspective." *Journal of Ethnic and Migration Studies* 35 (8): 1315–1334.

Lindqvist, Galina. 2002. "Healing Efficacy and the Construction of Charisma: A Family's Journey Through the Multiple Medical Field in Russia." *Anthropology and Medicine* 9 (3): 337–358.

Ma, Grace Xueqin. 1999. "Between Two Worlds: The Use of Traditional and Western Health Services by Chinese Immigrants." *Journal of Community Health* 24 (6): 421–437.

McCrone, P., K. Bhui, T. Craig, S. Mohamud, N. Warfa, S. A. Stansfeld, G. Thornicroft, and S. Curtis. 2005. "Mental Health Needs, Service Use, and Costs among Somali Refugees in the UK." *Acta Psychiatrica Scandinavica* 111: 351–357.

Menkhaus, Ken. 2002. "Political Islam in Somalia." *Middle East Policy* 9: 109–123.

Messias, DeAnne K. Hilfinger. 2002. "Transnational Health Resources, Practices, and Perspectives: Brazilian Immigrant Women's Narratives." *Journal of Immigrant Health* 4 (4): 183–200.

Mogensen, Hanne O. 2005. "Finding a Path through the Health Unit: Practical Experience of Ugandan Patients." *Medical Anthropology* 22: 209–236.

Mölsä, Mulki, and Marja Tiilikainen. 2007. "Potilaana somali. Auttaako kulttuurinen tieto lääkärin työssä?" *Duodecim* 123: 451–457.

Mölsä, Mulki, Karin Harsløf Hjelde, and Marja Tiilikainen. 2010. "Changing Conceptions of Mental Distress Among Somalis in Finland." *Transcultural Psychiatry* 47 (2): 276–300.

Pelizzari, Elisa. 1997. *Possession et thérapie dans la Corne de l'Afrique.* Paris: L'Harmattan.

Rebuilding Somaliland, Issues and Possibilities. 2005. *WSP International Somali Programme.* Lawrenceville, N.J.: The Red Sea Press.

Rousseau, Cécile, Taher M. Said, Marie-Josée Gagné, and Gilles Bibeau. 1998. "Between Myth and Madness: The Premigration Dream of Leaving among Somali Refugees." *Culture, Medicine, and Psychiatry* 22 (4): 385–411.

Safran, William. 1991. "Diasporas in Modern Societies: Myths of Homeland and Return." *Diaspora* 1 (1): 83–99.

Samatar, Ahmed I. 2001. "The Somali Catastrophe: Explanations and Implications." In *Variations on the Theme of Somaliness*; Proceedings of the EASS/SSIA International Congress of Somali Studies, Turku, Finland, Aug. 6–9, 1988; ed. Muddle Suzanne Lilius, 7–30. Turku, Finland: Centre for Continuing Education, Åbo Akademi University.

Serkkola, Ari. 1994. *A Sick Man Is Advised by a Hundred: Pluralistic Control of Tuberculosis in Southern Somalia.* Kuopio University Publications D, Medical Sciences 40. Kuopio, Finland: University of Kuopio, Department of Public Health.

Silveira, Ellen, and Shah Ebrahim. 1995. "Mental Health and Health Status of Elderly Bengalis and Somalis in London." *Age and Ageing* 24: 474–480.

Slikkerveer, Leendert J. 1990. *Plural Medical Systems in the Horn of Africa: The Legacy of "Sheikh" Hippocrates.* London: Kegan Paul International.

Statistics Finland. 2011. "2011 Population Structure. Language according to age and gender by region 1990–2010." Electronic Document: http://pxweb2.stat.fi/database/StatFin/vrm/vaerak/vaerak_en.asp.

Tiilikainen, Marja. 2001. "Suffering and Symptoms: Aspects of Everyday Life of Somali Refugee Women." In *Variations on the Theme of Somaliness*; Proceedings of the EASS/SSIA International Congress of Somali Studies, Turku, Finland, Aug. 6–9, 1988; ed. Muddle Suzanne Lilius, 309–317. Turku, Finland: Centre for Continuing Education, Åbo Akademi University.

———. 2003. *Arjen islam: Somalinaisten elämää Suomessa.* Tampere, Finland: Vastapaino.

———. 2005. "Suffering, Social Memory, and Embodiment: Experiences of Somali Refugee Women." *Pakistan Journal of Women's Studies: Alam-e-Niswan* 12 (2): 1–16.

———. 2010a. "Spirits and the Human World in Northern Somalia." In *Milk and Peace, Drought and War: Somali Culture, Society and Politics,* ed. Markus V. Hoehne and Virginia Luling, 163–184. London: Hurst and Company.

———. 2010b. "Sitaat as Part of Somali Women's Everyday Religion." In *Perspectives on Women's Everyday Religion,* ed. Marja-Liisa Keinänen, 203–218. Stockholm Studies on Comparative Religion 35. Stockholm: Stockholm University.

Tiilikainen, Marja, and Peter H. Koehn. 2011. "Transforming the Boundaries of Health Care: Insights from Somali Migrants." *Medical Anthropology* 30 (5). 518–544.

Vertovec, Steven. 2001. "Transnationalism and Identity." *Journal of Ethnic and Migration Studies* 27 (4): 573–582.

Wahlbeck, Östen. 1999a. "Flyktingforskning och begreppet diaspora: Att studera en transnationell social verklighet." *Sosiologia* 1999 (4): 269–279.

———. 1999b. *Kurdish Diasporas: A Comparative Study of Kurdish Refugee Communities.* Basingstoke, U.K.: Macmillan Press in association with Centre for Research in Ethnic Relations, University of Warwick.

ELEVEN

Mobility and Connectedness: Chinese Medical Doctors in Kenya

Elisabeth Hsu

Since the late 1980s, Kenya has seen a constant coming and going of Chinese medical doctors. These traveling medical experts have not been excessively numerous (during the last 20 years their numbers have ranged between only 20 and 40 persons at any point in time), and they are not exactly a public health issue, but the complexities of their situation are worthy of anthropological investigation. During my fieldwork, one of the most pressing questions that local patients, health personnel, acquaintances on the bus, or colleagues at the university asked was: who are these Chinese medical doctors and why have they come to us?

In order to answer this question asked by one set of actors during my fieldwork, I elicited the individual life stories of another set of actors, the Chinese doctors themselves. The question was simple; it came from the grassroots. The stories were moving, and they stand for themselves. However, their analysis points out important blanks in the medical anthropological literature.

First, while medical anthropology has seen a flurry of studies on patients' illness narratives (e.g., Kleinman 1988; Good and Good 1994; Mattingly 1998), practitioner narratives that highlight their vulnerability, and how it affects their medical practice, are few and far between (e.g., Katz 1985 and Hunter 1993).[1]

Second, only a few medical anthropologists have researched complementary and alternative medicines (CAM) in the urban centers of Third World countries (e.g., Napolitano 2002), and Chinese medicine in Africa belongs into this under-studied category. It appears as though medical anthropologists consider the First World to have CAM and the Third World to have TM, traditional medicines (the latter have been widely discussed in Kenya, see, e.g., Beckerleg 1994; Parkin 1995; Giles 1999; Geissler and Prince 2010).[2]

Third, particular patterns of mobility emerged from these narratives, patterns which—in good medical anthropological fashion—put the individual center-stage. They also highlight how little researched these patterns of mobility are.[3] Importantly, South–South relations, or more precisely, East–South relations have only recently attracted the interest of social scientists,[4] and even though China–Africa relations have now become a hot topic in the political sciences, ethnographic studies are still fairly limited (but see Haugen and Carling 2005; Dobler 2008; Hsu 2002, 2007, 2008). With regard to Chinese patterns of mobility, the finding that in Tanzania Chinese medical doctors mostly originated from northeastern China (Hsu 2002), rather than from the old sending areas of southeastern China (e.g., Pieke 2007: 83), pointed to a newly emerging sending region (Xiang forthcoming). The finding that in Kenya many Chinese medical doctors came from Shandong province, by contrast, falls into another well-known pattern of migratory flows between defined areas of origin and destination[5]: one Chinese medical doctor, who formerly had worked as a medical expert in one of the many Shandong medical teams sent on two-year missions to Tanzania and who shortly after his return to China had chosen to emigrate to Kenya, invited many Chinese medical physicians to work with him on his Kenyan premises, most of whom thereafter independently set foot elsewhere in the country.

The narratives reveal what could be interpreted as push and pull factors. On the one hand, they concern individuals who not infrequently had enjoyed a secure livelihood in the People's Republic of China (PRC) during the Cultural Revolution (1966–1976) but lost it due to the economic reforms that have taken place from 1978 until today.[6] On the other hand, they highlight certain conditions of the Kenyan health system that have facilitated the incursion of Chinese medical health provision. They touch on well-known problems within Kenyan biomedicine, where overwork, burnout syndromes, and an excess of red tape mutually reinforce each other in a downward spiral (Iliffe 1998: 169–199; Raviola et al. 2002), and where the profession is weakened by a relentless exodus of trained medical and paramedical personnel. However, to speak of push factors in the PRC and pull factors in Kenya would oversimplify the issue. Rather, this East–South medical transfer testifies to dynamics that recently have affected global health at large.

The medical experts interviewed openly declared of themselves that they made their living as business people, a finding that can be understood only in the light of the economic reforms in the PRC and of the current global trend toward the commercialization of health care. Biomedical ideology has it that health care is a service to humanity, not primarily a business, and in line with this ideology that is critical of those practitioners who make their living as entrepreneurs, some medical anthropologists have tended toward a condescending tone when highlighting the entrepreneurial skills of traditional medical doctors. The livelihood of biomedical health professionals who receive a salary from a state institution has not been a central anthropological theme of research. Since many of my interlocutors for this study previously were state-employed biomedical professionals before becoming medical entrepreneurs in Kenya, frequently as a consequence of early retirement schemes, this chapter makes inroads into barely discussed terrain in this respect as well.

After World War II, health care became a responsibility of the state, not only in Europe and North America, but also in the many nation-states that declared their independence in the following decades. The WHO made it its mission to work through these nascent bureaucratic structures of the nation-state (Fee, Cueto, and Brown forthcoming). However, as world economies turned to neoliberalism, health care was among the sectors affected. The media has perhaps commented on this neoliberal turn most loudly (see, e.g., the film *Sicko* by Michael Moore, released in 2007); while medical anthropology highlighted the increased reliance on the purchase of pharmaceuticals, not least for treating mental health problems (e.g., Luhrmann 2001). The shift in jargon from "international health" to "global health" hints at this shift away from health care delivery as a point of pride of national sovereignty (aided by the WHO) to health care as globally interlinked entrepreneurship (Brown, Cueto, and Fee 2006).

The worldwide trend toward liberalism weakened the WHO and allowed the World Bank to gain the center stage in health policies.[7] Diverse efforts to reduce the red tape-ism in the bureaucracies of the nation-state by encouraging direct bilateral relations between health institutions and foreign donors, along with other market driven considerations, have led to the unregulated activity of entrepreneurial organizations in health care (often NGOs and other private enterprises), among which the recently opened Chinese medical clinics in Kenya belong. In a world where the sovereignty of the state is increasingly encumbered by interdependencies between global assemblages,[8] health care appears to be slipping out of the remit of the state's responsibilities. In medical ethics, these developments have received a critical appraisal (e.g., Pellegrino 1999), but in 2001, when this research began, medical anthropologists had only just started to become interested in how this neoliberal order has affected global health at large and the individual therapeutic encounter in particular.

The above should make clear that a simple question from the grassroots on a curious phenomenon in contemporary health care—Chinese medicine in Kenya—has highlighted a dearth of medical anthropological research in several areas: namely, on narratives of health professionals, on CAM in the Third World, and on the East–South medical transfer. Is it that medical anthropology has become too (bio)medicalized? Is its research too much defined by Western public health agendas? The questions raised above suggest that medical anthropology needs to broaden its agenda to include, in particular, research on health issues in the urban centers of the developing world, and the commercialization of health on the global scale. Furthermore, medical anthropology needs to understand itself as a discipline that in its social critique dares also to explore taboo areas of biomedical ideology. The livelihood of biomedical professionals affects the care they deliver. Health professionals are human beings with a life history, with narratives about it, and with a culture, which in the case of traveling medical experts often is alien to the recipients of their medical care.

Notes on the Sociology of the Chinese Medical Doctors in Kenya

Chinese medical doctors in Kenya have in common that they are Chinese from the PRC, that they advertise themselves as competent in delivering Chinese medicine, and that they make a livelihood of it. They furthermore have in common that they all have moved into Kenya since the late 1980s and 1990s, and they are, as are many other Chinese in Kenya, entrepreneurs. Most are men, who came on their own (whether single, married, or divorced), or with a partner, and/or with family. In April 2003, they numbered about 20 in Nairobi (of whom about five were women), three in Mombasa, one in Kisumu, one in Eldoret, and one in Nakuru. Africa (*Feizhou*) as a concept did not merely invoke the foreign, but also racist prejudice, fuelled by recurrent media accounts in the PRC of African students raping Chinese women.[9] All Chinese I interviewed knew about this stereotype. Even if they did not embrace it, they all considered Africa underdeveloped and backward (*luohou*). Nevertheless, they had moved to Africa and built up a living. Why?[10]

Chinese medical doctors in Kenya and in Africa at large are generally not held in high esteem in the PRC; they are not considered "real" (*zhengui*) Chinese medical doctors with "deep" (*shen'ao*) insight into Chinese medicine. Indeed, their educational levels varied, although all, even those who had had exposure to Chinese medicine within a family tradition, claimed to have undergone training in Traditional Chinese Medicine (TCM), the revived form of Chinese medicine taught at government institutions in the PRC (Farquhar 1994; Hsu 1999; Scheid 2002; Taylor 2005).

In the sample of the approximately 20 doctors I interviewed in 2001 and 2003, only one practitioner had a post-graduate degree (*shuoshi*). Four had been regular students at a TCM college with five years of training in Chinese (and also Western) medicine. Two had three years of vocational training in TCM (and Western medicine). Two had attended, as full-time students, special classes in either acupuncture or "integrated Chinese and Western medicine" (*zhongxiyi jiehe*) for four years. Several had only attended evening classes at a

TCM college, between one to four years. Among the latter were biomedically trained doctors (two who had five years of training), biomedically trained health workers (five), and members of non-medical professions (three). Some had many years of work experience, some none. Regardless of their education, they all advertised themselves as competent in "Chinese medicine" or "Traditional Chinese Medicine," but the various forms of medicine that they delivered are probably more accurately described as manifestations of "integrated Chinese and Western medicine" (*zhongxiyi jiehe*).

The questions I asked, apart from the sociological ones on family background and education, centered on the motivations that instigated the dislocation from their homelands, the difficulties encountered in the recipient country, and the cultural differences perceived. I also asked my interlocutors about the nature of their separation from the homeland. The dual experiences of "separation and reunion," according to Charles Stafford (2000), form a theme that, if not unique to Chinese cultures, is definitely a dominant in them, and Chinese medical doctors in Kenya play on this theme in interesting ways: on the grounds of their life stories and self-presentation, I emphasize their "mobility and connectedness," and the continuous state of ambiguity in which they live. This quality of ambiguity became particularly evident from the question I asked at the end of the interview, which was whether they thought of moving back to China in the future. It put their voluntary dislocation into perspective: almost none considered spending old age in Kenya. One doctor commented: "None of these doctors has bought property here." She herself was using Kenya as a stepping-stone to get to Canada. This observation is in line with others that Chinese migratory processes since the 1990s are not only driven by an unusually overt economic zest but also by heightened mobility (Pieke et al. 2004). The contacts to the home country are not given up, but cultivated, not least for business. Integration into the recipient country is minimal. One hesitates to speak of these Chinese migrants as "settlers."[11]

Having said this, three out of my sample of 21 Chinese doctors did speak of settling into Kenya. One was a Cantonese woman, a Western medical doctor by training who had married a Kenyan whom she had met in medical school in Canton and with whom she founded a family in Nairobi. The other was also a biomedical doctor, who on his first visit back home after seven years in Kenya realized that it was most unlikely he would ever settle again in China. In the era of the economic reforms, his colleagues had acquired new biomedical knowledge and skills to such an extent that he had no chance of catching up with them again. The third was one of the first Chinese medical doctors to emigrate to Kenya, in 1988. He hoped to accumulate enough money in Nairobi to be a pensioner in China but, well aware that life among the middle classes was in the meantime more modernized and more expensive in China than it was in Kenya, and that the Chinese economy was rising while the Kenyan one was decreasing, he said: "If I am constrained to stay here long-term, I can do it, but I can't eat African food." For him, as for many of the other doctors and their families, the geographical separation from China did not fundamentally alter their culinary culture.

Forms of Mobility

The mobility of some doctors was rather remarkable. It was sometimes pendular, and involved a moving back and forth between the PRC and Kenya; sometimes it was more web-like, with points of connectedness all over the globe; finally, it could also involve shifting across different stations within Kenya. In what follows I will describe examples of these three modes of mobility.

STAR-LIKE FORM OF MOBILITY

Dr. Qiao, after working 17 years at the Railway Central Hospital in Harbin, took advantage of an early retirement scheme in 1992. In the late 1980s and 1990s such early retirement schemes made it possible for work units (*danwei*) to free positions held by victims of the Cultural Revolution, whose schooling was not as reliable as that of young professionals trained in the 1980s after the Dengist reforms. Dr. Qiao emphasized that he had passed the entrance examinations to medical school in 1965. Although he did not mention it, it is clear that anyone at university between 1966–1969 would not have received much formal training, because during those years universities were closed and academics persecuted. In the early 1990s, many work unit members undertook entrepreneurial activities (*xiahaile*); in northeastern China (Dongbei) there was a fashion (*you re*) to emigrate to post-Gorbachev Russia. Dr. Qiao had work experience as a Western medical doctor, but worked as an acupuncturist at a Lada car factory. He said he liked the Russians—they were honest (*laoshi*). He soon returned to China to divorce his wife in order to marry a Russian woman, whom he divorced, however, a few years later, in 1998, when he returned to China. He said this with a laugh (which sounded sad to me). While it is often the case that Chinese Western-trained doctors offer their services as Chinese doctors (*zhongyi*) and acupuncturists (*zhenjiu shi*) outside their home country, usually after taking one to four years of evening classes, only a few get married to locals. Dr. Qiao said that it was a "young and beautiful girl" who wanted to marry him, and that this also enabled him to get a residence permit. Romantic feeling was thus coupled with overcoming the administrative problems of the migrant. Dr. Qiao did not explain why he returned to China in 1998. Given that his first wife was the daughter of a high-ranking military commander, he said he now encountered increased difficulties in his home province. He bought property in Dalian, a resort place on the shores of Bohai, but soon became bored as a pensioner at only 52 years old. So, he emigrated to Ghana.

Dr. Qiao explained that he had worked for two years as a member of a Chinese medical team for the Tanzanian railway in 1977–1979.[12] In the 1970s, he had become quite fond of Africans—they too were honest (*laoshi*)—but times had now changed, he commented. "African people today," he said in broken English, "they give you many traps, they are very tricky, I was cheated many times." In the late 1990s, there were, according to Dr. Qiao, about four to five Chinese doctors in Accra, among them himself as an acupuncturist. As explanation for his return from Ghana to China after only two years, he said that four Chinese had died of malaria (he said "cerebral malaria") within a space of six months. He bought another house in China, this time in a popular resort place in the south, on Hainan Island. However, at 54 years of age, he felt he was "not yet so old" and could still "make money," although he quickly added, "I have not come here only to make money." He now moved into East instead of West Africa. He first visited Tanzania, but Tanzania was too poor, he said, not a suitable place for making money. A chance encounter with a native (*laoxiang*) from northeastern China brought him to Nairobi. However, within a few weeks of living there, he was robbed at 7:00 AM in the morning,[13] and anyway, "Nairobi was too crowded." So, he moved to a town on the periphery of Kenya.

Dr. Qiao's narrative draws out a pendulum movement of inward and outward mobility, to and from China. It is not exactly an oscillating mobility in that Dr. Qiao did not move back and forth between one place and the other, but into different places inside and outside of China. If one takes the PRC as the center, it was a star-like movement. Although Dr. Qiao had residences in different places, the far north and the far south, he referred to the PRC as the center of his movement. Naturally, he was physically "separated" from his homeland, but in his narrative his sense of being "mobile" was more pronounced.

One could also say that Dr. Qiao's narrative testifies to the fate of the "lost generation": his marriages failed and his entrepreneurial achievements were only temporary. His mobility could be viewed as the response to such failure. The seed of his failures, one could say, was the fate of being enrolled in medical school during the Cultural Revolution. On the other hand, he was also an agile navigator of adverse situations: he had married the daughter of an important military commander, and although he only mentioned the disadvantages of the divorce, there must have been advantages in professional life and general livelihood during the marriage; he experienced love in Russia, and once he put his mind to "making money" was able to buy two houses in highly desired Chinese resort places. In the PRC those who migrate to Africa are likely to be viewed as losers, due to the above stereotypes about Africa and a general bias against the foreign as barbaric, but even if to a certain extent he was a "loser" because he did not win out in the competitions within the PRC, his mobility was that of a skilful entrepreneur who liked life with a tint of adventure.

WEB-LIKE FORM OF MOBILITY

The other form of mobility is more complex, in that it involves more than one central point of inward and outward movement. It may not be coincidence that several doctors engaged in this form of mobility were a generation younger than the Cultural Revolution cohort (to which Dr. Qiao belonged). Nevertheless, like most life histories of PRC citizens, those of these young doctors suggested that they too were victims of political circumstance. Dr Chen explained that he had been among the active student demonstrators in 1989 and that he had a file with the police. Neither Dr. Qiao nor Dr. Chen presented themselves as victims of political movements, however, and they did not consider themselves political refugees. They spoke in a matter-of-fact manner of political movements, as though these were part of the geographic landscape into which they were born. Dr. Chen was at the time studying English at an inferior university in Chengdu (he had failed the entrance exams to study history at Sichuan University), and already before the 1989 movement had the desire to go abroad. He worked as a tour guide in Tibet, set out to learn the art of Chinese cuisine from an acquaintance who was a cook, and enrolled in evening classes on Chinese medicine.[14] Finally, in 1994, he seized the opportunity to go abroad as an interpreter for a Sichuanese firm involved in a project at the electric power station of Owen Falls in Uganda.

Dr. Chen generally was vague about his past movements in China and Africa; I pieced the above information together from different conversations with him and his wife, and also from comments other doctors made about him in passing. However, he was articulate about future movements. In 2001, when I visited his clinic for the first time, he had just married his girlfriend from Sichuan, but shortly after their wedding in Kenya she had moved to Chile, because, as he explained, a friend working at the Chilean Chinese embassy had told them that Chilean citizenship could be easily acquired once one had been resident there.¹⁵ So, the couple moved between China, South America, and Africa, and before long, his wife became pregnant. In December 2001 the future father declared that he intended to prevent his child from becoming a "banana" (*xiangjiao*), outside yellow and inside white (meaning with the yellow skin color of a Chinese person but a Westernized mind). He wished his wife to give birth in the PRC. Eventually, however, their daughter was born in Kenya. "The Indian doctor we had was so competent," Dr. Chen's wife chided.

During my visit in spring 2003, the three were enjoying the dream of the nuclear family living in a one-family house in a chic suburb, with an African nanny, a quality car (air-conditioned), and special access to a beach resort. They were adamant that they intended to make "big money," and this, according to them, was possible only in Third World countries, not in the First World with its tight tax regulations. They spoke of moving on, not to the U.S.A. nor to Europe, but to Chile and perhaps eventually to Canada. Their minimally furnished house was tangible testimony to their commitment to mobility.¹⁶ Unlike the pendular movement to and from a center, the movement of this couple appeared more like a web, spread out over the globe, with various points of contact.

"SHIFTING," BUT STAYING PUT

Most doctors did not work in the same medical practice they had originally started in. Most had moved around the suburbs of Nairobi, and their clinics opened and closed at a fairly high rate. Of the 11 clinics I visited in December 2001, two had moved from one place to another within the same suburb, two had closed, and three had opened or re-opened in a new place by April 2003.¹⁷ Ever since the late 1980s, when the first practice opened in Nairobi, there has been a constant to-ing and fro-ing of Chinese medical doctors. However, as a visit in 2006 revealed, more instances of shifting practices had been observed among those who stayed in Kenya between 2001 and 2003 than between 2003 and 2006. Regardless of how often practitioners shifted within Nairobi or Kenya initially, once they had come to terms with making their livelihood in Kenya, at least for the foreseeable future, they stayed put. This did not usually diminish their close connection to the PRC, which was easy to maintain electronically through internet, email, and Skype, whereas the mobile phone was used mostly for local communication. They also upheld their home connections physically: one commuted for business purposes on a biweekly schedule; others at longer regular and irregular intervals; some because their spouse, or their child, or their spouse and child, or their parents required their care. Some returned for Chinese New Year—but not necessarily every year, and many would choose not to buy the airline tickets during the festive period when they were particularly expensive.

Motives for Mobility

No doubt, the above forms of mobility were motivated largely, but not only, by economic zest. One of my interview questions was what had motivated the interviewee to come to Kenya, and many of the answers included mention of one individual, Dr. Ru. He had been a member of the prestigious medical teams from Shandong province that were sent to Tanzania in the 1970s. He had treated Julius Nyerere, then the president of Tanzania, in person, as large photos in the spacious waiting room of his practice showed. He had become involved in local politics, other doctors told me, was sent back to Shandong, and then emigrated from there to Nairobi in the late 1980s. He was not the first doctor from the PRC to emigrate to Nairobi, but he was the best known among the expatriate community. Between 2001 and 2003, he was involved with a research project funded by the Ford Foundation to evaluate the efficacy of his brand of an herbal tea with which he treated HIV / AIDS patients.

When I asked Dr. Ru why he had moved to Kenya, he said one word: "Freedom" (*ziyou*). It implied that he knew that people in Kenya considered democratic states to have more freedom than socialist ones. He disagreed when I mentioned to him that other Chinese medical doctors had told me they had moved to Kenya to do "medicine as business." "Not only," he said. However, he could not deny that he was a good businessman. In March 2003, he was the director of a successful Chinese medical clinic and a "factory" for making herbal pills, tablets, capsules, and gels, and he apparently employed over 30 staff. His intentions of expansion had brought several other Chinese medical doctors from Shandong to Kenya. He had invited them to work in his clinic, and several of them later set up their own clinics. One doctor had worked in Burundi for 18 months; another had tried for four months to set up a clinic in Sudan before moving to Nairobi; both had been well received by Dr. Ru and also briefly worked for him. Dr. Ru's practice thus represented the gateway to Kenya for the majority of Chinese medical doctors working in Nairobi. As already noted, this pattern of migration is well documented (Levitt and Glick Schiller 2004: 1009). Shandong was the province in charge of the neighboring nation of Tanzania; other provinces had similar relations to other African nations (Yunnan to Uganda, Sichuan to Zambia). Kenya had never had such close political relations with the PRC, and thus a doctor who had fallen into disgrace with the Socialist regime had no problem setting foot in Nairobi.

While Dr. Ru's move to Kenya may have been politically rather than economically motivated, the doctors he attracted seemed to be a different story. They stated, often with a disarming candor, that they were "doing business" as though they had no sense that medicine is considered an altruistic or humanitarian service. It appeared as though they had learnt in the PRC of the 1990s that "doing business" was a laudable activity and required no further explanation. However, other motivations also surfaced in the course of our conversations; they were political, ideological, idealistic, and, in particular, educational.[18]

There is more to be said about the motives prompting people into mobility than can be said in this space. It would be wrong to say that Kenya attracted the losers of the Dengist reforms, just as it would be wrong to say that it attracted dissidents. Nevertheless, although the life histories of Chinese medical doctors in Kenya do show traits of both, these were never presented to me as being as relevant as education. Several Chinese medical doctors had teenage children for whom they aspired to procure a better education than their own. For instance, one couple, of the Cultural Revolution cohort, had emigrated to Kenya in the early 1990s and managed to pay for the education of two sons at a U.S. university. Two other Chinese women doctors were mothers who had moved to Kenya with their teenage children, a daughter and a son, respectively, intent on sending the child later to an American university. Their medical practices in Kenya were not exactly thriving, but their husbands ran lucrative businesses in the PRC.

The most moving personal life histories came to the fore when I asked the Chinese medical doctors about their motivations for the move from China to Africa. These revealed connectedness to their kin in the PRC, to Chinese food, and to Chinese cultural values in general. Their efforts striving for their offspring's good education was a cultural aspect of life that, in their minds, was intrinsically Chinese. In this way, they remained deeply connected to China and to what they considered essential to Chinese culture.

Mobility and New Encounters

The Chinese medical doctors mentioned three groups of people in Kenya with whom they made connections: their fellow Chinese, representatives of the Kenyan authorities, and their patients.

ENCOUNTERS WITH FELLOW CHINESE

Some doctors had fairly close relations to other Chinese, fellow practitioners or other business people, others had barely any. Some would phone each other on a regular basis, they might have lunch together in a cyber cafe, or their spouses would visit each other for a chat. Most were involved with some kind of transaction of material goods with each other, be it a computer or a car, books, magazines, newspapers, or videos. Some also cooked for each other, particularly if someone fell ill. Emotions were expressed through the idiom of food; the gift of food expressed polite and/or heartfelt care, and comments on its quality reflected on the quality of the friendship. Some wrote letters for business people with lesser educational backgrounds, including, for instance, love letters to a prospective partner found in cyberspace. In general, the interviewees emphasized, however, that they enjoyed the relative autonomy they had in Kenya, and they were not eager to tighten their relations with other Chinese. Having said this, most doctors in Nairobi were in touch with a representative of the Ministry of Commerce at the Chinese Embassy. Apparently, one of them had put forth the idea that this representative should write letters of recommendation to facilitate their access to the necessary Kenyan authorities (the City Council and the Department of Culture or, more recently, the Ministry of Health) so they could be green-lit for opening a medical practice. However, at the time this happened several other doctors were already well established, and they had not depended on such a letter of recommendation from the embassy; some of those made clear to me that they did not wish to have any relations with Chinese officials at all.

ENCOUNTERS WITH KENYAN AUTHORITIES

Chinese medical doctors did not openly complain about the attitude of the Kenyan government toward their practice, perhaps because of their uncertainty about my status, perhaps out of habit, but it was clear that there were problems. Many Chinese medical doctors (but not all) were selling a very small number of Western medical drugs that had been produced in China (aspirin, penicillin, and sulfonamids, in particular), and they knew that the government disapproved of and criminalized this activity. Throughout the period of my yearly fieldwork stints, the Kenyan government was increasing its efforts to regulate the health care market. In September 2002, there had been a meeting of both Chinese medical doctors and Kenyan healers and diviners with representatives of the Ministry of Health. Certificates for opening practices of "traditional medicine" in the past had been issued by the Department of Culture, but in future were to be issued by the Ministry of Health. This was for some Chinese medical doctors a veritable worry, although it was a development similar to that in other nation-states, including the PRC, where until the mid-1950s Chinese medicine was under the jurisdiction of the Ministry of Commerce before it came under the Ministry of Health's. The difference was that the government in the PRC had been more favorable to the development of traditional medicines then (Taylor 2005: 75ff.) than the Kenyan government was now.

A Chinese doctor commented:

> There are three points that the biomedical doctors of the Kenyan authorities do not understand: first, they have not had firsthand experience of our traditional medicine, and have prejudices against it; second, they think Western medicine can solve all health problems, without the help of traditional medicines; third, there is also a question of competition between traditional and modern medicine on the health market, that should not be underestimated.

At the meeting in question, health officials had declared that each "traditional medical" ingredient in a drug should be tested for its efficacy in Kenya before coming onto the market, according to Kenyan rather than PRC standards. Given that Chinese medical doctors were selling up to hundred and more different ready-made formula drugs, each constituted by several ingredients, it is clear that such a decision would make all their business illegal. In a series of smaller follow-up meetings, it also became clear that the Kenyan government did not have the facilities to carry out the necessary tests. The debate about the regulation of traditional and complementary and alternative medicines is still ongoing.

Although Chinese medical doctors felt marginalized, none was keen on setting up an association. First, the mere idea of becoming part of a politically active organization was unappealing. Second, any regulatory body would have to include some but exclude others. The extreme variations in educational background were one reason for this. Furthermore, opinions about each others' competence were strong and not always good. So, despite the obstacles they faced from the Kenyan government, and the advantages that a union might have brought, all Chinese medical doctors interviewed in 2001 and 2003 upheld the motto that each should care for his or her own business.

ENCOUNTERS WITH PATIENTS

The people Chinese medical doctors encountered on a daily basis were their patients. They were mainly Kenyans, of Kikuyu and other ethnicity, and also, quite frequently, refugees from Somalia or Sudan. Chinese medical doctors treated their patients with respect, and they also told me that they valued the respect that their patients gave them (some maintained that in the First World CAM practitioners would not be treated with the same respect, and they gave this as a reason why they chose to go to Africa). Based on participant observation, it is fair to say that the practitioners interviewed were genuinely interested in trying to help and care for their patients. Simultaneously, they also were interested in selling their medicines. As in other traditional medical settings, prescriptions and the prices of prescriptions depended partly on the doctor's evaluation of the patient's spending power. Many encounters with patients were warm and friendly, and some doctors had known certain of their clientele for over a decade.

A few doctors had made one or two close Kenyan friends. When asked about them, they commented that they were unpretentious and true (*shizai*), praised their good heartedness (*xin hao*) and humor, and said they were good company. Most Chinese medical doctors, however, barely had any local friends. "Africans," a Chinese doctor commented, "what should I say about them, I don't really know them . . .." He pointed to the lack of social responsibility he felt they had, in particular the government's complete lack of social responsibility: government authorities just would not care about the people. He expressed admiration for the optimism with which the common people encountered difficult life situations; with no money, no job, no anything, yet they knew how to be happy. Although he said this with a certain admiration, it reminded me of the paternalistic view colonizers once held toward Africans whom they had stereotyped as happy-go-lucky. The doctor concluded, "They make no plans, all happens in the moment." This made it difficult to form friendships with them. Perhaps long-term friendships were rare, but romantic involvements, if more short-lived, were known to occur with slightly more frequency. Despite the AIDS scare, several male doctors were said to have had local girlfriends, generally without marriage being a considered option. Two doctors were exceptions, having become married to Kenyans in the course of my fieldwork. Moreover, some of the Chinese teenagers dressed like their schoolmates and insisted on wearing Kenyan hairstyles, and there were prospects of these second-generation Chinese having intimate friends who were locals.

In general, the medical anthropological literature emphasizes the services in a direction going *from* doctors *to* their clientele; it explores the relationship between doctor and patient in this light and discusses treatment evaluation from this perspective. My research among Chinese doctors in Africa demonstrates, however, that patients can also have lasting effects on their doctors. Doctors, just like patients, sometimes need to come to terms with difficult life situations. More importantly, the patient–practitioner relationship may often be more marked by a mutual give and take than is generally assumed. My interviews accounted for an aspect of life that had a lasting effect on Chinese medical doctors, and sometimes resulted directly from the encounters with their clientele: this is religiosity.

One doctor, a party member, confided in me that she was impressed with the faith of her patients in God and by the inner strength this gave them to cope with their illness. "Africans are simple-minded (*pushi*)," she commented, "they got a Christian education." She implied with this that Christianity provided guidance for them. She herself was complicated (*fuza*), like Chinese generally are, and therefore, it was impossible for her to believe in God. However, she was impressed by the physical and psychological strength that the belief in God engendered in her patients.

Another doctor commented: "I think the church is good, if there were no African church, the Africans would develop into bad people, just like the Chinese have in recent years." He explained to me that if I was to go to China again now: "You would not be able to adapt, I myself cannot adapt. Can you imagine, young Chinese people now think the elderly ought to die, they have no conscience whatsoever (*genben meiyou liangxin*)." His outrage reflected deeply engrained Confucian filial piety, although he was not an intellectual (*zhishifenzi*) who would say of himself that he adhered to Confucian morals. Rather, he identified himself as a Buddhist. He had read the bible, he had been given many booklets by Christian missionaries, he had heard his patients speak of God, but he decided against converting. Unlike another Chinese medical doctor, he had not reserved a spot for incense burning on the floor in the waiting room of his practice in front of a painted scroll depicting the deity Guanyin, nor did his ideas strike me as particularly Buddhist. Yet in his case the Christianity of his patients had reinforced his awareness of, and adherence to, his own religion, which he said was Buddhist. Considering that he was from a modest rural background, and (along with many others of similar social standing) due to the Cultural Revolution had received a very basic form of medical education, there is little doubt he adhered to what the literature calls "Chinese popular religion" (Shahar and Weller 1996: 1).

In 2001, there was a fellowship of about 20 Chinese Christians who met at least once weekly, on Sunday afternoons, in central Nairobi. By 2003, two of the 21 Chinese doctors I interviewed had converted to Christianity and were members of this fellowship. They had made the most visible steps away from the values they were familiar with before moving to Kenya. One had fallen in love with a local Kenyan lady, and for this reason had become Christian; they first had a child, then another one, and only years later got married. The other claimed to have been saved from being a gambler due to his conversion; he had plans of leaving Africa to be trained in pastoral work in Southeast Asia.

In summary, encounters in Kenya with fellow Chinese, Kenyan authorities, and patients opened up new avenues for these mobile medical experts to become connected to their recipient country, although the overall trend among them was toward self-reliance and self-containment. New forms of connectedness appear to have arisen, in particular, through their work with patients whose Christian faith moved them. The widely acknowledged power that patients drew from their faith encouraged two Chinese doctors to join a Christian fellowship, within a time span of just about a year. This fellowship itself was Singaporean, and offered not merely Kenyan but also transnational forms of connectedness.

This chapter concerns the narratives of Chinese medical doctors who are migrant entrepreneurs in Kenya. Two themes that recurrently emerged in these narratives were the speakers' "mobility" and their "connectedness." For almost all doctors old age was to be spent in China; their venture into Africa was thus temporary, their separation from the PRC not final. Some regularly returned for reunions with family and friends at the Chinese New Year before separating again for a year, but most returned to China only once in several years. Rather than enacting periodic reunions, their connectedness consisted in a "way of being" (Levitt and Glick Schiller 2004: 1010), through the importation of material goods like medicines and foods; Chinese (and Taiwanese) pop music and videos; and continued adherence to Confucian morals or Buddhist religious practice.

The themes of "mobility and connectedness" elaborate on the themes of "separation and reunion" (Stafford 2000). This chapter comments on these themes through the actors' own narratives. Agility or flexibility (*ling*) is a cherished quality in Chinese cultures, particularly in religious contexts (Sangren 1987), but also in medical ones (Farquhar 1994 renders it as "virtuosity"). Connectedness, *tong,* is a quality that the ancient sages sought: they aimed to be connected with the universe (Sivin 1991 renders *tong* as "continuity"), and in medicine there is a saying that if there is connectedness, then there is no pain—*tong bu tong.* Although the Chinese doctors I interviewed did not mention these terms, their narratives conveyed a sense of being alive through *ling* (being flexible) and *tong* (being connected). An interesting aspect for further analysis would be how this understanding of their own lives shaped their medical practice and encounters with their clientele.

John Bowlby's attachment theory applies to humanity in general. The "mobility and connectedness" of these Chinese should not be ethinicized, but rather understood to be features common among migrants who wish to entertain continuing ties to their home country. "Mobility and connectedness" may accordingly also be a sociocultural idiom that captures the situation of many migrants in the current neoliberal world order.

In their narratives, only a few practitioners presented their profession as a vocation. Instead they spoke about the problems of making a livelihood while carrying out responsibilities for a family—parents, in-laws, and children. One of their main concerns was securing the future of their offspring, mainly in the form of a good education, ideally in the U.S. (entry into Europe was considered unobtainable). One of their main problems was their status as TM/CAM practitioners, which to them was more worrying than their immigrant status. It relegated their practice into the realm of the unregulated if not the illegal (Adams 2002). However, no one supported any initiative of organizing themselves into a social body of any kind, even if it would result in an association that might ameliorate their professional standing. This attitude is best understood in light of past experiences in the PRC. All practitioners upheld the ethos of not excessively inquiring into or interfering in each others' business (which did not, however hinder some individuals in developing close friendships).

Ong (2006) argues that governments of nation-states are active agents who navigate neoliberalism in their own interest. Indeed, the Kenyan state could consider improving its primary care by regulating the status of Chinese health professionals, not least through working with the Chinese authorities, and then aim to attract well-trained TCM experts from the PRC for specific health care tasks into Kenya. Instead, the state-approved biomedical establishment is entrenching its position through the protracted non-regulation of CAM. Prospects are that well-trained TCM professionals will avoid immigrating into Kenya, and that some of those who are there, while they may once have received a reasonable education, are not maintaining their professional standards. While a few doctors will survive as protégés of rich and politically powerful clientele, the current neoliberal order fosters a climate conducive to attracting minimally educated Chinese medical entrepreneurs into the informal sector—that is, not well-trained medical practitioners, but drug sellers who are jacks of all trade.

Acknowledgments

This article represents part of ongoing research on Chinese medicine in East Africa funded by the British Academy; British Institute of Eastern Africa; Chiang Chingkuo Foundation for International Scholarly Exchange; the Oppenheimer Fund of Queen Elizabeth House; and the Institute of Social and Cultural Anthropology, University of Oxford. For valuable comments on earlier versions of this manuscript, originally written in 2002, I thank David

Parkin, Frank Pieke, Charles Stafford, and Ellie Vasta; for advice in 2008 on how to finalize it for publication, I thank the editors of this volume.

Notes

1. Shimazono (unpubl.) made this point most forcefully.

2. On WHO policies toward the combined categories TM/CAM, see Bodeker et al. (2005).

3. While it is the case that there are studies on the health of immigrants, particularly within applied medical anthropology, those focus mainly on patients as migrants and not on practitioners. Even within migration studies, the mobility of health professionals barely has been researched. A recent publication on physician migration undertaken by medical researchers is based merely on questionnaires (Astor et al. 2005).

4. When this study began, these had as yet barely been researched. Howell (1995: 172) had mentioned in passing flows "between non-western societies" in her discussion on flows of religion and art into the West.

5. "There may be one individual who maintains high levels of homeland contact and is the node through which information, resources and identities flow" (Levitt and Glick Schiller 2004: 1009).

6. They thus throw light on the recent economic reforms from an as-yet barely discussed angle that complements research into contemporary China.

7. I draw here on personal communications with foreign health officials in Tanzania in 2001 and with medical historians at a workshop on the history of the WHO in Arribida, Portugal, 2007.

8. Hörbst and Wolf (2003), inspired by Appadurai (1990), speak of "medicoscapes."

9. Students from many African countries have been sent to socialist China on a regular basis to receive higher education, mainly in the sciences, medicine, and engineering.

10. The life stories of the Chinese medical doctors were elicited in two semi-directed interviews, usually in Chinese: once in December 2001 without a tape recorder and once in April 2003 with a tape recorder. A Kenyan anthropologist, Mwenda Ntarangwi, had located these doctors and their clinics, often in wealthy suburban supermarket complexes, and had carried out a preliminary survey in English a month before the first interviews. Some other doctors were found through the snowball method. For the evaluation of their narratives, I draw heavily on participant observation in multi-sited fieldwork during yearly one-month visits from 2001–2008.

11. Cohen (1997: 85–89), based on Wang Gongwu's reasearch, described the Chinese of Late Imperial China who migrated from Fujian and Guangdong to Southeast Asia as "sojourners" rather than "settlers." Similar traits seem to apply to the Chinese migrant doctors in Kenya in the post-Mao era.

12. He used the word "medical team" (*yiliaodui*), because that invoked prestige, but he was not one of the government-selected Shandong physicians who established the high reputation of the "medicine of the Chinese" (*dawa ya*

Kichina) in Tanzania; he was a member of a medical team working for Tazara, the Tanzania-Zambia railway, which also continues to be remembered for their competent medical services. See Hsu (2002).

13. He was not the only Chinese doctor to have been robbed at gunpoint; it had happened to almost all the Chinese medical doctors I interviewed in Nairobi.

14. Chinese immigrants often spread themselves thin as they aim to make business out of their exoticness, e.g., the exotic food or medicine they offer (Jørgen Carling, personal communication, 2005).

15. On the gender role of women as earners of residence permits, see Ong (1999: 127–129). Ong describes men as "astronauts" in midair shuttling across borders on the trans-Pacific business commute, whereas the movements of Dr. Chen and his wife are more web-like.

16. Parkin (2002) points out the minimal objects owned by refugees, and also by migrants, who engage in a more general process of "self-inscription in non-commodity."

17. There were a handful of other doctors who had moved in and out of Nairobi and who returned to China before I had a chance to interview them.

18. They are spelled out in Hsu (forthcoming).

References

Adams, Vincanne. 2002. "Randomized Controlled Crime: Postcolonial Sciences in Alternative Medicine Research." *Studies of Social Science* 32 (5–6): 659–690.

Appadurai, Arjun. 1990. "Disjuncture and Difference in the Global Cultural Economy." *Public Culture* 2 (2): 1–24.

Astor, Avraham, Tasleem Akhtar, María Alexandra Matallana, Vasantha Muthuswamy, Folarin A. Olowu, Veronica Tallo, and Reidar K. Lie. 2005. "Physician Migration: Views from Professionals in Colombia, Nigeria, India, Pakistan, and the Philippines." *Social Science and Medicine* 61 (12): 2492–2500.

Beckerleg, Susan. 1994. "Medical Pluralism and Islam in Swahili Communities in Kenya." *Medical Anthropology Quarterly* 8 (3): 299–313.

Bodeker, Gerard, Chi-Keong Ong, Christopher Grundy, Gemma Burford, and Kin Shein, eds. 2005. *WHO Global Atlas of Traditional, Complementary, and Alternative Medicine.* Kobe, Japan: World Health Organization.

Brown, Theodore M., Marcos Cueto, and Elizabeth Fee. 2006. "The World Health Organization and the Transition From 'International' to 'Global' Public Health." *American Journal of Public Health* 96 (1): 62–72.

Cohen, Robin. 1997. *Global Diasporas: An Introduction.* London: UCL Press.

Dobler, Gregor. 2008. "Solidarity, Xenophobia, and the Regulation of Chinese Businesses in Namibia." In *China Returns to Africa: A Rising Power and a Continent Embrace,* ed. Chris Alden, Daniel Large, and Ricardo Soares de Oliveira, 237–255. London: Hurst.

Farquhar, Judith. 1994. *Knowing Practice: The Clinical Encounter of Chinese Medicine.* Boulder, Colo.: Westview Press.

Fee, Elizabeth, Marcos Cueto, and Theodore Brown. Forthcoming. *Global Health: A History of the World Health Organization.*

Geissler, Paul W., and Ruth Prince. 2010. *"The Land is Dying": Contingency, Creativity, and Conflict in Western Kenya.* Oxford: Berghahn.

Giles, Linda L. 1999. "Spirit Possession and the Symbolic Construction of Swahili Society." In *Spirit Possession, Modernity, and Power,* ed. Heike Behrend and Ute Luig, 142–164. London: James Curry.

Good, Byron J., and Mary-Jo DelVecchio Good. 1994. "In the Subjunctive Mode: Epilepsy Narratives in Turkey." *Social Science and Medicine* 38 (6): 835–842.

Haugen, Heidi, and Jørgen Carling. 2005. "On the Edge of the Diaspora: the Surge of Baihuo Business in an African City." *Ethnic and Racial Studies* 28 (4): 639–662.

Hörbst, Viola, and Angelika Wolf. 2003. "Globaliserung der Heilkunde: Eine Einführung." In *Medizin und Globaliserung: Universelle Ansprüche— Lokale Antworten,* ed. Angelika Wolf and Viola Hörbst, 3–30. Münster, Germany: Lit Verlag.

Howell, Signe. 1995. "Whose Knowledge and Whose Power? A New Perspective on Cultural Diffusion." In *Counterworks: Managing the Diversity of Knowledge,* ed. Richard Fardon, 164–181. London: Routledge.

Hsu, Elisabeth. 1999. *The Transmission of Chinese Medicine.* Cambridge: Cambridge University Press.

———. 2002. "'The Medicine from China Has Rapid Effects': Patients of Traditional Chinese Medicine in Tanzania." Special Issue: "Countervailing Creativity: Patient Agency in the Globalisation of Asian Medicines," *Anthropology and Medicine* 9 (3): 291–314.

———. 2007. "Zanzibar and its Chinese Communities." Special Issue: "New Chinese Diasporas," *Populations, Space, and Place* 13: 113–124.

———. 2008. "Medicine as Business: Chinese Medicine in Tanzania." In *China Returns to Africa: A Rising Power and a Continent Embrace,* ed. Chris Alden, Daniel Large, and Ricardo Soares de Oliveira, 221–235. London: Hurst.

———. Forthcoming. *Chinese Medicine in East Africa.* Oxford: Berghahn.

Hunter, Kathryn M. 1993. *Doctors' Stories: The Narrative Structure of Medical Knowledge.* Princeton: Princeton University Press.

Iliffe, John. 1998. *East African Doctors.* Cambridge: Cambridge University Press.

Katz, Pearl. 1985. "How Surgeons Make Decisions." In *Physicians of Western Medicine: Anthropological Approaches to Theory and Practice,* ed. Robert A. Hahn and Atwood D. Gaines, 155–175. Dordrecht, the Netherlands: Reidel.

Kleinman, Arthur. 1988. *The Illness Narratives: Suffering, Healing, and the Human Condition.* New York: Basic Books.

Levitt, Peggy, and Nina Glick Schiller. 2004. "Conceptualizing Simultaneity: A Transnational Social Field Perspective on Society." *International Migration Review* 38 (3): 1002–1039.

Luhrmann, Tanya M. 2001. *Of Two Minds: An Anthropologist Looks at Psychiatry.* New York: Vintage Books.

Mattingly, Cheryl. 1998. *Healing Dramas and Clinical Plots: The Narrative Structure of Experience.* Cambridge: Cambridge University Press.

Napolitano, Valentina. 2002. *Migration, Mujercitas, and Medicine Men: Living in Urban Mexico.* Berkeley: University of California Press.

Ong, Aihwa. 1999. *Flexible Citizenship: The Cultural Logic of Transnationality.* Durham, N.C.: Duke University Press.

———. 2006. *Neoliberalism as Exception: Mutations in Citizenship and Sovereignty.* Durham, N.C.: Duke University Press.

Parkin, David. 1995. "Latticed Knowledge: Eradication and Dispersal of the Unpalatable in Islam, Medicine, and Anthropological Theory." In *Counterworks: Managing the Diversity of Knowledge,* ed. Richard Fardon, 143–163. London: Routledge.

———. 2002. "Mementoes as Transitional Objects in Human Displacement." *Journal of Material Culture* 4 (3): 303–320.

Pellegrino, Edmund D. 1999. "The Commodification of Medical and Health Care: The Moral Consequences of a Paradigm Shift from a Professional to a Market Ethic." *Journal of Medicine and Philosophy* 24 (3): 243–266.

Pieke, Frank N. 2007. "Editorial Introduction: Community and Identity in the New Chinese Migration Order." Special Issue: "New Chinese Diasporas," *Population, Place, and Space* 13: 81–94.

Pieke, Frank N., Pál Nyíri, Mette Thunø, and Antonella Ceccagno. 2004. *Transnational Chinese: Fujianese Migrants in Europe.* Stanford, Calif.: Stanford University Press.

Raviola, Giuseppe, M'Imunya Machoki, Esther Mwaikambo, and Mary Jo DelVecchio Good. 2002. "HIV, Disease Plague, Demoralization, and 'Burnout': Resident Experience of the Medical Profession in Nairobi, Kenya." *Culture, Medicine, and Psychiatry* 26 (1): 55–86.

Sangren, P. Steven. 1987. *History and Magical Power in a Chinese Community.* Stanford, Calif.: Stanford University Press.

Scheid, Volker. 2002. *Chinese Medicine in Contemporary China: Plurality and Synthesis.* Durham, N.C.: Duke University Press.

Shahar, Meir and Weller, Robert P. 1996. "Introduction: Gods and Society in China". In *Unruly Gods: Divinity and Society in China,* ed. Meir Shahar and Robert P. Weller, 1–36. Honolulu: University of Hawai'i Press.

Shimazono, Y. 2003. "Narrative Analysis in Medical Anthropology." MPhil diss. in Medical Anthropology, University of Oxford.

Sivin, Nathan. 1991. "Change and Continuity in Early Cosmology: The Great Commentary and the Book of Changes." In *Chugoku kodai kagaku shiron (On the History of Ancient Chinese Science, 2),* 3–43. Kyoto: Institute for Research in Humanities.

Stafford, Charles. 2000. *Separation and Reunion in Modern China.* Cambridge: Cambridge University Press.

Taylor, Kim. 2005. *Medicine of Revolution: Chinese Medicine in Early Communist China 1945–1963.* London: Routledge.

Xiang, Biao. Forthcoming. *Making Order from Transnational Migration: Labor, Recruitment Agents and the State in Northeast China* (working title). Princeton: Princeton University Press.

TWELVE

Guinean Migrant Traditional Healers in the Global Market

Clara Carvalho

West African traditional therapists, healers, and ritual experts have crossed national and continental borders, spreading their therapeutic knowledge and worldview along their migrant itineraries. Nowadays, in every southern European capital, West African therapists act professionally in different contexts and for a varied clientele, including African and non-African, immigrant and local patients. Being migrant workers themselves, they become cultural brokers, mediating circuits of information and power amongst their patients. Although this process is not a new one, it changed in scope and vitality in the 1990s, a decade marked by the imposition of structural adjustment plans (SAPs) on indebted southern economies, a measure that led to the liberalization of the markets but also increased the impoverishment of both the working class and the emerging middle class in Africa, contributing to the flow of migrants from the global South to the global North. Amongst these migrants seeking better lives were therapists, religious experts, and other professional healers practicing local traditions. The mobility of such traditional workers has long been noticed in different African settings at a regional level, as has their capacity to adapt their knowledge to different challenges and situations (Feierman 2006; West and Luedke 2006). In 1992, Feierman and Janzen drew attention to the changing patterns of health and healing in Africa. Nowadays patients have a varied set of options for diagnosis and treatment, and it is the reasons behind their choices that anthropologists try to understand when studying the concepts of health and disease from the patients' point of view. Patients can choose amongst local healing traditions, both religious and biomedical, which have their own distribution in time and space. These different systems have their own dynamic, and (as medical anthropologists have stressed) so-called "healing traditions" have changed according to the new conditions of health and disease of their patients (Feierman and Janzen 1992; Nichter and Lock 2002). Different living conditions resulting from changes in political control and economic production, as well as new or newly widespread diseases (especially tuberculosis, malaria, and now HIV / AIDS), have led healing practices to change accordingly. This is particularly true for migrant populations, both within Africa and beyond. The intensification of the flow of migrants from Africa to Europe has made the movement of both people and ideas, including healing practices, along the migration routes more obvious, and created a new challenge for traditional healers.

My claim in this chapter is that the new migration circuits act as a parallel and inverse movement to the diffusion of both biomedicine and pharmaceutical products, and should be understood in the context of the transnational flows that characterize the modern age—as well as being appreciated as one of the best examples of cultural globalization (Whyte, van der Geest, and Hardon 2002). Globalization is a multilevel phenomenon, and the dissemination of multiple therapeutic practices brought into Europe by migrant populations is a good example of the dual circulation of healing practices. In order to obtain an insight into the complexity of this process, I will present a multi-sited ethnography, following traditional therapists through the migrant circuits that have led them to cross not only physical borders but cultural ones marked by distinct meaning systems and contrasting cosmogonies. The practices, actions, and interpretations of these therapists are better understood as answers to the challenges of life experiences in which clashing events, different labor markets, and sociogeographical contexts have to be integrated by both the therapists and their patients into daily practices.

The focus of this chapter is Guinean traditional therapists working in Portugal and France who participate in a wider migration movement that originates in Guinea-Bissau and Senegal and is directed toward Portugal, Spain, and France. It has long been stressed in the literature that local or traditional therapists deal with affliction problems broadly understood (classified as misfortunes in classic works by Edward Evans-Pritchard or Jeanne Favret-Saada). This category includes occupational, familiar, affective, and sexual troubles, besides dealing with health problems. Currently there are two categories of professionals dealing with affliction problems amongst Guinean immigrants in Portugal: *mouros* or *marabouts*, and *jambakus*. *Marabouts* are part of a widespread movement that has been acting in Europe for decades and has achieved some public recognition (Kuczynski 2002). *Jambakus*, on the other hand, represent a local form of cult, performing as diviners, ritual experts, and healers in local areas of Guinea-Bissau and southern Senegal. Their recent integration into the transnational market has to be understood within the international migratory circuit of which they are part.

Creation of the Guinean Diaspora

For centuries Guinea-Bissau has been a source country for migrant work-ers, giving rise to a true diaspora whose influence has become even stronger in the past decade.[1] This diaspora may be characterized in three historical periods.

The first migratory movement witnessed from this area involved young people from coastal groups in Guinea who worked seasonally in European concessions or on merchant ships from the eighteenth century onward. This led to the establishment of intercontinental Guinean communities of Manjaco origin[2] composed of merchant sailors who gathered in French ports during the nineteenth century (Gable 1990; Diop 1996). Throughout the twentieth cen-tury migratory movements in Guinea-Bissau became more pronounced, par-ticularly from rural areas, heading toward Senegal and Gambia and following on to France and England (Hochet 1983; Diop 1996). These were composed of rural workers who settled in communities in bordering countries, generally Senegal or Gambia, and still maintain strong identity ties with a regional eth-nic base. This early migration was initially composed exclusively of men, who were later followed by women. It arose from the appeal of better economic conditions and political freedom in the neighboring countries and led to the establishment of numerous Manjaco communities in Casamance, Dakar, and the outskirts of Paris during the colonial period (Diop 1996; Teixeira 1996; Trincaz 1981). Initially, migration was limited to coastal populations, but in the 1980s it extended to other settings, particularly the northern and eastern areas, while maintaining the same characteristics of rural migration with an economic motivation (Hochet 1983). Even the transcontinental movements observed up through the 1980s were a continuation of the early rural migra-tion to Senegal and Gambia, as the Guinean immigrants to those countries who were able to generally preferred to move on to the former colonizers, France and the United Kingdom. This early migration included rural work-ers who earned a living from the cultivation of peanuts, as well as artisans and traditional therapists who often traveled to neighboring countries on a seasonal basis.

Over the past two decades the introduction of the SAP and economic lib-eralization have been the direct causes of a new, more differentiated migrant flow. This new movement is multiethnic and includes a majority of people of urban origin, most of them with schooling (Machado 2002: 79). The eco-nomic and political pressure experienced in recent decades in Guinea-Bissau has affected salaried groups in particular, who are generally employed in pub-lic services and have middle- and even higher-level education. This middle class, who attended high school or university abroad with scholarships, were the first to see their ambitions in their own country thwarted and to find themselves in a weaker position as a result of the progressive impoverishment of the domestic economy. Entirely dependent on their salaries, as opposed to the rural population and those who make a living in the informal economy, following the SAP in 1987 they found themselves in a context of extreme fragility due to galloping inflation and an ongoing scenario of limited and unpaid wages, a situation which accession to the African Financial Community in 1997 further intensified. Migration from rural areas has also become more pronounced, heading directly for European destinations by both air and sea via Cape Verde or the Canary Islands. The final destinations are varied, with Portugal, Spain, France, and England being the most sought-after European countries, with immigration channels that have been open to Guineans for some time. These immigrants are employed as an unskilled workforce, mainly in public works in Portugal or as rural workers in Spain.

Transcontinental migration, which originally headed for England and France via Gambia and Senegal, is currently directed at Portugal, from where it is easy to cross to Spain and France. The contingent of immigrant Guineans in Portugal comprises three distinct groups, the largest composed of unskilled workers who arrived in the last 20 years. A second group, which Fernando Luís Machado calls Luso-Guineans (Machado 1994), includes a significant part of the former national elite who after independence opted for Portuguese or dual nationality. Most of the members of this group belong to wealthy or influential families and experienced easy social integration in the host country, albeit while maintaining their networks of relationships in their country of origin. They played an important role in the integration of the Guinean elite who abandoned the country after the coup d'état of 1998, often with refugee status (see below).

A third migratory movement is made up of highly qualified officials who had initially lived abroad as students before looking outside of Guinea for more suitable living conditions. Since the 1950s, the Guinean elite have been sending their children to conclude their studies overseas, the best-known example being Amílcar Cabral, the leader of the Guinean liberation struggle. During the colonial period the obvious destinations included Portugal, as well as Eastern Europe for those who participated in the nationalist war.[3] After independence the number of students abroad grew as most Guinean senior government officials completed their education in Eastern European countries, which were the main donors of scholarships before the fall of the Berlin Wall. Only a limited number of students went on to Brazil, or, sporadically, to the U.S.A. These graduates and PhDs comprised the majority of the government elite and senior officials of Guinea-Bissau. However, the poor conditions and instability in Guinea-Bissau, or the attractiveness of the host countries, drove many members of this group to emigrate from very early on, creating a network of transcontinental immigrants who maintain their ties—through family, friendship, or interest—with their country's elite. In this respect, Guinea-Bissau is part of a general trend that has affected the whole of sub-Saharan Africa, where a "flight of senior officials" was witnessed in the late twentieth century. This movement became more pronounced after the coup of June 7, 1998, which led to the removal of President Nino Vieira from power after a military conflict in which the majority of the Guinean army opposed the Senegalese forces who came in aid of the former ruler. The armed struggle that took place in Bissau's streets; the deterioration of living conditions in the city; and the political instability that led to the prudent withdrawal of many international organizations and NGOs which decided to set up their headquarters in safer bordering countries all turned Bissau into an unstable city. Many members of the government, along with the local elite, preferred to withdraw at this stage and, availing themselves of their international contacts, sought the support of other countries.

These different motivations to emigrate created a Guinean diaspora heterogeneous in terms of its social origin, its objectives, and its forms of action, reflecting the country's social diversity. It has gained some visibility and intervention capacity due to the activity of the former senior officials and members of the local elite. Portugal, as the former colonial power, became the most significant host country for these new migrants, and one where the numerous networks organizing the diaspora are very often centered, contributing to a stronger presence of the Guinean community in the country.

Ritual Experts Abroad: The Marabouts

My focus in this chapter is the traditional Guinean therapists working in Europe, who form part of a wider migration movement just described. While this movement was originally of migrants from the countryside who had previous experience of working in Senegal, as mentioned above it now includes urban migrants from Bissau in a flow that has increased over the last two decades. In Portugal there are currently two categories of professionals dealing with affliction problems: *mouros* or *marabouts,* and *jambakus.* Although they share a common geographical origin, these professionals are marked by striking differences, as the *marabouts* from Guinea-Bissau belong to Islamic brotherhoods based in Senegal, whereas the *jambakus* are representatives of a cult native to an area of Guinea-Bissau and southern Senegal. The latter act as local diviners, ritual experts, and therapeutic professionals in local areas, and come mainly from the Manjak-speaking populations of the Bissau and Cacheu regions.

Marabouts—or *mouros* in current Guinea-Bissau terminology—are ritualists and religious specialists who act through the reading of the Qur'an, or as diviners and producers of talismans. The largest of the Islamic brotherhoods to which they are related is the Mouride congregation based in Touba (Senegal) (Bava 2005). Mourides form hierarchical and literate congregations and have long been integrated in transnational networks that both support and encourage the transnational migration movements. Their public image is well known in European cities, as they publicize their activities through newspapers, flyers, and the internet.[4] In a recent study based in Lisbon, Portugal, Eduardo Costa Dias (2007) profiles *marabouts* who have migrated to that country. Usually they come from the countryside, from the Mandinga and Fula regions, where the seasonal migration of these specialists was common throughout the twentieth century. Most *marabouts* aim to be community leaders as well as religious ones and they continue to be the polarizing centers of their communities in the migratory context just as they were in their homeland. Operating in downtown Lisbon or on the outskirts of the city, they receive their patients in a professional space, consisting of a room for their healing activities and a waiting room for their customers, located in leasehold apartments for domestic use. Surrounding the *marabouts* are other categories of individuals, such as their assistants—generally enlisted from among their relatives—and their clientele, defined by Costa Dias as the "friends from the *tabanca*," people that claim a family or neighborly relationship with the *marabouts*. These leaders identify themselves with a definite lineage or school, as they always refer to a previous *marabout* (father, uncle, or grandfather) or to their Qur'an teacher or *karamo* as their initiator.

Marabouts find their customers either by advertising in periodicals, by distributing flyers in the streets, or through individual recommendations, their most common resource. Their clientele is diversified in terms of gender, religion, and nationality. It includes a clear predominance of women and of Africans, particularly Guineans and Cape Verdeans, but there are also Portuguese and Brazilians amongst their patients. Their individual prestige depends on their *baraka*, a divine blessing genealogically transmitted, but they also draw their authority from their knowledge, from their student period at a Qur'anic school, and from their family ties with other *marabouts*. They are also supposed to fulfill the five obligations or pillars of the Islamic faith, including the pilgrimage to Mecca (*Hajj*).

As noted by Costa Dias, in African and particularly in Guinean Islam, religious and magical-therapeutic knowledge is transmitted primarily through oral rather than written tradition and is essentially a malleable practice adapted from numerous local traditions (Dias 2007: 193). Its transcontinental path is generally multi-sited, and the passage of its practitioners through Portugal (generally headed to Lisbon) is never considered definitive. Endowed with great mobility, these professionals circulate between Guinea-Bissau and neighboring countries, especially Gambia and Senegal, and along the main migratory circuits of their peers, namely to France, Portugal, and Spain. Their connection to the multinational Islamic community in Portugal is weak, and they prefer to maintain ties with their native region or village as their practice falls within the context of the Guinean migrations. The most successful *marabouts* set up their own development organizations or local associations. The best-known example is that of Kausso Baldé, one of the first *marabouts* to come to Portugal in the 1970s and a leader of the immigrant community. The Master, as he is known, has created an association and clearly has political influence in his native country, acting as a mediator in national politics and a businessman, besides having influence as a prestigious *marabout*. His varied activities enhance each other and give the Master prestige—and success.

The *marabouts* define themselves as religious professionals and therapists integrated in networks with a lengthy tradition of activity in Europe. To acquire the necessary knowledge and skills to work as a *marabout* requires a long training period (six years or longer) in a Qur'anic school and represents a form of social ascension both for the *marabout* and for his family. His migratory path stems from his professional practice: as demonstrated by Costa Dias, most of the *marabouts* included in his survey do not pursue their activity in their village of origin. As professionals, their genealogical status (their proximity or distance from the *imam* or religious leader, and their genealogical subordination to other *marabouts*) leads them to seek areas other than their community of origin in which to work. It should be noted that their economic power and, particularly, the religious and political prestige obtained in the migratory context are also vital aspects in their process of religious and political capitalization. The main *marabouts* are not limited to a single place of work, but carry out their activity in different countries. Often traveling with only a tourist visa, they stay for a few months in each location with the support of numerous individuals and complex logistics involving several places of action and different residences. Their great mobility also enables them to become successful brokers between different communities, particularly their village (or region, or even country) of origin and the communities of immigrants with whom they come into contact, acting as vehicles for the transmission of goods and ideas among different groups and disparate political and cultural settings.

Affliction Cults in the Cacheu Region

Besides *marabouts,* the other ritualists acting as transcontinental migrants are the ones generally known as *jambakus.* While this Creole term of Floup (Djola) origin has several local and ethnic interpretations, it always designates ritualists worshiping at local or individual shrines (Einarsdóttir 2000, 2005). Compared to *marabouts, jambakus* act at a more secretive level, as they do not advertise their activities and are not identified with a universal religion. On the contrary, *jambakus* always refer to a precise ethnic identity (Floup, Manjaco, Pepel, Balanta, Mancanha) and to local shrines where they have to worship, even when working at a transnational level. Another important difference concerns the acquisition of ritual status. *Marabouts* have to endure formal education lasting at least six years, besides having to be members of a *marabout* family. *Jambakus,* on the other hand, have both to be members of a family of *jambakus* and to undergo initiation in obedience to a particular sign. This sign (contact with certain kinds of ants, meeting large snakes, hearing voices, etc.) is interpreted as the wish of an ancestor, himself a *jambakus,* that his offspring shall become a ritual performer. Generally the new *jambakus* is only nominated after having dealt with an affliction problem that leads him or her to worship different spirits and consult local ritualists. The initiatory process is conducted by the other *jambakus* of his/her congregation, during which he/she acquires secret, esoteric knowledge. This is not a male-gendered process as it is with *marabouts,* for both men and women are able to become *jambakus.*

Jambakus working in Europe are originally from Bissau or the Cacheu region and identify themselves as belonging to the local ethnic categories (Floup, Manjaco, Pepel, Balanta, Mancanha) related to the Manjak group of languages. In the Cacheu region, north of Bissau, *jambakus* are merely one of the various categories of ritual professionals working locally who all share some basic cultural features. These include the obligation to undergo initiation in order to become a diviner and a ritual expert, for in this region every cult is an affliction cult connected to a local shrine controlled by a priest or ritual performer. All the shrines in a particular region are hierarchically related to the sacred grove were the male initiation shrine stands. This fact encouraged Wim van Binsbergen to propose a topographical classification of this area as divided into initiation regions, each corresponding to a shrine complex related to the same central initiatory shrine or *kambaç* (van Binsbergen 1984, 1988). Every ritual leads to a system of individual promises or "contracts with the spirits" (Crowley and Ribeiro 1987; Crowley 1990). Spirits (called *iran* in Creole or *usai* in Manjak) are dubious figures, recalling the Yoruba *Esu*[5] or trickster who has to be worshiped both to guarantee his protection and to avoid his revenge. Failure to keep a promise may put both the contractor and his family at risk of being attacked by a spirit that has not been properly appeased. From then on, any problem faced by the individual or family, be it related to money, work, health, or anything else, is interpreted as the spirit's revenge. Both rituals and ritualists are part of a hierarchical system, including the shrines and local congregations. The main forms of affliction cult in the Cacheu region include *kansaré*,[6] *ussái fankas*,[7] and *defunto*[8] in addition to *jambakus*. Ritualists have to undergo an initiatory process in order to acquire a "shell" or protection that will serve them in their interaction with the spirit world. For male ritualists this represents their second initiation, and they are locally known as "two times initiated" (Carvalho 1998, 2001). Migrants have circulated some of these forms of affliction cult, and the worship of the *kansaré* shrine is now widespread in southern Senegalese communities (Teixeira 1996). Nevertheless, of all the local cults only *jambakus* have adapted to the transcontinental flow of migrants. In what follows, I will stress that this phenomenon is due to certain characteristics of the *jambakus* ritual process. In order to understand their particularities, I will examine the cases of three *jambakus* (or *jambakus*-to-be), two men and a woman, who represent disparate experiences of migration, initiation, and empowerment.

Jambakus: The Ritual Process

The first *jambakus* I met, in 1992, was an immigrant in France called Sábor, who returned to his native village in Jeta, an island north of Bissau, in order to embark on the initiatory process that would turn him into a ritual expert. Sábor's experience was particularly striking because he had refused for a long time to become a *jambakus*. As a young boy, Sábor had left Jeta for Dakar in Senegal, where he followed his father, himself a well-known Manjaco migrant *jambakus* who worked in that town. From Senegal he went to France, following a migration pattern common in the region until the 1980s. After finishing his secondary education, Sábor stayed in Argenteuil, near Paris, were he worked and settled with his wife and children. He located his troubles in the late 1980s, when he faced some health problems and a period of unemployment. He tried the biomedical sector before consulting a *jambakus* working in France. The latter removed an object described as a stone from his abdomen, which was considered a sign of witchcraft or spirit persecution, and prescribed Sábor the sacrifices he should offer to the initiation shrine on his native island.

Sábor returned to Jeta for the first time during his adult life in order to "settle his obligations," for the *jambakus*'s interpretation was that either he or a relative had a contract with the spirits there that must be fulfilled. During this ceremonial act he confronted a snake, which was seen as an undoubted sign that he should follow in the footsteps of his late father as a *jambakus*. Sábor rejected that explanation at the time, as he did not want to endure the expensive and dangerous initiation ritual or to become an active *jambakus* himself. On returning to France he was hospitalized again and eventually decided to return to Jeta and to negotiate an expeditious initiation with his father's congregation.[9] He was helped by his cousin, herself a migrant *jambakus* operating in Bissau, who organized the ceremony down to the last detail in order to fit into the new neophyte vacancy period. When the day came, the members of the congregation built him, in his matrilineage compound, a *pubol* or libation place where he was to work later. During the first night he was given a narcotic beverage that was said to "kill" him and then he had to run away from the other *jambakus*, to be found, eventually, unconscious near the initiation shrine. In the morning, protected by his congregation, he woke up (or was reborn) on the legs of an old woman *jambakus*,[10] in simulation of a delivery or a funeral. He was given gifts and saluted by all those present, including his relatives and neighbors. For the next few days he acted as a newborn, hesitant and almost speechless. He did not leave his *pubol* during the day, protected day and night by the *jambakus* of his congregation. For two weeks he stayed in his *pubol* while older members of his congregation taught him the secrets of the *jambakus*, the art of divining, and the correct way to worship both the initiation spirit and his own shrine, where an emanation of that spirit stayed (represented by materials removed from the original shrine). He was then given a necklace that he should wear for the rest of his life as a sign of his new condition, and joined his congregation in the initiation of a new *jambakus*. Nevertheless, he was only able to leave the island after the first rains, when his cousin and initiation protector washed the white cloth that protected him during his rebirth as a *jambakus*. Next, the new *jambakus* gathered in a collective celebration (*kadjika bapene*) where, in a kind of masquerade, they sang and danced in their ceremonial white outfits supplemented with Western goods like sunglasses and hats. Only then was Sábor able to leave behind his *pubol* and private shrine, carrying with him, in a horn, materials taken from all the shrines at which he had worshiped, including his own, and set off for France, where he would start receiving patients as a *jambakus* diviner.

Sábor is now part of a *jambakus* congregation, a secret, hierarchical society whose members are obliged to share their income and to act together in initiating others and in ceremonial eating and feasting. The initiatory pro-

cess described above includes elements common to other secret societies in
Western Africa, such as the symbols of death and rebirth, feelings of fear and
danger, neophyte reclusion, group commensality, and, particularly, the secrets
shared by all the members. As Jean La Fontaine points out, this kind of association "creates the boundaries which separate outsiders from members, for
it emphasizes in dramatic form the distance that separates the two statuses
between which initiated must pass. Experience of the ritual and knowledge of
its meaning both constitute secrets, possession of which is the right of every
member and is denied to non-members" (La Fontaine 1985: 58). Secrecy and
the protection of the esoteric knowledge of the group are essential as markers
of group differentiation, and all its members are united by a sermon of secrecy
(Jamin 1977; Zempléni 1993).

The new *jambakus* starts working as a ritualist after the first rains (May /
June) in a private shrine built during the initiatory process in his family compound's backyard, or in a shrine he builds himself in his migrant settlement,
but which is always regarded as an emanation of the original location. This
shrine includes a pot containing blood and alcohol from every sacrifice and
beverage offered during the initiation process, bits of cotton, the horns of
sacrificed animals, and finally shells, representing his condition as a "shell person," a two-times initiated. *Jambakus* are able to diagnose an affliction problem
and give instructions about the therapeutic process. The diagnosis is always
confirmed by reading the gonads of a sacrificed rooster. Among the most
famous *jambakus* are those who have built local hospitals to receive patients
during the long therapeutic process, which includes physical care, administration of herbs, and worship at specific shrines. Every therapy obliges the patient
to make a sacrificial offering in the sacred grove and to participate in (or donate
food for) the congregation's annual celebration.

The initiation ritual of Sábor in the *jambakus* society was simultaneously
a therapeutic performance.[11] For Sábor, this was understood as a moment—
perhaps the final moment—in a long process involving the use of a variety
of therapies, including biomedicine: Sábor interpreted the hospitalization to
which he had been subjected as a "sign" from his father. His path was marked
out by the *jambakus* he consulted in France and locally, who established the
diagnosis in conjunction with the patient and set out the therapeutic process
to be followed. Throughout this process several solutions were negotiated and
tried out: therapeutic experiments, discursive practices, and different causal
explanations, from biomedicine to the local cosmological system. For Sábor,
the different nosological discourses were heterogeneous yet complementary
explanations that would enable him to deal with his pain and suffering. A char-

acter that was key in Sábor's path was Mamé Có, a relative of his, a *jambakus* and migrant like him, who lived in Bissau, where she carried out her practice. She represented the figure of therapy manager described by Feierman and Janzen (1992: 18), seeking out ritualists, organizing the initiation process with them, and negotiating its timing while protecting the neophyte. As mentioned, the nosological discourse appears to the patient as a heterogeneous set of causalities within which he seeks the solution to his own suffering through experimentation. The role of the therapy manager is vital, as, besides indicating the treatment and negotiating the conditions under which it is going to take place, it adds legitimacy to the process.

In the local nosological system, the notion of disease is not isolated; it is not understood merely as a consequence of a pathogenic cause. Quite on the contrary, the concept of disease is included in a much wider notion of evil—*le sens du mal,* in the opportune definition of Marc Augé (Augé and Herzlich 1986)—of misfortune, and of disorder at a personal, social, and cosmological level. That is why only the Manjaco nosological discourse (as opposed to that of biomedicine) was able to respond to the anguish felt by Sábor, in that it related his health complications to his working difficulties. Once he had identified himself as a patient suffering first of all from an attack of witchcraft (confirmed by the malicious object removed from his body by a *jambakus* in France), therapeutic alternatives were suggested to him. Such therapies can be varied and are seen as practices that lead to a new social or even cosmological equilibrium: they are ritualized processes in which the patient becomes a neophyte and which are very often aimed at changing his personal status, as in Sábor's example. In a more explicit way than in biomedical practices, immediate efficacy is not expected, nor are unidirectional causalities invoked. Consequently, these paths are negotiable and adaptable by the patient or sufferer.

The initiation ritual, as a therapeutic performance, draws its efficacy from the fact that it involves not only the neophyte or patient, but also his relatives and the entire community. Furthermore, this ritual establishes a relation between the suffering individual and the cosmological (and social) order, generally represented by the spirit of an ancestor that has chosen this particular individual to become a *jambakus* in his turn. During the initiation ritual the neophyte is guided day and night in such a way that all his initial reservations and fears end up being forgotten, and the individual, little by little, becomes capable of assuming his new social role. The fear and anguish felt by the neophyte also has to be seen as part of the therapeutic process of initiation, as already argued by several authors. In the words of Carol Laderman and Marina Roseman: "The healing effects of performance are, on one level, caused by the catharsis that occurs when a patient's unresolved emotional distress is reawakened and confronted in a dramatic context" (Laderman and Roseman 1996: 7). The ritual process itself plays dexterously with the patient's involvement, literally starting with his funeral and working toward control of the body and of the knowledge given, and ending with the exuberant collective feast of the *kadjipa jambakus* described above. As seen in other contexts, the efficacy of this process is directly related to the patient's belief and his ability to adopt a different—positive—attitude to his individual tribulations.

These different forms of relationship between humans and spirits form part of several other alternative affliction cults. Some of these cults emphasize qualities of adaptability and integration, which in the context of extensive emigration promote their exportation to new places and ways of life. Professional *jambakus* have a greater capacity to adapt and respond to the different recurrent problems characteristic of the migration context. As they themselves are migrants who master a nosological discourse that relates disease, suffering, and misfortune to the cosmological and cultural references of their patients, they are particularly capable of indicating a significant therapeutic path for those who seek them out.

Exporting Local Therapies

Our aim is to understand how a primary local affliction cult has adapted to the migratory process, even if it always obliges practitioners to return to make offerings to local shrines and to join a local congregation, as seen in Sábor's initiation. The second story presented here, that of Luis Kapol, demonstrates the adaptation of the *jambakus* cult and the professional practice of the migratory circuit particularly well. When I first met Luis Kapol in 2005, he was a migrant worker in Portugal from Caió, near Canchungo, north of Bissau. As he was the eldest sibling, his family had supported him in his migrant adventure by paying for his travel expenses to Europe. Kapol had been successful; he had worked in the Portuguese public construction boom of the 1990s as a manual laborer and was able to send a large amount of money back home. His father, a well-known *jambakus* and the head of a local Caió congregation, chose him to become his successor in his congregation—which in itself is a remarkable adaptation of the system, for typically only the ancestors were able to choose new *jambakus*. Kapol believed that this choice had been sanctioned by the ancestors, because he came across some red termites while making his offerings to the sacred grove. So, with his father and the members of his congregation he organized the initiation ritual to fit in with his annual vacation. He was initiated in 1999 and has since been acting as a *jambakus* in his lodgings, a room in a house he shares with other migrants in Bairro do Fim do Mundo, a slum in Estoril, near Lisbon. During the week he works as a manual laborer on construction sites; on Saturdays and Sundays he receives his patients in his lodgings. Sacrifices are performed over a horn container, where some of the sand and blood from the original shrines of his homeland are kept. He then prescribes the therapeutic process to be followed, indicates future sacrifices to be held, and, when required, administers herbal preparations he usually makes himself with plants from his homeland. Sacrifices to the spirits used to be performed in Caió by his late father, and are nowadays offered by his successor at the head of the *jambakus* congregation. Patients in Portugal pay for the animals and beverages to be consumed during the ritual offerings to the sacred grove, and the money is sent back to Caió. Kapol's patients are mainly Guineans, but include occasional Cape Verdeans, Angolans, Brazilians, and sometimes Portuguese who are recruited in the work and social circles in which he or his patients move. These correspond to the main nationalities of the unskilled workers who have come to Portugal during different periods of economic growth: Cape Verdeans since the early 1960s, and Brazilians and Angolans in the 1980s and '90s (Matos 1997; Machado 2002). These are also the main immigrant groups who speak Portuguese and are more prone to share a belief in the action of spirits amongst humans. It is worth noting that most of the non-Guineans are women, and, according to Kapol, their main complaints are related to "belly troubles," a general term for a diverse set of conditions concerning reproduction and affective relations as well as specific gynecological disorders. Although this multinational clientele reveals an acceptance of Kapol's discourse that transcends national borders, his main patients are Guineans and it is amongst this group that the more complex healing or protective processes are undertaken.

Kapol is a successful case of an integrated *jambakus,* and his experience highlights the way these practices are becoming transnational, a phenomenon that has also been noticed by Saraiva (2008). *Jambakus* are creating an alternative way for goods, money, and people to circulate between local congregations and transcontinental migrant destinations. As seen in this case, they are doing so actively in an organized circuit. And while they facilitate this material circulation, they also spread a certain idea of body, disease, and therapy. As has been stressed in other studies, traditional therapies correspond to a holistic ontological concept and are able to give a more integrated interpretation of illness. However, the spirits and shrines that Kapol worships are not universal:

it is his interpretation, his ability to listen, and his patients' thirst for a global explanation that may explain his success as a transnational ritualist.

Confronting the Hospital

Sábor's case is a particularly happy one in that he benefitted from his family's help and support from his congregation and community. Also remarkable was the neophyte's easy adaptation to his new role. The process of producing a *jambakus* requires not only capital investment of financial resources, but also the social capital represented here by his family environment and his genealogical legitimacy, as well as the ability to draw on a syncretic symbolic repository which combines varied possible responses to misfortune (misfortune in the classical sense used in anthropology of the repetition of elements considered to be harmful to the individual). This lengthy, slow, and expensive process is only accessible to individuals who, besides their genealogical legitimacy and the pertinence of the prognoses made by other ritualists, are able to come up with the material and social capital required for the initiation ritual. In the Guinean context, these practices are facilitated by the support of communities and families, and several initiations in the various congregations take place during the dry season, ending with the ceremony that celebrates the new *jambakus*. In a migratory context, the costs of this process are drastically increased. Those individuals who face the greatest difficulties as migrants and who enjoy less family or community support in their migratory context may find it extremely difficult to fulfill the requirements of a treatment proposed by traditional healers with regard to the Guinean cosmogony when the treatment implies an elaborate plan of ritual offers and sacrifices in specific local shrines. The ritual also depends on the social and financial capital the neophyte is able to gather, and not every patient who is diagnosed as having received an ancestral mandate is able to undertake it, as we shall see below. When Guineans are in this situation, their lack of adaptation to their new lives may land them in a hospital, and from there they are generally confined to psychiatric institutions. They display various symptoms that they understand in cultural terms as signs of their need to take part in an initiatory process. The health professionals that attend them in hospitals do not share this cultural interpretation, and doctors, particularly in the psychiatric sector, interpret these same "signs" as hallucinations or even symptoms of mental disorder. Lisbon psychiatric hospitals include cases of Guinean women diagnosed as suffering from persecution delirium, auditory-verbal hallucinations, and bewilderment. Our third story concerns Rose (pseudonym) and illustrates the difficulties faced by those who cannot mobilize enough capital to undertake the initiation ritual and find themselves trapped between different diagnoses and nosological interpretations.

Rose was born in Bissau and moved to Portugal in her early twenties to do occasional domestic and agricultural work there and in Spain. Without regular work she found herself in a situation of near poverty, unable to support herself as a single parent with two small children. She started to behave erratically, hearing voices and getting lost during long periods of total absence from reality. Her relatives had her admitted to a psychiatric hospital in Lisbon (Hospital Júlio de Matos) in order to deal with her immediate problems. She was diagnosed with schizophrenia and had "depression, auditory-verbal hallucinations, visual hallucinations and persecutory delusions" (Tavares, Pires, and Carvalho 2009: 40). However, in her own interpretation, she was in the process of undergoing several rituals that would lead her to become a *jambakus* and bearer of a *defunto,* an ancestral spirit. Her inability to sustain the long and expensive ritual process aggravated her depressive state, and she saw her problems as countless further trials brought about by the spirits who demanded her attention. It seemed impossible to find common ground between her discourse and that of the health professionals in their search for different meanings, despite the commitment of both to reach a mutual understanding.

Rose's case poses the question of the extent to which dialogue is possible in a migratory context of therapeutic practices, particularly regarding behavior patterns that are considered psychopathological in a clinical and hospital environment. The search for dialogue is limited by the need felt by medical professionals to classify standards of behavior that they see as deviating from the norm into previously defined nosological categories; by the fact that their discourse and authority are not acknowledged by the patients; and by the very restrictions created by the institution and its prison-like nature. These factors result in apathy and disinterest in the patients, who must struggle to interpret not only their illness but also the incomprehensible discourse of the therapists who treat them. The psychiatric response, which interprets the issues of members of minorities in terms of "culture-bound syndromes" (Pussetti 2006; Fassin 2000), and their behavior as deviating from the norm, merely reflects a widespread attitude in the power circles of the host societies whereby each individual is defined essentially in cultural terms, and "culture" is a term referring to a set of irreducible, closed practices. The cultural determinism presented in these interpretations overlooks the individual's capacity to react, translate, and manipulate different signs and symbols, as well as the adaptability of groups and individuals. As Littlewood and Dein note, "It is not that psychiatry's inevitable grid, pathology, is necessarily inappropriate for different societies, but pathology is just one possible grid and one that carries with it particular assumptions about normality and abnormality, which explicitly ignore considerations of power and of context of observation, and what is observed, and how 'observation' itself might shape it" (Littlewood and Dein 2000: 23). Rose's case is a clear example of therapeutic misunderstanding and of a power relation maintained by the medical institution. Although from the medical perspective she was receiving treatment for a depressive state, from her own point of view she had to undergo hospitalization and drug dependence as a result of not having enough social and economic capital to undertake the therapeutic process of becoming a *jambakus*. The explanation and treatment that could be given in a hospital environment were not those that Rose required, and she quickly decided to abandon both the treatment and the dialogue that the doctors tried to establish.

Migrants are subject to stressful life conditions that favor not only the development of several pathological states, but also experimentation with new therapies, new cultural creations, new nosological explanations, and new therapeutic circuits. In the case of the *jambakus,* these circuits are a counter-movement to the hegemony of globalization, and particularly to the transnational flow of both biomedicine and pharmaceutical products. As mediators between different sociocultural environments, migrants are the main agents of transnational exchanges, defined by Basch, Glick Schiller, and Blanc (1994: 7) as "the processes by which immigrants forge and sustain multi-stranded social relations that link together their societies of origin and settlement." Migrants must be understood not only as transnational agents but also as transcultural brokers and creators circulating a variety of cultural practices and symbolic interpretations. The cases presented in this chapter are an illustration of such circulation. By forcing people to recreate their social identities and supporting networks, migration and dislocation precipitate unaccommodating behavior, inducing pain and suffering. As Kleinman et al. have stressed, the human experience of pain is also an extreme experience of resistance and reaction to uncontrolled and stressful social and individual experiences. The authors point out that pain has a role in resisting "domination in family relations, in political and economic structures, and in the often alienating activities of medical diagnosis and treatment. At times it enables the sufferer to resist such oppressive structures more eloquently than any available discourse" (Kleinman et al. 1992: 18). Expressing suffering is the first step in actively seeking a solution. In the cases presented in this paper, the patients acted within a set of multiple symbolic possibilities, seeking a meaning for their or others' suffering within a culturally accepted frame of reference. These references are negotiable and malleable, even if they are ultimately attached to a local (Guincan and spiritist) worldview. Sábor's initiation can be understood as a multilevel action, acting both as a therapeutic process and a space for the symbolic re-creation of his social identity as a *jambakus* and a migrant worker. This action demands strong social capital and the control of local networks that are not always available, as seen in Rose's case. Local congregations also organize their members' movements and include multi-sited rituals in their practice, expressing their resilience and malleability—and reproducing what the *marabouts'* congregations have been doing for decades. The experience of suffering and its absolute demand for an explanation and resolution offer the space for the creation of new symbolic meanings and referents. As transcultural brokers, both *marabouts* and *jambakus* are acting as agents for the creative integration of heterogeneous cultural referents that every migrant is obliged to accomplish.

Acknowledgments

This paper is based on ongoing research that started in Guinea Bissau in 1992 and continues in Paris and Lisbon. In preparing it I am particularly grateful to the editors of this volume, Hansjörg Dilger, Stacey Langwick, and Abdoulaye Kane for their support and insightful comments; to the healers mentioned, and particularly Mario Sábor, Luis Kapol, and Kausso Balde for their trust and interest; and to graduate students Maria Isabel Aguiar and João Tavares for opening up new perspectives for this research.

Notes

1. In a survey carried out in 1996, sociologist Fernando Luís Machado opined that the protracted migration tradition of Guinea-Bissau had not yet given rise to a true diaspora (Machado 2002: 76). In this article I endorse the belief that the rise in the migratory flow, particularly after the coup in 1998, has led to the creation of an active Guinean diaspora.

2. Because of its geographical and topographical characteristics, Guinea-Bissau has long been a refuge for groups fleeing the expansionist movements of the Sahelian powers. As a direct result, Guinea-Bissau is nowadays characterized by its ethnic diversity. Besides the urban population of Creole origin that settled in coastal towns from the sixteenth century onwards, there are the rural peoples of the coastal regions, who mainly speak Balanta and Manjak dialects (Balanta, Manjaco, Mancanha, and Pepel), and the Muslim groups that identify themselves

as Mandé (Mandinga) or Fulbe (Fula) in the northern and eastern parts of this tiny country (Forrest 1992; Carvalho 2008).

3. The national struggle began in Guinea-Bissau in 1963 at the initiative of the PAIGC (African Party for the Independence of Guinea and Cape Verde) and only ended in 1974.

4. Advertisements by *marabouts* have long been known in French cities and are widespread on the internet. See, for example, http://www.math.jussieu .fr/~cochet/marabouts/marabout.html or http://www.echolaliste.com/1199 .htm.

5. Margaret Drewal mentions that both the Yoruba *Esu* and his counterpart, the *Exu* of the Brazilian Umbanda religion, are manifestations of a change of frame: "Frame slippage is dangerous because it destabilizes a situation and throws it into a zone of ambiguity. At the same time, it sets up opportunities for alterations" (Drewal 1992: 16).

6. *Kansaré* is a community spirit cult represented in every village in the northern coastal region in Guinea Bissau and in Manjaco villages in the Casamance region.

7. *Ussai Fankas* is a "speaking spirit" based in the Caio sector, north of Bissau, that attracts numerous patients from neighboring countries.

8. *Defunto* is a Creole term that means literally "the dead one" and designates people that have incarnated former ancestors and participate in ritual life representing their possessing entities.

9. Membership in secret societies, as opposed to groupings based on the rites of maturity which include all members of the community of the same age group and gender, is always formal (La Fontaine 1985).

10. This is a woman from the same congregation of *jambakus* who is past childbearing age, as otherwise this "birth" would prevent her from having other children.

11. The therapeutic characteristics of the initiation processes in the congregations of *jambakus* and of the *kansaré* ritualists were also mentioned by Maria Teixeira in the case of the Manjaco emigrants in Ziguinchor (Teixeira 1996, 1998).

References

Augé, Marc, and Claudine Herzlich, eds. 1986 [1984]. *Le Sens du Mal. Anthropologie, histoire, sociologie de la maladie.* Paris: Éditions des archives contemporains.

Basch, Linda, Nina Glick Schiller, and Cristina Szanton Blanc. 1994. *Nations Unbound: Transnational Projects, Postcolonial Predicaments, and Deterritorialized Nation-States.* Amsterdam: Gordon and Breach Science Publishers.

Bava, Sophie. 2005. "'Reprendre la route': les relais mourides des migrants sénégalais au Niger." In *Entreprises religieuses transnationales en Afrique de L'Ouest,* ed. Laurent Fourchard, André Mary, and René Otayek, 73–88. Paris: Karthala.

Carvalho, Clara. 1998. "Ritos de Poder e a Recriação da Tradição. Os régulos manjaco da Guiné-Bissau." PhD diss., Lisbon, ISCTE.

———. 2001. "De Paris a Jeta, de Jeta a Paris. Percusos migratórios e ritos terapêuticos entre França e a Guiné-Bissau." *Etnográfica* 5 (2): 285–302.

————. 2008. "Local Authorities or Local Power?" Special Issue: "Local Experiences of Conflict Management," ed. Georg Klute, Birgit Embaló, Anne-Kristin Borszik, and Idrissa Embaló, *Soronda Especial*: 39–55.

Crowley, Eve L. 1990. "Contracts with the Spirits: Religion, Asylum, and Ethnic Identity in the Cacheu Region of Guinea-Bissau." PhD diss., Yale University.

Crowley, Eve, and Rui Ribeiro. 1987. "Sobre a medicina tradicional e formas da sua colaboração com a medicina moderna." *Soronda* 4: 95–112.

Dias, Eduardo Costa. 2007. "Les Musulmans Guinéens Immigrés de Lisbonne. Évitement et fascination ambiguë pour 'l'autre musulman'." *Lusotopie* 14 (1): 181–203.

Diop, Amadou Moustapha. 1996. *Société Manjak et migration*. Paris: Publications Puce et Plume.

Drewal, Margaret Thompson. 1992. *Yoruba Ritual: Performers, Play, Agency*. Bloomington: Indiana University Press.

Einarsdóttir, Jonina. 2000. *Tired of Weeping: Mother Love, Child Death, and Poverty in Guinea-Bissau*. Stockholm: Stockholm Studies in Social Anthropology.

————. 2005. "The Restoration of Social Order Through the Extinction of Non-human Children." In *Managing Uncertainty: Ethnographic Studies of Illness, Risk, and the Struggle for Control*, ed. Richard Jenkins, Hanne Jessen, and Vibeke Steffen, 31–52. Copenhagen: Museum Tusculanum Press.

Fassin, Didier. 2000. "Les politiques de l'ethnopsychiatrie. La psyché africaine, des colonies africaines aux banlieux parisiennes." *L'Homme* 153: 231–250.

Feierman, Steven. 2006. "Afterword: Ethnographic Regions—Healing, Power, and History." In *Borders and Healers: Brokering Therapeutic Resources in Southeast Africa*, ed. Tracy J. Luedke and Harry G. West, 185–197. Bloomington: Indiana University Press.

Feierman, Steven, and John M. Janzen. 1992. "Introduction." In *The Social Basis of Health and Healing in Africa*, ed. Steven Feierman and John M. Janzen, 1–24. Berkeley: University of California Press.

Forrest, Joshua. 1992. *Guinea-Bissau: Power, Conflict, and Renewal in a West African Nation*. Boulder, Colo.: Westview Press.

Gable, Eric. 1990. "Modern Manjaco: The Ethos of Power in a West African Society." PhD diss., University of Virginia.

Hochet, Anne-Marie. 1983. *Paysanneries en attente: Guiné-Bissau*. Dakar, Senegal: ENDA.

Jamin, Jean. 1977. *Les lois du silence. Essai sur la fonction sociale du secret*. Paris: Maspero.

Kleinman, Arthur, Paul E. Brodwin, Byron J. Good, and Mary-Jo DelVecchio Good. 1992. "Pain as Human Experience: An Introduction." In *Pain as Human Experience: An Anthropological Perspective*, ed. Marie-Jo DelVecchio Good, Paul E. Brodwin, Byron J. Good, and Arthur Kleinman, 1–28. Berkeley: University of California Press.

Kuczynski, Liliane. 2002. *Les marabouts africains à Paris*. Paris: CNRS Edtitions.

La Fontaine, J. S. 1985. *Initiation: Ritual Drama and Secret Knowledge Across the World*. London: Pelikan.

Laderman, Carol, and Marina Roseman. 1996. "Introduction." In *The Performance of Healing*, ed. Carol Laderman and Marina Roseman, 1–16. New York: Routledge.

Littlewood, Roland, and Simon Dein, eds. 2000. *Cultural Psychiatry and Medical Anthropology: An Introduction and Reader.* London: The Athlone Press.

Machado, Fernando Luís. 1994. "Luso-africanos em Portugal: nas margens da etnicidade." *Sociologia—Problemas e Práticas* 16: 111–134.

———. 2002. *Contrastes e Continuidades. Migração, Etnicidade e Integração dos Guineenses em Portugal.* Oeiras, Portugal: Celta Editora.

Matos, Ana M. S. M. C. 1997. *Identidades Reconstruídas.* Oeiras, Portugal: Celta Editora.

Nichter, Mark, and Margaret Lock, eds. 2002. *New Horizons in Medical Anthropology: Essays in Honour of Charles Leslie.* London: Routledge.

Pussetti, Chiara. 2006. "A patologização da diversidade. Uma reflexão antropológica sobre a noção de *culture-bound syndrome.*" *Etnográfica* 10 (1): 5–40.

Saraiva, Clara. 2008. "Transnational Migrants and Transnational Spirits: An African Religion in Lisbon." *Journal of Ethnic and Migration Studies* 34 (2): 253–269.

Tavares, João, Ana Matos Pires, and Clara Carvalho. 2009. "Entre a Baloba e o Hospital." *Saúde Mental* 10 (6): 38–42.

Teixeira, Maria. 1996. "Dynamique des pouvoirs magico-religieux des femmes manjak de Canchungo (Guinée-Bissau) émigrées à Ziguinchor (Senégal)." *Soronda* 1 (1): 121–157.

———. 1998. "Bouleversements sociaux et contre-sorcellerie manjak (Guinée-Bissau/Senégal)." *Cahiers de Sociologie Économique et Culturelle (Ethnopsychologie)* 30: 63–87.

Trincaz, Jacqueline. 1981. *Colonisations et religions en Afrique noire. L'exemple de Ziguinchor.* Paris: L'Harmattan—CNRS.

van Binsbergen, W. M. J. 1984. "Socio-ritual Structures and Modern Migration Among the Manjak of Guinea-Bissau: Ideological Reproduction in a Context of Peripheral Capitalism." *Antropologische Verkenningen* 3 (2): 11–43.

———. 1988. "The Land as Body: An Essay on the Interpretation of Ritual Among the Manjak of Guinea-Bissau." *Medical Anthropology Quartely* 2 (4): 386–401.

West, Harry G., and Trady J. Luedke. 2006. "Introduction. Healing Divides: Therapeutic Border Work in Southeast Africa." In *Borders and Healers: Brokering Therapeutic Resources in Southeast Africa,* ed. Tracy J. Luedke and Harry G. West, 1–20. Bloomington: Indiana University Press.

Whyte, Susan Reynolds, Sjaak van der Geest, and Anita Hardon, eds. 2002. *Social Lives of Medicines.* Cambridge: Cambridge University Press.

Zempléni, Andras. 1993. "L'invisible et le dissimulé. Du statut religieux des entités initiatiques." *Gradhiva* 14: 3–14.

CONTRIBUTORS

Clara Carvalho is Professor at the Department of Anthropology and chair of the Center of African Studies (CEA-ISCTE) at the Lisbon University Institute. She is currently conducting research on health and migration among African migrants in Europe and directing a project on women's access to private health care in Africa.

Hansjörg Dilger is Junior Professor of Social and Cultural Anthropology at Freie Universität Berlin. He is co-editor (with Ute Luig) of *Morality, Hope, and Grief: Anthropologies of AIDS in Africa* and has published articles in a range of journals, including *Medical Anthropology, Anthropological Quarterly, Afria Today,* and *African Diaspora.*

Viola Hörbst is an investigator at the Center of African Studies (CEA-IUL) at the University Institute of Lisbon (ISCTE-IUL). Recent publications in English include "Reproductive Disruptions: African Perspectives" in *Curare* and "Focusing Male Infertility in Mali: Kinship and Impacts on Biomedical Practice in Bamako" in *Muslim Medical Ethics: Theory and Practice.*

Elisabeth Hsu is Professor of Social Anthropology at the School of Anthropology, University of Oxford, and a Fellow of Green Templeton College. Publications include *The Transmission of Chinese Medicine; The Telling Touch: Pulse Diagnosis in Early Chinese Medicine;* and *Chinese Medicine in East Africa.*

John M. Janzen is Professor of Anthropology at the University of Kansas. He is guest curator of the exhibition project "African Healing Journeys" for the Penn Museum, a preview version of which was shown at the University of Kansas in connection with the conference "Medical Anthropology in Global Africa."

Abdoulaye Kane is Associate Professor in Anthropology and the Center for African Studies at the University of Florida. He is author of *Tontines, caisses de solidarité et banquiers ambulants: L'univers des pratiques financières informelles en Afrique et dans le milieu immigré africain en France,* along with many articles and book chapters in both French and English on the transnational practices of Senegalese living in Europe and the United States.

Stacey A. Langwick is Associate Professor in the Department of Anthropology at Cornell University. She is also an associate in the Law, Organization, Science, and Technology Project at the Max Planck Institute in Germany. She has published articles in a range of journals, including the *American Ethnologist, Medical Anthropology,* and *Science, Technology, and Human Values.* She contributed to *Borders and Healers* (IUP, 2006) and is author of *Bodies, Politics, and African Healing* (IUP, 2011).

Adeline Masquelier is Professor of Anthropology and chair of the Department of Anthropology at Tulane University. She is author of *Prayer Has Spoiled Everything: Possession, Power, and Identity in an Islamic Town of Niger* and *Women and Islamic Revival in a West African Town* (IUP, 2009), which won the 2010 Melville J. Herskovits Award for best scholarly book on Africa. She is editor of the *Journal of Religion in Africa* and of *Dirt, Undress, and Difference: Critical Perspectives on the Body's Surface* (IUP, 2005).

Adam Mohr is a Senior Writing Fellow at the University of Pennsylvania's Critical Writing Program. He is currently writing a book titled *Enchanted Calvinism: Labor Migration, Afflicting Spirits, and Christian Therapy in the Presbyterian Church of Ghana.*

Kristin Peterson is Assistant Professor of Anthropology at the University of California, Irvine. She is currently finishing a book project on pharmaceutical markets in Nigeria, which analyzes the politics of pharmaceutical distribution in the aftermath of the 1980s economic crisis and structural adjustment.

Marja Tiilikainen is Postdoctoral Researcher at the Department of Social Research, University of Helsinki. Publications include *Arjen islam: Somalinaisten elämää Suomessa* [Everyday Islam: The Life of Somali Women in Finland] and chapters in *Milk and Peace, Drought and War* and *Spirit Possession and Trance.* Her current research project entitled "Suffering, Healing, and Healthcare: The Transnational Lives of Somalis in Exile" is being funded by the Academy of Finland).

Angelika Wolf is Instructor at the Institute of Social and Cultural Anthropology at the Freie Universität Berlin. She is co-founder of the working group "Medical Anthropology" within the German Anthropological Association and was its president for seven years. Currently she is preparing a book on health insurance in the context of globalization.

INDEX